Facial Pain:
Living Well with
Neuropathic Facial Pain

Including Trigeminal Neuralgia

Edited by

Anne Brazer Ciemnecki, MA

and

Jeffrey A. Brown, MD, FACS

With Guest Editor, Beth Darnall, PhD

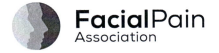

Facial Pain: Living Well with Neuropathic Facial Pain–Including Trigeminal Neuralgia

Copyright © 2024 by the Facial Pain Association

For more information, contact the Facial Pain Association, info@facepain.org or 800-923-3608.

Disclaimer: The information in this book is intended to help readers understand the diagnosis and treatment of pain that is associated with the trigeminal nerve and other facial pain conditions. This book does not provide specific medical advice and is not intended as a substitute for the advice of qualified medical practitioners. If you have trigeminal neuralgia or other neuropathic facial pain, seek advice from a medical professional.

ISBN (paperback): 979-8-9912283-0-5

(ebook): 979-8-9912283-1-2

(audio): 979-8-9912283-2-9

Library of Congress Control Number: 2024919933

The Publishing Portal
Los Angeles, California

Printed in the United States of America

Dedication

"Look for the helpers. You will always find people who are helping." Fred Rogers (alias Mr. Rogers) always remembered what his mother taught him. In times of trouble, there is always someone who will help. Helpers abound for us also. Who are our helpers? They are doctors, nurses, and hospital and medical office staff. They are the people who advocate for you: the staff, boards, and volunteers at the Facial Pain Association (FPA). Most important among the helpers are your friends and family. Friends who stay by your side are like precious gems. Family, especially family members who live with you, are treasures. They may not be perfect, but neither are we. If their intentions are good, they are on our side. Whether they accompany you on medical appointments, call to check in, bring you a meal, or sit by your side as you stream Netflix, they are there for you. I have been on both sides of the facial pain abyss. Frankly, I would rather have the pain than see someone I love (or even know casually) in pain that I cannot make go away. With all that said, Dr. Brown, Dr. Darnall, and I dedicate this book to all the helpers in whatever capacity they function. THANK YOU FROM THE BOTTOM OF OUR HEARTS.

As we think about helpers, we need to give a special shout out to the coeditor of this book and *Facial Pain: A 21st Century Guide* (Lulu, 2020). In 2023, Dr. Jeffrey Brown retired from the active clinical practice of neurosurgery. This is a well-deserved retirement. Patients from around the world depended on Dr. Brown for relief of trigeminal neuropathic pain (TNP). Dr. Brown still has his hands in the facial pain world. He maintains a teaching position as Assistant Clinical Professor at NYU Winthrop Long Island School of Medicine. He is a member and the immediate past chair of the Medical Advisory Board of the FPA. He served unselfishly in that chair position for six transformative years.

Dr. Brown is so much more than his professional accomplishments. He is a mensch. Mensch is a Yiddish term that means a person whom one can trust to act with honor and integrity. The term also suggests someone who is kind and who fuses responsibilities with compassion. He never gave up on a patient. Dr. Brown's favorite expression, and one that he earned the right to say repeatedly, is "I can help you." He has an interesting sense of humor. While working on the 2020 book, I asked Dr. Brown for a picture for the back cover. He sent me a picture of himself throwing axes. This year, he sent me a picture proving that he can tie his own bow tie. Fortunately, he did not bring axes into his operating rooms. As for the bow ties, his surgical knots are impeccable. It has been a privilege to work with Dr. Brown. From the bottom of our hearts, we sincerely appreciate his continuing contributions to the facial pain community and wish him a long, healthy, happy retirement from clinical practice.

Acknowledgments

Many thanks to all the authors and readers who contributed to making this book a reality. We especially thank the Facial Pain Association (FPA) staff, Board of Directors, Young Patient's Committee, and Medical Advisory Board. Special appreciation goes to Melissa Baumbick, CEO, and Brandi Underwood, Manager of Development, Research, and Advocacy, who helped with many aspects of this publication. We also appreciate John Temple, a reviewer extraordinaire, who provided invaluable early feedback. In addition, we thank Jack Nestor and Anali North Martin of Technica Editorial. We also appreciate Erica Ellison's expert and careful editing, and acknowledge Sarah Winner, Natalie Merrithew, and Harry Nestor for the updated cover design.

We would also like to thank Regina Gore, volunteer coordinator, for assembling a team of "white glove" readers, Melissa Anchan, David Meyers, Mary Rice, Rachel Scherer, and Brandi Underwood. A special shout out goes Jeffrey Fogel, MD whose meticulous attention to detail, extensive medical knowledge, and playful sense of humor pushed us over the finish line.

Table of Contents

Foreword 1

Jeffrey A. Brown, MD, FACS, FAANS, Editor

Six hours after attending a recent fundraiser for local police and first responders, I became acutely nauseated. I'd been poisoned and was suffering all the nasty effects of it. After repeated bouts of this, I surrendered my pride of self-sufficiency and agreed to call on those first responders for a different reason—a 10-minute trip to the local hospital.

Packed into the tight ambulance, speaking to two calmly speaking men whom I'd determined to be quite competent at their jobs, I realized something important to this preface.

I no longer felt ill.

Had I been wrong to seek help?

Eight hours and 3 liters of intravenous fluid later, when I had awakened long enough to contemplate my situation, I realized this:

The simple effect of finding *someone who could help me, someone in whose knowledge and competency I had faith, someone who could guide me through the process of recovery* made me better, calmed my suffering.

Was it real?

I certainly felt it.

This is my hope for each of you by providing you with this guidebook.

It is neither a prescription, nor a referral, exercise, or diet. It is meant to be a guide through the dense entanglement that those who experience trigeminal neuropathic pain (TNP) all find themselves caught up in.

When should you seek help? How should you evaluate the help you receive? What kind of medicines should you take, or not take? What kind of health care provider will know enough to help? Are there others like you to whom you can relate?

Each chapter in this book is preceded by a summary introduction, but here is the overall picture:

We begin with facial pain 101: back to the beginning and the first twinge of pain. How should you proceed in the best of worlds?

Dr. Liedtke then presents his lifelong experience with the medical treatment of neuropathic facial pain. His compendium of information cannot be digested in one reading. Use it as a reference guide or perhaps as a resource for your physician who may be stuck on what to do next. Ensuing chapters delve in greater detail into topical medications and ketamine use.

The psychology of chronic pain is also discussed. There are many innovative approaches to quiet a mind that is otherwise embroiled in the heat of painful experience. Some of them involve short training exercises. The most exciting is the use of virtual reality to transport you to a place of peace and tranquility in three dimensions and brilliant color. Imagine walking on an empty beach with blue waves lapping on the shore with the regularity of a metronome; no one there to disturb you; no drugs required. Does it relax you? No limit to the duration of use. Addictive? A news article described the experience as "digital fentanyl," of course without the threat to tumbling into its spell. Worthwhile? Research says so.

One of our themes is an effort to demonstrate that you are not alone with your pain. Several individuals experiencing trigeminal neuropathic pain tell their stories and describe their journeys toward a positive outlook and good health.

What should you do in a dire emergency? We update the outline of medication options presented in our last book.

Is there an option to declare full disability and be reimbursed? It is possible, but the route can be fraught with expense and frustration.

Finally, we discuss the possibility of inherited trigeminal neuropathic pain. Your mother had it—could you also be at risk?

I would like to quote the words of Sir Winston Churchill. We know him for his wartime British oratory designed to save a country. But in his life, four times he faced his own adversity. As an adolescent, he plunged 30 feet from a bridge to the ground, leaving him in coma for days. He nearly drowned from a foolish lake swim off a small boat that kept drifting away from his reach. Later, as a young British soldier, he led the last of the great cavalry charges into enemy lines and faced Dervish swords seeking those weakened by dropped weapons, torn stirrups leaving an uncontrollable mount, or bleeding wounds of either the soldier or the horse. Finally, later in life, he was struck by a car on Fifth Avenue in New York City when he exited a cab and, like all civilized Brits, assumed that the traffic would part ways for him while he crossed the street.

> ... the message I bring back from these dark places is one of encouragement. I certainly suffered every pang, mental and physical, that a street accident or, I suppose, a shell wound can produce. None is unendurable. There is neither the time nor the strength for self-pity. There is no room for remorse or fears. If at any moment in this long series of sensations a grey veil deepening into blackness had descended upon the sanctum I should have felt or feared nothing additional. Nature is merciful and does not try her children, man or beast, beyond their compass. It is only where the cruelty of man intervenes that hellish torments appear. For the rest— live dangerously; take things as they come; dread naught, all will be well.

Foreword 2

Beth Darnall, PhD, Guest Editor

I am delighted with I am delighted with Facial Pain: Living Well with Neuropathic Facial Pain and its progressive inclusion of many chapters that address the "whole-person" experience of pain.

The role of the mind in the experience of pain has long been misunderstood. Today, more people than ever know that the mind matters for pain relief—and for our quality of life. Ongoing pain presents clear challenges to every person. Medical advances offer new treatment approaches to help address those challenges, and this book includes exciting and important medical updates. Targeting the mind and the psychosocial dimensions of pain can provide other critical avenues to reduce pain and its impacts. Accordingly, you will notice that this book contains multiple chapters that elucidate the experience of pain and its various dimensions, including social, emotional, and cognitive dimensions. Although not widely appreciated, pain itself is defined as a negative sensory and emotional experience, as described in detail in key chapters of this book. Better appreciation of the psychosocial dimensions of pain can help shape a person's willingness to engage in treatments that might otherwise have seemed unimportant or like something that could only work for other people. Many psychological treatment approaches involve learning proven techniques that engage one's central nervous system to gain relief. In this book, you will find several chapters that serve as a foundation for understanding how the mind and body react to pain—and what that might mean for pain relief. You will read content from clinical, scientific, and experiential experts, with the latter being people with lived experience who provide messages of connection and hope, as well as pathways to engage with a community of patient-peers.

It is my hope that these chapters provide you and others with new and deeper understandings and ways to think about whole-person pain relief. In this whole-person model, medical and nonmedical treatments work together to help people gain maximal relief and quality of life. May you be inspired to continue a journey of learning and connection!

Preface

Anne B. Ciemnecki, MA,
Secretary of the Board of Directors of the FPA, Editor

Welcome to Facial Pain: Living Well with Neuropathic Facial Pain. This book is intended to accompany Facial Pain: A 21st Century Guide that was published in 2020. All of the material in this volume is new. We are fortunate to have so many professionals who contributed their time and knowledge to bring this volume to the facial pain community. Highlights include an updated and expanded chapter on medications for trigeminal neuropathic pain (TNP) and 10 chapters on various presentations of TNP. We address current topics that people with facial pain have been hearing about, including Teflon-free microvascular decompression and the clinical trials of Basimglurant. If the U.S. Food and Drug Administration approves Basimglurant, it will be the first drug approved specifically for TNP since carbamazepine in the 1960s. This volume also addresses preliminary work on the NRF2 network, familial facial pain, and virtual reality for pain relief.

If you must have TNP, 2024 is a better time to have it than 30 years ago, when mine started; 60 years ago, when my mother first felt pain; or longer ago, when my grandmother was afflicted. We have come a long way since the time when the only options were painful alcohol injections and/or Dilantin, a difficult drug to take that caused acne for me and did not touch my pain. Imagine feeling the shocks of TNP without access to the internet. Imagine the days before magnetic resonance imaging and microvascular decompression. Imagine not having the resources of the Facial Pain Association. It was a lonely journey. People with TNP were discredited. They were often told the pain was "all in their heads." How ironic is that?

The dentist who performed my root canal at the beginning of my TNP journey was a close friend. I was sure he believed that I was in constant pain and that he would be supportive. He referred me from one dental professional to another, none of whom knew much about TNP. He became frustrated (not as frustrated as I was), and in a fit of arrogance and ignorance, told my husband that I was like the princess in the *Princess and the Pea*, a classic fairy tale written down by Hans Christian Andersen in 1835.

In the *Princess and the Pea*, a prince wishes to marry a princess. He goes on an extensive search to find his royal bride, but he cannot be completely sure that any of the women he meets are *bona fide* princesses. One dark and stormy night, a young woman arrives at his castle, asking to take shelter inside. The woman claims to be a princess, so the prince's mother takes a pea and places it under 20 mattresses in the bed where the princess will sleep. In the morning, the young princess recounts that she passed an awful night because there was something hard underneath her in the bed, and her body was black and blue by the time morning came. The prince and his mother take this as proof that this young woman is a real princess, as only someone of truly royal blood could be so tender and sensitive to have been troubled by a pea concealed under 20 mattresses. The prince and the princess get married, and the pea is put on display in a museum.

Let me shatter that myth. I am not a princess. I never was. I do not keep vegetables under my mattress. I never did, not even as a midnight snack. In addition to my husband, I have shared my bed with sleepless babies, tossing toddlers, talkative teens, homesick campers, my BFF, a dog in diapers, a snoring doxle, a licking poodle, and a cat that needs to be in the crook of my arm and paws at me if I do not pat him during the night. That pea would not keep me awake. It probably would not keep you awake either.

What might keep us awake is not a pea. It is a gigantic, evil, painful boulder. Our task is to smash that boulder to smithereens. Imagine yourself as a superhero with Thor's hammer. Every step you take to care for yourself destroys a piece of that boulder. Make connections with providers from the Facial Pain Association's (FPA's) "Find a Doctor" list. Swing your hammer. Go to an FPA conference. Smack that boulder again. Join a support group. Strike it harder this time. Speak with a peer mentor. Visit the FPA's website (https://www.facepain.org). Download the patient guide. Make some more fragments. Check in with a mental health professional. Two swings for that one. Sign up for the newsletter. Look for the next webinar. Punch it. Thump it. Hit it harder. Oh, of course, read this book. Soon your boulder will be dust. You will not lose sleep or be a prince or princess. You will be a superhero or heroine. Superman? Wonder Woman? Batman? Hercules? Xena? Popeye? Who will you be?

One final thought: When you reach out and help another person with TNP, you have turned your pain into power. Care for yourself. Volunteer for the FPA. Care for someone else. Live your best life despite TNP. Take back your power to be yourself, not your pain.

Read this book in good health and accept my sincere wishes for love, peace, and no pain.

Editor's Note: This book has 42 subchapters written by 57 authors or coauthors. The authors come from around the world and are experts in a myriad of fields. I was not surprised to see that the authors use different nomenclature to refer to facial pain. Try not to let the variety of names confuse you. In the end, the pain is neuropathic facial pain (NFP), also called trigeminal neuropathic facial pain (TNP), or the pain is a neuropathy.

- Neuropathic pain is pain originating in a nerve, usually due to injury or disease.
- Neuropathy happens when the nerve is damaged or malfunctions. Neuropathy causes numbness when it occurs in a sensory nerve. Beyond the neuropathic/neuropathy distinction you will see the following terms throughout the book:
  - Classic trigeminal neuralgia is extreme, intermittent, sudden burning or shock-like pain. The pain lasts anywhere from a few seconds to a few minutes per episode. The attacks can occur close together, in stretches that can last for prolonged periods. It is also called Type 1 trigeminal neuralgia.
  - Atypical facial pain is a term that refers to a constant burning or aching sensation rather than overwhelming jolts of pain. It lasts for a long time and encompasses a wide area of the face. Classic trigeminal neuralgia is called atypical if the atypical type of pain is present more than half of the time. This type of pain has also been called idiopathic facial pain (or persistent idiopathic facial pain). "Idiopathic" means without a clear cause. It has also been called Type 2 trigeminal neuralgia.

Besides these classifications you will also read about many subtypes of neuropathic facial pains including glossopharyngeal, geniculate, occipital, and post herpetic neuralgia. You will also see chapters on bilateral facial pain, autonomic effects, and migraine.

Dog-ear or flag this page and come back to these definitions if you must. I hope you do not let the different terms used to define pain bog you down as you read.

On another topic, we all know that doctors and other health care professionals come in all genders and gender-identities. We did our best to use gender-neutral language throughout the book. If we missed a few references, please excuse the errors and know that our heads and hearts meant well.

Last comment. This book is chocked full of valuable information that could help ease your pain and your mind. It is not, however, a substitute for your own doctor. Please do not make any changes to your medical regime based on what you read in this (or any) book. Consult with your own health care team. Bring the book along to the visit if you think that will enlighten your provider.

Chapter 1
Medication for Trigeminal Neuropathic Pain

Anne B. Ciemnecki, MA

If you are like most people with trigeminal neuropathic pain (TNP), medications will be a significant part of your life. You will probably spend more time taking medications than not taking them.

Almost everyone tries to control pain with medication before turning to surgeries. If you have had surgery, you may need to supplement it with some medication afterwards. Integrative medicine uses conventional medication along with disciplines such as acupuncture, massage, meditation, tai chi, and reiki, as well as products including vitamins, minerals, and dietary supplements.

Whether you are taking a lot of medications or a little, it is important to learn as much as you can about them. This chapter of the book will help you do just that.

After an introduction to TNP by Jeffrey A. Brown, MD (Section 1.1), Wolfgang Liedtke, MD, PhD, reflects on his more than 25 years of clinical practice to provide a critical update of approaches that worked for his patients. He discusses maintenance medication, as-needed or rescue medications, injectable medications, and medications to manage brain fog. He also provides critical insight on the importance of controlling hypertension for those with neuropathic facial pain (Section 1.2). In Section 1.3, Gary Heir, DMD, a world-renowned orofacial pain specialist, discusses the benefits of topical, specially compounded medications that have few to no side effects and do not require titration. Ketamine infusions are growing in popularity in the facial pain community. In Section 1.4, Xiang Qian, MD, and his colleagues present information about ketamine infusions for pain relief. Section 1.5 presents an update of the protocol developed by Mark E. Linskey, MD, for what to do when pain requires urgent or emergency care.

As you begin to read and learn from this first chapter of the book, I will share my top 10 medication tips:

1. Unless your doctor tells you otherwise, keep a steady stream of medications in your body. Maintenance medications for TNP are not to be used only as needed.

2. Do not give up on a prescribed medication too quickly. It may take a few days or a few weeks for your body to adjust to side effects such as "brain fog" or dizziness.

3. Along the same lines, do not change medication routines too frequently. Give each medication plenty of time to relieve pain (or not). If you make too many changes at once, you will not know which medication is working and which is not. My doctor's recommendation is to wait 3 weeks before making a change.

4. That said, everyone is different. If one medication is not working, do not despair. Give another medication a chance. Finding the right medication or combination of medications can take time.

5. You must titrate off most medications slowly. Dropping a medication suddenly can cause rebound or other effects. Follow your doctor's orders.

6. When your doctor prescribes a medication, ask for a plan for titrating up and for titrating down, if necessary.

7. Create a system that works for you so that you do not forget to take your medications regularly. You can take medications at meals or at bedtime or set an alarm on a phone or smart watch for another time of day. There is nothing worse than being in pain and realizing that you forgot to take your medications.

8. Carry spare medications in a purse or pocket. They are like a security blanket. If you are unexpectedly caught away from home, it is helpful to have a dose on hand. Likewise, do not wait for the last minute to refill medications. You do not want to be caught short. Before embarking on a work trip or vacation, be sure you have enough medication on hand to last through the time away from home.

9. Some pharmacies offer medication packets that are organized by dose, date, and time; securely sealed; clearly labeled; and easy to open. This is often a free service and is very convenient.

10. Make friends with your pharmacist. Many of your medications will be taken off-label i.e., for non FDA approved purposes. It can be helpful for your pharmacist to understand why you are taking the particular mix of medications you are. Your pharmacist can also advocate for you with your insurance companies.

1.1
Facial Pain 101
Jeffrey A. Brown, MD, FACS, FAANS

Author's Note: The information contained in this section is not intended to provide individual medical advice, diagnosis, or treatment or to induce the reader to seek care with any specific physician. Always seek the advice of your physician or other qualified health care provider with any questions you may have regarding a medical condition or treatment and before undertaking a new health care treatment, and never disregard professional medical advice or delay in seeking it because of something you have read in this book.

You have a frightening pain in your face. It happens once. You hope it does not reappear. It does. Is it because of that darned dental work you just had? Maybe it is something wrong after that sinus surgery?

Back to the dentist or the ear, nose, and throat (ENT) surgeon.

Here's the first pitfall: If the dentist is not positive that it is a nerve root issue but would like to proceed with a root canal, ask them to hold off. Too many patients have gone through the progression of a root canal, and when that doesn't work, an adjacent root canal, and next a tooth extraction and on and on.

Trigeminal neuralgia (let's call it trigeminal neuropathic pain or TNP) often presents after a dental procedure. It is not because anything was amiss or because a nerve was injured by the "novocaine" injection. (Most dentists do not use Novocain anymore. They often use short-acting Lidocaine or longer-acting Bupivacaine.) TNP can be "kindled" by a surge of electricity that can occur during routine dental work. That spark kindles the ongoing fire of TNP. The pain is most often intermittent at first. Why? The short circuit that elicits the stab of pain needs a bit of extra electricity to get it going.

This can be provided by a touch to the face or by chewing or talking—or it may not be clear what sets it off.

Why does the pain occur from something as simple as a gentle touch to the face and not necessarily from something intrinsically painful itself?

Once set in motion, TNP is repeatedly triggered by normal sensations that travel through the nerve to the short circuit. The fibers that trigger this pain are normal sensory fibers of the nerve, not pain fibers. This is important in understanding at least one of the surgical treatments: balloon compression rhizotomy.

How does the dentist diagnose a dental origin for the pain? Of course, by examination and by office imaging. Tooth decay is a "nociceptive" pain, meaning that the pain results from inflammation in the dental pulp that "upsets" the normal sensory nerves, which, in turn, transmit the injury to the brain. Nociceptive pain is aching and throbbing—like a "toothache." Pain is not "neuropathic" unless a nerve is injured. Neuropathic pain is tingling, burning, stabbing, or prickling—all electrical sensations. An already-injured nerve doesn't like to be bothered. The dentist will do a "tap test" to investigate nerve injury. By tapping a diseased tooth, the dentist can elicit pain. Another approach is to blow cold air on the suspect tooth. Exposed nerves don't like that. It hurts. This suggests that the nerve root is involved, and a root canal might be indicated. Bacterial infections, if extensive, can involve the nerve root as well. This should show up in dental imaging.

No infection?

Beware of that root canal, then.

If TNP is suspected, the dentist, if well informed, will suggest a neurology consultation.

Most neurologists know "something" about TNP, but very few neurologists are experts in the condition. They should know enough, however, to offer a trial of an anticonvulsant drug.

Why? Anticonvulsant drugs (ACDs) are not pain medications, so why use them?

By definition, ACDs slow electrical conduction in the brain and the whole nervous system. That is how they inhibit or stop seizures, as seizures are surges of too much electricity in the brain. Similarly, ACDs work in TNP because flooding the whole body with the drug also reduces the amount of electricity passing through the trigeminal nerve, reducing it enough to stop the surges that set off the stabbing pain of short circuits. That is, they "turn off the switch."

The problem is that ACDs also reduce the normal function of the brain and nervous system if too much is given too quickly, before the body can get used to it. ACDs need to be started at low doses and gradually increased (if needed); otherwise, people feel foggy, can't think clearly, are clumsy, may trip and fall. So, beware of side effects and of taking too much medication too fast.

The safest of the ACDs is called gabapentin and should be started at as low a dose as 100 mg at night (so it doesn't make you drowsy during the day). "Fancier" drugs are not necessarily better drugs. Increases in dosage can be made every 3 days if the dose used is not adequate to stop the stabbing pains. However, if the increased dose causes additional (not really "side") effects that are bothersome, then the dose should be dropped back.

If the medicine works, then great—but it likely won't work forever, and the dose will need to be increased as time goes by. TNP tends to be progressive once it commences.

What else needs to be done?

Of course, the neurologist or internist must do a careful examination. There are many disease entities that can cause TNP. The most common is an injury to the trigeminal nerve inside the brain caused by the unhappy circumstance of an otherwise-normal artery or vein bumping repeatedly against the trigeminal nerve until it has stripped the insulation off thousands of the wires that compose the cable that is the trigeminal nerve.

Hold on to that thought for a moment.

Other diseases that are associated with TNP include multiple sclerosis and some other immunologic entities: scleroderma, Sjögren's syndrome, and lupus. Some blood tests will help sort these out. Temporomandibular joint (TMJ) disorders cause jaw pain. Parotid gland (salivary gland) disease can cause facial pain. These need to be sorted out as well, but they tend to cause aching, throbbing, nociceptive pain not neuropathic pain. Understand, for example, that TMJ pain occurs because of inflammation in the TMJ joint. Inflammation usually causes throbbing and aching, not stabbing.

If the physician's evaluation does not turn up anything, then it is time for a magnetic resonance imaging (MRI) exam.

Not all MRI scans are equal. Not all neuroradiologists are equal. The doctor may say that MRI is important to make sure that there is no brain tumor causing the pain. This would be extremely rare. What is important is that the MRI ordered be performed using one of the special techniques known by the acronyms FIESTA and CISS. It is not the power of the MRI scanner that is important as much as it is the technique used to acquire the images and the knowledge base of the neuroradiologist viewing the images.

FIESTA or CISS MRI scans allow the doctor to see the trigeminal nerve, arteries, veins, spinal fluid, and brain tissue distinctly. Such detailed images can then show whether there is a causative blood vessel in contact with the trigeminal nerve. Often, the neuroradiologist will say that the nerve is "normal." Because MRI scans can't detect disease in the nerve, the nerve will most often look "normal" when there is TNP. The radiologist may not know to consider whether there is an artery or vein in contact with the nerve and, therefore, may not comment on it. Other times, the radiologist will say that no "compression" of the nerve can be seen. TNP does not require compression by an artery or vein. If there is contact, the blood vessel may be "stuck" to the nerve through arachnoid adhesion. If so, then the blood vessel's pulsations are transmitted to the nerve enough to injure it. Understand that MRI scans cannot detect injury. They are just pictures of the nerve and brain and are not detailed enough to show actual anatomic disruption. That would require a biopsy. However, doctors don't like to take bites out of nerves to look for disease. That would likely injure the nerve and make things worse.

Okay. You have had your MRI scan. Perhaps it was read as "normal." Perhaps it was read as showing something of concern. Perhaps your pain is under control. What next?

Neurosurgeons who are experts in TNP can be of enormous help at this point. Why not consult one? An expert in this arena will not pressure you into surgery that is not indicated or not wanted. However, an expert can best inform you of what to expect and what to consider as the condition inevitably progresses.

Not all neurosurgeons are experts in TNP.

What makes a neurosurgeon an expert in TNP? See Section 3.1, "What Makes a Neurosurgeon an Expert?", for a detailed explanation of the most important qualifications.

The important point is that one should consult an expert neurosurgeon as soon as the diagnosis of TNP is suggested. It can't "hurt."

It is beyond the scope of this Introduction to go into detail about the varied surgical options for the treatment of TNP. These can be gleaned in the surgical sections in this book and in its companion, Facial Pain: A 21st Century Guide.

The takeaway from this Introduction is to consider consulting a neurosurgeon with expertise in the arena of TNP as soon as the diagnosis of TNP has been offered to you. Make use of the Facial Pain Association to find one, and you will be well served.

Editor's Note: Orofacial pain dentists are also experts in diagnosing TNP quickly and accurately. They offer treatments with medications and can refer you to an expert neurosurgeon when necessary. Although orofacial pain dentists have been practicing for a long time, the area of orofacial pain diagnosis and treatment was recognized as a dental specialty only in 2020. The Facial Pain Association website lists orofacial pain specialists along with other doctors who specialize in TNP.

1.2
Traditional Medical Treatments
Wolfgang Liedtke, MD, PhD

Author's Notes: The information contained in this section is not intended to provide individual medical advice, diagnosis, or treatment or to induce the reader to seek care with any specific physician. Always seek the advice of your physician or other qualified health care provider with any questions you may have regarding a medical condition or treatment and before undertaking a new health care treatment, and never disregard professional medical advice or delay in seeking it because of something you have read in this book.

In this section, I am sharing my own opinions, experiences, and impressions based on long-standing clinical practice, not those of my affiliations, namely, Regeneron Pharmaceuticals, Duke University/Duke Health, and New York University College of Dentistry.

Medical treatment with appropriate, safe, and effective therapeutics will be needed for many people with TNP and other forms of craniofacial pain mediated by the trigeminal sensory system. This update on medications is a critical review of what has worked during my more than 25 years of clinical experience. Now a biotech-pharmaceutical executive, I also provide comments on the rational basis of medical treatments and what I believe is a promising future with new medicines to meet the continuing, severe, unmet need for medical treatment of TNP.

This primer for medical treatments is divided into three subsections: (1) as-needed treatments (often called rescue medications) for early intervention; (2) baseline-continuous regular medications for ongoing management and prevention, including medications to manage side effects such as "brain fog"; and (3) injectables for maintenance management as well as the diffusion of pain crises. The therapeutics include oral formulations, topically applied medicines (e.g., skin creams, orally dissolving lozenges, nasal sprays), and both subcutaneous and intravenous injectables.

Introduction. Pain is a survival instinct, and the accelerating pace of scientific discovery in recent decades has led to clarification of its neural basis. We have learned that trigeminally mediated pain mechanisms are connected to brain areas that are important for emotional processing, regulation of mood, and autonomous function. Such functions include day–night rhythms, hunger, thirst, and hormonal regulation. In chronic facial pain, if the trigeminal sensory system has malfunctioned, the devastation can have a greater impact than pain that is not mediated through the trigeminal system.

These insights emphasize the need to view different forms of trigeminal pain under one umbrella. This umbrella of entities includes

- Trigeminal neuralgia;
- Trigeminal neuropathic pain (TNP);
- Other forms of trigeminal pain, such as
  - Those associated with eye, ear, sinus, dental, oral, and orofacial pain, as well as skin disease,
  - Head pains and headaches,
  - Migraine,
  - Cluster headaches,
  - Other headaches, and
  - Temporomandibular joint pain; and
- Glossopharyngeal, geniculate, and occipital nerve pain.

Medical treatment for TNP and trigeminally-mediated pain will be needed for many patients on their journey to better health. I will present here my understanding of what will be helpful on that journey. These views represent my personal experiences as a treating physician over many years. They are real-world insights, gained together with my patients. Although they may differ from currently published guidelines and "textbook knowledge," they are based on an understanding of the trigeminal system and human physiology that I have acquired over many years as a molecular biologist, physiologist, and clinical physician.

As-Needed Treatments (Also Called Rescue Medications). What can you do when the pain becomes intolerable? With forms of TNP that present with episodic attacks, patients need potent treatments that work immediately. Regular tablets will not be enough, because their action onset is too slow. As-needed medications should be orally dissolvable, liquid, or chewable; nasal sprays; or topical gels or jellies. Most of these medications can also be used for maintenance treatments, however the formulation will have to be adopted for specific purposes (e.g. orally-disolving is for as-needed treatment and regular or slow-release tablets are for maintenance. Because they have varied mechanisms of action, these medicines can also be combined for added benefit. Diligent use of such medications can be the difference between a mere flare-up and a malicious attack that spirals out of control. Table 1-1 lists the available compounds with high-level comments on dosing and practical qualifiers.

For TNP with clinically dominating exacerbations, hypertensive blood pressure needs to be controlled in a timely manner. High blood pressure can exacerbate pain. Assume that blood pressure goes up with TNP attacks. Take a blood pressure measurement when pain is severe. Report it to your doctor. Consider antihypertensive as-needed treatment (listed in Table 1-2) when blood pressure exceeds 160 systolic and 95 diastolic provided that resting blood pressure has been normal (less than 140 mmHg systolic and 90 mmHg diastolic). If these normal thresholds are exceeded, blood pressure management needs to be discussed with a family physician and possibly a hypertension specialist.

Early as-needed analgesic treatment for pain attacks is prioritized over antihypertensive treatment. These analgesics can be combined for increased effectiveness when managing TNP or rapidly worsening

Table 1-1. Rapid-Acting, As-Needed Medications for Trigeminal Neuropathic Pain[a]

Drug Type	Compound	Formulation and Dose	Comments and Links to RxList.com and Wikipedia or Journal Article
Sodium-channel blocker	Carbamazepine	Chewable,[b] 50–200 mg (100 mg tablet Rx)	Can be repeated 5–10 min later, up to 400 mg total per attack. Long-standing first-line experience. Tegretol (Carbamazepine): Side Effects, Uses, Dosage, Interactions, Warnings (rxlist.com) Carbamazepine - Wikipedia
Sodium-channel blocker	Oxcarbazepine	Liquid, 50–200 mg (variable doses possible with liquid)	See chewable carbamazepine. Can also be used as "swish-and-spit" treatment; exclusively intra-oral effect with minimal systemic absorption; chewable carbamazepine alternative. Trileptal (Oxcarbazepine): Side Effects, Uses, Dosage, Interactions, Warnings (rxlist.com) Oxcarbazepine - Wikipedia
Benzodiazepine	Clonazepam[c]	Orally dissolving tablet, 0.125–0.25 mg	Can be repeated up to 1 mg total (soft limit). Balance with mild sedation (which will not kick in at lower doses because of the TNP attack). Other benzodiazepines are not analgesic. Long-standing first-line experience. Synergistic combination with carbamazepine. Klonopin (Clonazepam): Side Effects, Uses, Dosage, Interactions, Warnings (rxlist.com) Clonazepam - Wikipedia
Gabapentinoids	Gabapentin	Liquid, 100–300 mg	Alternative if carbamazepine/oxcarbazepine works poorly or if the patient has a known gabapentin/pregabalin response to maintenance medication. Neurontin (Gabapentin): Side Effects, Uses, Dosage, Interactions, Warnings (rxlist.com) Gabapentin - Wikipedia

NMDA-receptor blocker	Ketamine[c]	Nasal spray, 10–15 mg/puff (100–150 mg/mL)	2–4 puffs per nostril; can be used bilaterally (on both sides), depending on laterality of the pain and laterality of the effect. Soft limit of 100–200 mg/attack and 200–400 mg/day. Dose-limiting effects are psychotropic effects (feeling weird); higher doses can be hallucinogenic (which many individuals have tolerated when facing TNP attacks). Some individuals are very responsive to lower doses; most need higher doses. Nasal irritation can be overcome by pretreatment with 1% lidocaine liquid or jelly. One of the most rapid onset medications against TNP. Newer approach, possibly promising. Ketamine Hydrochloride (Ketamine HCl): Side Effects, Uses, Dosage, Interactions, Warnings (rxlist.com) Ketamine - Wikipedia
NMDA-receptor blocker	(S)-Ketamine,[c,d] Esketamine[c,d]	Nasal spray, 28 mg/puff	Brand name Spravato (controlled substance, high insurance hurdle). If an individual uses this drug, medication for a mood disorder is recommended. Spravato (Esketamine Nasal Spray): Side Effects, Uses, Dosage, Interactions, Warnings (rxlist.com) Esketamine - Wikipedia
Gepant (CGRP-receptor blocker)	Rimegepant[d]	Orally dissolving tablet, 75 mg	1 tablet; can repeat with sufficient supply. Patients need to have a sufficient supply of tablets to engage in repeat applications as-needed. Because it is officially covered through the migraine indication, there will be limits on monthly supply, such as 4 or a maximum of 8 tablets per month. Patients need to "budget" with what they have so they have enough until the next refill. This is an important practical consideration that can cause stress. Newer approach, with limited experience: some patients experience a high-impact beneficial response; for most, it is a suitable combination with carbamazepine and/or clonazepam. Nurtec ODT (Rimegepant Orally Disintegrating Tablets, for Sublingual or Oral Use): Side Effects, Uses, Dosage, Interactions, Warnings (rxlist.com) Rimegepant - Wikipedia

(Continued)

Table 1-1. Rapid-Acting, As-Needed Medications for Trigeminal Neuropathic Pain[a] (Continued)

Drug Type	Compound	Formulation and Dose	Comments and Links to RxList.com and Wikipedia or Journal Article
Gepant (CGRP-receptor blocker)	Zavegepant[d]	Nasal spray, 10 mg/puff	1 puff; can have second. Very recent approach; possibly equally effective as Rimegepant. No practical experience. Possibly use Rimegepant for third-branch pain and Zavegepant for second- and first-branch pain. Both gepants suitable for trigeminal pain that facilitates migraines (or cluster headaches). Zavzpret (Zavegepant Nasal Spray): Side Effects, Uses, Dosage, Interactions, Warnings (rxlist.com) Zavegepant - Wikipedia
Sodium-channel blocker	Lidocaine	1–2% jelly, spray	Intra-oral use for third-branch triggered trigeminal pain. Nasal spray for second-branch triggered pain. Add-on to carbamazepine/clonazepam. Premedication for nasal ketamine in cases where ketamine has nasally irritant properties, which would defeat its powerful action on the trigeminal system. Lidocaine HCl Mucous Membrane: Uses, Side Effects, Interactions, Pictures, Warnings & Dosing - WebMD (rxlist.com) Lidocaine - Wikipedia
Oxytocin	Oxytocin[b]	Nasal spray, 24 IU/puff (240 IU/mL)	2 puffs per nostril, bilateral (both sides). Limited experience; however, great safety and adjunct to any partially effective, as-needed rapid-onset medication. Pitocin (Oxytocin Injection): Side Effects, Uses, Dosage, Interactions, Warnings (rxlist.com) Oxytocin (medication) - Wikipedia

[a]Abbreviations: CGRP, calcitonin gene-related peptide; IU, international unit; NMDA, N-methyl-d-aspartate; Rx, prescription; TNP, trigeminal neuropathic pain.
[b]Requires formulation by a compounding pharmacy.
[c]Controlled substance.
[d]Insurance approval hurdles; expensive.

Table 1-2. As-Needed Medications Against Hypertension Associated with Trigeminal Pain Attacks[a]

Drug Type	Compound	Formulation and Dose	Comments and Links to RxList.com and Wikipedia or Journal Article
ACE inhibitor	Captopril	Tablet, 25 mg	Can be repeated 30 min later if lack of effect on pain-associated hypertension. Expect onset of action within 15–20 min; fastest acting ACE inhibitor. Coordinate the as-needed pain-hypertension therapy with family physician and/or hypertension specialist. Capoten (Captopril): Side Effects, Uses, Dosage, Interactions, Warnings (rxlist.com) Captopril - Wikipedia
α_2-Adrenoceptor agonist	Clonidine	Tablet, 0.1 mg	Lowers blood pressure by acting on the α_2-adrenoceptors in the brain. Onset of action >30 min. Can be synergistic in situations of withdrawal symptoms of abuse or menopausal flushing. Coordinate the as-needed pain-hypertension therapy with family physician and/or hypertension specialist. Perspective: Clonidine nasal spray awaiting development for pain-associated hypertension. Catapres (Clonidine): Side Effects, Symptoms, Uses, Dosage, Interactions, Warnings (rxlist.com) Clonidine - Wikipedia
Benzodiazepine	Clonazepam,[b] Lorazepam[b]	Clonazepam: Orally dissolving tablet, 0.5 mg Lorazepam: Liquid, 2 mg	NOT antihypertensives, but sedating, muscle-relaxing, and anti-anxiety effects will indirectly reduce hypertensive blood pressure values. Advantageous to use if mild sedation and anxiolysis are desirable, e.g., when pain episodes/attacks trigger panic attacks or are critically driven by feed forward of stress→pain→stress and so forth. Clonazepam also has an analgesic impact on the trigeminal system. Klonopin (Clonazepam): Side Effects, Uses, Dosage, Interactions, Warnings (rxlist.com) Clonazepam - Wikipedia Lorazepam is one of the most effective fast-acting anti-anxiety medicines. Ativan (Lorazepam): Side Effects, Uses, Dosage, Interactions, Warnings (rxlist.com) Lorazepam - Wikipedia

[a]Abbreviation: ACE, angiotensin-converting enzyme.
[b]Controlled substance.

episodes. Unfortunately, super-rapid-acting formulations for antihypertensive as-needed treatment are not available.

The vicious cycle of pain begetting pain needs to be defeated early. Using these safe as-needed medications when an attack seems imminent, yet does not ultimately manifest, is preferable. Do not let pain establish a foothold in the trigeminal system and engage the brain's stress response. When this happens, pain becomes refractory to the low-impact as-needed measures outlined here. Starting too late can lead to a need for the emergency room, with all its unfortunate possible outcomes, including delayed attention; exposure to noise, light, and smells; inappropriate treatments; discrimination; and bullying.

Have as-needed medications available in your purse or pocket, on your night table, in your bathroom at home, and while traveling. This provides invaluable reassurance, as it reduces stress and anticipatory anxiety, which can worsen the disease for virtually all patients.

Regular Maintenance Medications. Maintenance medications for the control of TNP, listed in Table 1-3, are reviewed here, with a focus on empirically beneficial combinations, how to implement them, and how to make them work. Table 1-4 contains medications that oftentimes will be needed to combat the side effect known as brain fog brought about by the analgesic regimen.

Over the years, it has been my experience that balanced polypharmacy is preferable to individual medicines (or combinations of two medicines) at barely tolerable maximum doses, especially because of adverse effects including sedation, dizziness, and feeling depersonalized. There is no "one-size-fits-all" combination. I am sharing the experience that has guided my choices of combinations of drugs in Table 1-3. Ultimately, these options need to be trialed both in real life and in clinical practice. As combinations are tried, discontinue what does not work, and "go with the winners." In clinical research, trials are needed to demonstrate whether combinations are indeed more effective than their constituents while not impinging on safety. Biomarkers for forms of TNP that can help guide combination treatments need to be developed. Necessary monitoring is noted in Table 1-3, as are guidelines for long-term maintenance.

Injectables. Two types of injectable medications are described in Table 1-5. The first comprises injectable maintenance medications

Table 1-3. Maintenance Medications[a]

Drug Type	Compound	Formulation and Dose	Comments and Links to RxList.com and Wikipedia or Journal Article
Sodium-channel blocker	Carbamazepine	Regular tablet, extended-release form, 200–400 mg	Lower dose 100–200 mg/day; higher dose 800–1200 mg/day; extended release or regular tablet needs to be tried out; blood level monitoring not helpful. Unwanted effects: psychotrophic, cerebellar, low systematic sodium; rarer: hair loss, weight gain. Need to increase dose over days, response of trigeminal pain to carbamazepine a diagnostic category; Suitable for treatment of comorbid seizure disorder or bipolar disorder. Long-standing first-line experience. Tegretol (Carbamazepine): Side Effects, Uses, Dosage, Interactions, Warnings (rxlist.com) Carbamazepine Wikipedia
Sodium-channel blocker	Oxcarbazepine	Regular tablet, extended-release form, 150–600 mg	See carbamazepine. Some patients have better effectiveness with oxcarbazepine. Trileptal (Oxcarbazepine): Side Effects, Uses, Dosage, Interactions, Warnings (rxlist.com) Oxcarbazepine - Wikipedia
Sodium-channel blocker	Eslicarbazepine[b]	Regular tablet, 200–800 mg	See carbamazepine. Can possibly be more effective than carbamazepine/oxcarbazepine, one per day application. Not much experience for TNP. Aptiom (Eslicarbazepine Acetate Tablets): Side Effects, Uses, Dosage, Interactions, Warnings (rxlist.com) Eslicarbazepine acetate - Wikipedia

(Continued)

Table 1-3. Maintenance Medications[a] **(Continued)**

Drug Type	Compound	Formulation and Dose	Comments and Links to RxList.com and Wikipedia or Journal Article
Sodium-channel blocker, calcium-channel blocker	Lacosamide[c]	Regular tablet, 50–200 mg	More potent than carbazine compounds. Improved therapeutic window. Well-tolerated in terms of side effects. 50–200 mg/day in 2–3 doses. Rare side effect: obsessive thinking and negative thought content 2–3 months after onset of therapy at doses of >100 mg/day. Can be rescued by stopping with resumption at a lower dose (up to 100 mg/day) and combination with carbazine compounds. Suitable for comorbid seizure disorders and possibly also migraine. Caution warranted in cases of bipolar disorder and obsessive–compulsive disorder. Vimpat (Lacosamide Tablet and Injection): Side Effects, Uses, Dosage, Interactions, Warnings (rxlist.com) Lacosamide - Wikipedia
Sodium-channel blocker	Zonisamide	Regular tablet, 25–100 mg	25–200 mg/day Need to increase dose over days (weeks). Not as potent as carbazines or lacosamide; therefore, need to combine with another mainstay analgesic. Suitable for combination therapies where reduction of body weight is a goal. Also useful for migraine prevention. Zonegran (Zonisamide): Side Effects, Uses, Dosage, Interactions, Warnings (rxlist. com) Zonisamide - Wikipedia

| Gabapentinoids | Gabapentin | Regular tablet, extended-release form, 300–800 mg | From <300 mg/day to several grams per day.
Increase over days and weeks beyond 300 mg, 2–3 times/day.
Rarely completely effective by itself; in need of combination, first place with sodium-channel blocker and SNRI (see SNRI rows in this table); benign safety profile when slow initial and increased dosing.
Mild brain fog.
Extended-release formula helps some, but not of critical advantage for many/ most.
Suitable for comorbid seizure disorder and bipolar disorder.
Neurontin (Gabapentin): Side Effects, Uses, Dosage, Interactions, Warnings
Gabapentin - Wikipedia |
| Gabapentinoids | Pregabalin[c] | Regular tablet, capsule, extended-release form, 25–300 mg | See gabapentin.
For TNP, some patients have more effective analgesia with pregabalin; some with gabapentin.
Pregabalin is generally more troublesome, with adverse effects of weight gain, swelling/edema, and more difficulty weaning off than gabapentin, but an elusive pharmacogenetics element seems to play a decisive role. (A minority of patients show this, whereas others are completely unaffected by it.)
Lyrica (Pregabalin): Side Effects, Uses, Dosage, Interactions, Warnings (rxlist.com)
Lyrica CR (Pregabalin Extended-Release Tablets): Side Effects, Uses, Dosage, Interactions, Warnings (rxlist.com)
Pregabalin - Wikipedia |

(Continued)

Table 1-3. Maintenance Medications[a] **(Continued)**

Drug Type	Compound	Formulation and Dose	Comments and Links to RxList.com and Wikipedia or Journal Article
Phenyltriazine anticonvulsant	Lamotrigine	Tablet, 25–200 mg	May need to be part of a polypharmacy approach. Dosage must be increased very slowly at a rate of 25 mg per week or 14 days, with a target dose 100 mg. Can be a highly beneficial element of a polytherapy at 100 mg (to 200 mg), but slow dosing means it is not helpful for subacute analgesic needs. Relatively safe and benign with slow dosing. Any skin changes need acute medical attention to not evoke Stevens–Johnson syndrome, which can be dangerous and deadly. Suitable for comorbid seizure disorder, psychiatric comorbidity of bipolar disorder, as add-on to atypical antipsychotic in schizophrenia and schizoaffective disorder. Also used off-label in severe head pain disorders of cluster headaches and SUNCT (add-on). Lamictal (Lamotrigine): Side Effects, Uses, Dosage, Interactions, Warnings (rxlist. com) Lamotrigine - Wikipedia
GABA-B receptor agonist	Baclofen	Tablet, 5–20 mg	From 5 mg, 2–3 times/day to 20 mg, 3–4 times/day. Can be used as the dominant analgesic component in a polytherapy approach, e.g., in case sodium-channel blockers are not suitable. Meaningful combinations with other analgesic classes are feasible and potentially helpful. Overall benign safety profile. Useful with comorbid muscle spasticity or chronically tense muscles (e.g., neurogenic spasticity after stroke/neural injury, multiple sclerosis, chronic vertebrogenic pain with high muscular tension). Baclofen (Baclofen Tablets): Side Effects, Uses, Dosage, Interactions, Warnings (rxlist.com) Baclofen - Wikipedia

SNRI	Duloxetine	Capsule, 20–60 mg	Typically, 20–30 mg/day to 60–90 mg/day, in combination with gabapentinoids and/or sodium-channel blocker. Wean off over weeks or months, if needed, after longer-term therapy. Generally benign safety profile. Cymbalta (Duloxetine HCl): Side Effects, Uses, Dosage, Interactions, Warnings (rxlist.com) Duloxetine - Wikipedia
SNRI	Venlafaxine	Tablet, 25–100 mg Extended-release tablet, 37.5 and 75 mg	From 25 mg/day to 150 mg/day; regular tablet 2–3 times/day. Extended-release tablet 1 time/day. Can function as an analgesic where duloxetine works poorly or shows unwanted side effects (dizziness, sedation, sweating, and other autonomous dysfunction). Effexor (Venlafaxine Hydrochloride): Side Effects, Uses, Dosage, Interactions, Warnings (rxlist.com) Effexor XR (Venlafaxine Hydrochloride Extended-Release): Side Effects, Uses, Dosage, Interactions, Warnings (rxlist.com) Venlafaxine - Wikipedia
SSRI	Vortioxetine	Tablet, 5–20 mg	From 5 mg/day to 20 mg/day. Helpful in combination with gabapentinoids and/or sodium-channel blocker. Benign safety profile. Favorable combination in case of comorbid depressed mood. Brintellix (Vortioxetine Tablets): Side Effects, Uses, Dosage, Interactions, Warnings (rxlist.com) Vortioxetine - Wikipedia

(Continued)

Table 1-3. Maintenance Medications[a] (Continued)

Drug Type	Compound	Formulation and Dose	Comments and Links to RxList.com and Wikipedia or Journal Article
Atypical tetracyclic antidepressive	Mirtazepine	Tablet, 15–45 mg	From 15 mg/day to 45 mg/day. Suitable for combination with gabapentinoids and/or sodium-channel blocker; even balanced effects with SNRI. Mirtazepine can be a potent enhancer of weight gain. Remeron (Mirtazapine): Side Effects, Uses, Dosage, Interactions, Warnings (rxlist.com) Mirtazapine - Wikipedia
SNRI	Milnacipran	Tablet, 12.5–100 mg	From 25 mg, 1–2 times/day to 25 mg, 4 times/day. Similar to duloxetine, but increased effectiveness in fibromyalgia. Savella (Milnacipran HCl Tablets): Side Effects, Uses, Dosage, Interactions, Warnings (rxlist.com) Milnacipran - Wikipedia
NDRI	Bupropion	SR tablet, 100–200 mg XL tablet, 150–300 mg	From 100 mg/day to 200–300 mg/day. See duloxetine. Importantly, bupropion can help with weight loss and smoking cessation and can thus be an important element of combinatorial treatment of TNP polypharmacy. Wellbutrin SR (Bupropion Hydrochloride Sustained-Release): Side Effects, Uses, Dosage, Interactions, Warnings (rxlist.com) Budeprion XL (Bupropion Hydrochloride Extended-Release Tablets): Side Effects, Uses, Dosage, Interactions, Warnings (rxlist.com) Bupropion - Wikipedia

Cannabinoid	Dronabinol[c]	Capsule, 2.5–10 mg	From 2.5 mg/day to 10 mg, 2 times/day. Add-on to polypharmacy as third- or fourth-line agent. Can cause weight gain and/or sedation. Important complement for some patients, but rarely the critical component of a polypharmacy regimen. Barely analgesic by itself. Marinol (Dronabinol Capsules): Side Effects, Uses, Dosage, Interactions, Warnings (rxlist.com) Dronabinol - Wikipedia
Anti-inflammatory	Indomethacin	Tablet, 25–50 mg Extended-release tablet, 75 mg	25–50 mg, 2–3 times/day; extended release 75 mg, 1–2 times/day. Potent anti-inflammatory, pan-COX inhibitor with potentially hard unwanted effects on the GI tract (stomach, colon); need stomach protection and thorough hydration; aim for limited duration. If longer-term needed, use a 5/2 regimen (5 days on with stomach protection; 2 days off drug holiday, replace with 2–3 g of turmeric and 500–1000 mg of acetaminophen [e.g., Tylenol] per day). Of note, rapid resolution of severe craniofacial pain in response to indomethacin suggests a diagnosis of paroxysmal hemicrania. Tivorbex (Indomethacin Capsules): Side Effects, Uses, Dosage, Interactions, Warnings (rxlist.com) Indocin SR (Indomethacin Extended-Release Capsules): Side Effects, Uses, Dosage, Interactions, Warnings (rxlist.com) Indomethacin - Wikipedia
Anti-inflammatory	Meloxicam	Tablet, 7.5–15 mg	7.5–15 mg/day. If anti-inflammatory treatment needs to be added longer-term (e.g., comorbid TMJ, vertebrogenic neck pain), stomach protection and hydration are needed. Mobic (Meloxicam): Side Effects, Uses, Dosage, Interactions, Warnings (rxlist.com) Meloxicam - Wikipedia

(Continued)

Table 1-3. Maintenance Medications[a] (**Continued**)

Drug Type	Compound	Formulation and Dose	Comments and Links to RxList.com and Wikipedia or Journal Article
Atypical gliotropic	Low-dose naltrexone (LDN[d])	Tablet, 1–4.5–6 mg Capsule, also lipid formulation	At compounding pharmacy, can be formulated from 1–6 mg single dose. Final standard dose of 2–4.5 mg/day. Slowly increase dosing as follows: 1 mg/day for 2–4 weeks, 2 mg/day for 2–4 weeks, possible step up to 4.5 mg/day; can even go to 6 mg/day. A strict dose–response relationship has not been seen (awaiting more rigorous clinical trialing); perhaps 2–4.5 mg is more suitable for pure nerve pain, and 4.5–6 mg is more suitable for chronic pain with inflammatory component (e.g., in the context of autoimmune disorders). Aim for dose in the evening/before bed. Await effectiveness within weeks; can conclude futility after 2 months of use at full dose. Unique analgesic medication: slow onset of action. Can work in high synergy with sodium-channel blockers, gabapentinoids, SNRIs, and other well-balanced analgesic regimens that are partially effective and render them resoundingly effective upon addition of LDN. **Important:** LDN cannot work with concomitant opioid therapy. **Also important:** The side-effect profile of LDN is similar to placebo in clinical trials for various forms of chronic pain and inflammation. Sometimes, patients need ultra-low-dose naltrexone if they cannot tolerate LDN (GI, sleep, sedation). In these rare cases, try 0.1–0.5 mg/day, with a gentle and slow dose increase. The use of low-dose naltrexone (LDN) is a novel anti-inflammatory treatment for chronic pain – PMC Low-dose naltrexone - Wikipedia

Opioid	Hydrocodone[c]	Tablet, 5–7.5–10 mg, combined with 325 mg of Tylenol	First, patients should be weaned off marginally effective low-potency opioids so that LDN can be tried (an extraordinarily successful win–win for many patients). Up to 3 tablets/day in order to use less than 1 g of Tylenol. Drug holidays and irregular use are preferable to persistent medication in order to keep receptor systems susceptible. However, opioids for TNP and other forms of non-neuralgic pain should not be ruled out in all cases, as they have made significant differences for many patients and can be taken safely with proper medical guidance. They can also be combined with 0.25 mg of orally dissolving klonopin. There is no absolute counterindication for this approach. Some patients experience a particularly beneficial analgesic response to one specific opioid; although not yet completely explained scientifically, this clinical observation is undeniable. Patients metabolize opioid medications differently. "Hypermetabolizers" might experience less potent and shorter effects. This is genetically rooted. There are also individual variations in opioid receptor biology that likely contribute to individual opioid responses and need to be further elucidated. Vicodin (Hydrocodone and Acetaminophen): Side Effects, Uses, Dosage, Interactions, Warnings (rxlist.com) Hydrocodone/paracetamol - Wikipedia
Opioid	Oxycodone[c]	Tablet, 5–30 mg	In select cases for longer-term use, typically not exceeding 120 mg/day, including aiming for drug holidays (or short periods of lower dose) and practicing opioid rotation. For unavoidable longer-term use, consider methadone. Oxycontin (Oxycodone HCl): Side Effects, Uses, Dosage, Interactions, Warnings (rxlist.com) Oxycodone - Wikipedia

(Continued)

Table 1-3. Maintenance Medications[a] **(Continued)**

Drug Type	Compound	Formulation and Dose	Comments and Links to RxList.com and Wikipedia or Journal Article
Opioid/SNRI	Tramadol[c]	Tablet, 50–100 mg	50–100 mg, 2–3 times/day. Can be used for opioid rotation with hydrocodone or oxycodone. Can also be used as primary opioid in case it has improved analgesic effects. Same qualifiers and caveats as for hydrocodone and oxycodone. Ultram (Tramadol HCl): Side Effects, Uses, Dosage, Interactions, Warnings (rxlist.com) Tramadol - Wikipedia
Opioid/NMDA-receptor modulator	Methadone[c]	Tablet, 5–10 mg Liquid, 10 mg/mL	Many advantages for long-term use. Pretreatment electrocardiogram (ECG) officially recommended, but most meaningful in older patients and in those with any suggestion of cardiac comorbidity. Liquid form allows fine dosing as well as low or microdosing. Can interfere with wound healing. Dolophine (Methadone Tablets): Side Effects, Uses, Dosage, Interactions, Warnings (rxlist.com) Methadone (Methadone Oral Concentrate): Side Effects, Uses, Dosage, Interactions, Warnings (rxlist.com) Methadone - Wikipedia

| Opioid/ NMDA-receptor modulator, SNRI | Levorphanole[b,c] | Tablet, 2–3 mg | Soft upper limit of 12 mg/day. Can be preferable to methadone because it can be more analgesically effective, acting on multiple pain-relevant signaling systems. Overall higher potency and improved safety window compared to methadone. Possibly also higher psychotomimetic activity, but not practically relevant because patients are opioid-adapted before receiving levorphanol. Highest-level challenge involves supply and insurance coverage, as this drug is expensive, even though it was developed in the 1940s. Heavily underrated therapeutic in need of inexpensive generics and controlled clinical studies. Levo Dromoran (Levorphanol): Side Effects, Uses, Dosage, Interactions, Warnings (rxlist.com) Levorphanol - Wikipedia |

[a] Abbreviations: COX, cyclooxygenase; ECG, electrocardiogram; GABA, γ-aminobutyric acid; GI, gastrointestinal; LDN, low-dose naltrexone; NDRI, norepinephrine and dopamine reuptake inhibitor; NMDA, N-methyl-d-aspartate; PMC, PubMed Central; SNRI, serotonin and norepinephrine reuptake inhibitor; SSRI, selective serotonin reuptake inhibitor; SUNCT, short-lasting, unilateral, neuralgiform headache attacks with conjunctival injection and tearing; TMJ, temporomandibular joint; TNP, trigeminal neuropathic pain.
[b] Insurance approval hurdles; expensive.
[c] Controlled substance.
[d] Requires formulation by a compounding pharmacy.

Table 1-4. Medications to Manage "Brain Fog"[a]

Drug Type	Compound	Formulation and Dose	Comments and Links to RxList.com and Wikipedia or Journal Article
NMDA–receptor modulator	Memantine	Tablet, 5–10 mg	Final dose of 5 mg, 2–3 times/day or 10 mg, 2 times/day; can go up to 10 mg, 3 times/day. Extended dose escalation is recommended, e.g., increase by 5 mg/day per week. Treatment can be judged futile after 1 week on 10 mg, 2 times/day. Can also function as an ancillary analgesic. Overall, not a strong medication, so side effects not strong either. Namenda (Memantine HCl): Side Effects, Uses, Dosage, Interactions, Warnings (rxlist.com) Memantine - Wikipedia
DRI, orexin facilitator	Modafinil[b]	Tablet, 100–200 mg	Increase in 50-mg steps from 50 mg/day to 2x 100 mg/day. Can also facilitate effectiveness of a balanced analgesic regimen. Relatively benign drug; now generic. Needs to be taken in the morning and at the latest by noon/early afternoon. Provigil (Modafinil): Side Effects, Uses, Dosage, Interactions, Warnings (rxlist.com) Modafinil - Wikipedia
NDRI/CNS stimulant	Methylphenidate[b]	Tablet, 5–20 mg	From 2.5 mg, 1–2 times/day to 10–20 mg, 1 time/day. CNS stimulant needs to be balanced with sleep; thus, patient should take no more than 2 doses/day, one in the morning, one at noon/early afternoon. Inexpensive (low patient out-of-pocket expense), Schedule II controlled substance, but worth it for many patients. Ritalin (Methylphenidate HCl): Side Effects, Uses, Dosage, Interactions, Warnings (rxlist.com) Methylphenidate - Wikipedia

[a] Abbreviations: CNS, central nervous system; DRI, dopamine reuptake inhibitor; NDRI, norepinephrine and dopamine reuptake inhibitor; NMDA, N-methyl-ᴅ-aspartate.
[b] Controlled substance.

that are subcutaneously self-administered. These medications consist of anti-calcitonin gene-related peptide (anti-CGRP) neutralizing antibodies. The antibodies are known to be effective for the treatment of chronic migraines and have been repurposed for TNP. Clinical trials are currently in process to demonstrate sufficient clinical benefit for approval by the U.S. Food and Drug Administration for TNP treatment.

The second group of injectable medications consists of drugs used to obtain an analgesic impact in a pain crisis or more urgent situation. These hail from quite different classes of medicine and are also listed in Table 1-5.

Use of topically injected botulinum toxin (typically called "Botox") for the maintenance of analgesia will be reviewed separately in the future.

1.3
Treatment with Topical Medications
Gary M. Heir, DMD; Samin (Sami) Sarabadani, DDS; Bijal Shah, DMD; Hemamalini Chandrashekhar, MDS; and Sai Charitha Velamati, DMD

Administering medications topically is a viable alternative for treating trigeminal neuropathies. Topical medications are safe and exhibit minimal side effects and drug interactions. Topical medications are especially helpful for people who are medically compromised or who use a regimen of medications which could have potentially harmful interactions with other drugs.

The International Association for the Study of Pain (IASP) defines pain as "an unpleasant sensory and emotional experience associated with, or resembling that associated with, actual or potential tissue damage." (IASP Pain Terminology 1994) Pain is necessary for survival. It warns of actual and pending harm. IASP further identifies pain as "a personal experience that is influenced to varying degrees by biological, psychological, and social factors." (IASP Pain Terminology 1994)

Table 1-5. Injectables[a] (Not Including Botulinum Toxin)

Drug Type	Compound	Formulation and Dose	Comments and Links to RxList.com and Wikipedia or Journal Article
Anti-CGRP	Erenumab[b]	SC, 140 mg monthly	Subcutaneous self-injection. Can provide meaningful benefits against background chronic head/face pain, in particular that associated with migraines. TNP and migraine-related headaches coexist in many patients. Reducing the migraine burden typically benefits the TNP. This appears to be the benefit of anti-CGRP monoclonal antibodies. Decreased duration of action (shorter than 4 weeks) points toward higher doses with improved benefit, to be examined in future clinical trials. Of all anti-CGRP antibodies, erenumab is the only one directed against the CGRP receptor, not against the ligand. Most prominent side effects are injection-site irritation and pain, which are manageable in most cases. Less frequently, but at times challenging, is constipation. To date, no damage from long-term use has been seen. Aimovig (Erenumab-aooe Injection, for Subcutaneous Use): Side Effects, Uses, Dosage, Interactions, Warnings (rxlist.com) Erenumab - Wikipedia
Anti-CGRP	Galcanezumab[b]	SC, 240 mg loading dose; 120 mg monthly	See erenumab. 300 mg monthly is the approved dose for cluster headaches, suggesting a higher dose for craniofacial pain. To be examined in future clinical trials. Neutralizes CGRP (does not block receptor). Emgality (Galcanezumab-gnlm Injection): Side Effects, Uses, Dosage, Side Effects, Interactions, Warnings (rxlist.com) Galcanezumab - Wikipedia

Anti-CGRP	Fremanezumab[b]	SC, 225 mg monthly	See erenumab and galcanezumab. Ajovy (Fremanezumab-vfrm Injection): Side Effects, Uses, Dosage, Interactions, Warnings (rxlist.com) Fremanezumab - Wikipedia
Anti-CGRP	Eptinezumab	IV, 100 mg monthly	CGRP-neutralizing monoclonal antibody for IV use. Can be considered for urgent care use in case of therapy-refractory pain crises. In need of clinical trialing to further elaborate. Vyepti (Eptinezumab-jjmr Injection for Intravenous Use): Side Effects, Uses, Dosage, Interactions, Warnings (rxlist.com) Eptinezumab - Wikipedia
Sodium-channel blocker	Lidocaine	IV, 2.5–7.5 mg per kg of body weight	Pretreatment electrocardiogram (ECG) is mandatory, especially in patients with potential cardiac/cardio-circulatory cardiocirculatory risk factors and elderly. Treat with low dose first; if not effective, can go to 5 mg per kg of body weight; if partially effective, can go to 7.5 mg per kg body weight. Effective IV treatment can be given with a maximum frequency of once per week. The typical regimen for an analgesic response by the patient is application in intervals biweekly to monthly; importantly, this has to be perceived as a longer-term benefit by the patient. Suitable for urgent care application with intent to break through a vicious pain cycle. Intravenous Lidocaine for Acute Pain: A Systematic Review - PubMed Lidocaine - Wikipedia

(Continued)

Table 1-5. Injectables[a] (Not Including Botulinum Toxin) (Continued)

Drug Type	Compound	Formulation and Dose	Comments and Links to RxList.com and Wikipedia or Journal Article
High-dose steroid	Methylprednisolone	IV, 500–1000 mg/day for 3–5 consecutive days	High-dose steroid IV to break through pain exacerbations. Awaiting controlled trials, but clinical experience bespeaks of effectiveness to break through vicious, refractory migraine pain and other neuralgias. Overall beneficial experience with this IV regimen. Minimal commitment is 3 consecutive days; can be spread Mon–Wed–Fri or 5 consecutive days (Mon–Fri or start any weekday with weekend break). **Important:** Infuse in 500 mL of saline over 1 hour; latest start is 1:00 pm to prevent steroid insomnia. Steroid anxiety and other psychotropic effects can be prevented with 0.5–1 mg of clonazepam (anxiety, stress, also trigeminal analgesic) and 2–5 mg of haloperidol (paranoia, aggressive thinking), with one dose for each on the day of infusion. More severe psychotropic effects present a counterindication, but overall safe and manageable regimen. Intravenous (IV) Methylprednisolone (Solu-medrol) A-Methapred (Methylprednisolone Sodium Succinate): Side Effects, Uses, Dosage, Interactions, Warnings (rxlist.com) Methylprednisolone - Wikipedia
COX2 inhibitor	Meloxicam	IV, 30–60 mg/day	One-time IV, either injection (slow IV) or in 125–250mL 250 mL of saline over 20 min minutes. Particularly suitable for inflammatory co-component of the pain. For known NSAID-responsive pain that has exacerbated; overall milder and less abrasive IV-NSAID than ketorolac (see next). Still use stomach protection and pay attention to proper hydration. More of an urgent/emergency care medication. For regular use: add-on oral meloxicam instead. Anjeso (Meloxicam Injection): Side Effects, Uses, Dosage, Interactions, Warnings (rxlist.com) Meloxicam - Wikipedia

| Pan-COX inhibitor | Ketorolac | IV, 30 mg/day | One-time IV, either injection (slow IV) or in 125–250 mL of saline over 20 min. Need stomach protection and thorough hydration. Can be injected daily for a subacute pain crisis that has NSAID-responsive elements, e.g., TNP exacerbated by a dental, sinus, or eye event. Maximum duration of 5 days. Toradol (Ketorolac Tromethamine): Side Effects, Uses, Dosage, Interactions, Warnings (rxlist.com) Ketorolac - Wikipedia |
| Sodium-channel blocker, calcium-channel blocker | Lacosamide[b,c] | IV, 200 mg/day | One-time IV in 250–500 mL of saline over 1 h to jump-start a lacosamide oral therapy, or to combat a vicious trigeminal pain crisis, by selectively inhibiting pain-related sodium channels and calcium channels. Suitable for urgent/emergency care. Vimpat (Lacosamide Tablet and Injection): Side Effects, Uses, Dosage, Interactions, Warnings Lacosamide - Wikipedia |

[a] Abbreviations: CGRP, calcitonin gene-related peptide; COX/COX2, cyclooxygenase/cyclooxygenase-2; ECG, electrocardiogram; IV, intravenous; NSAID, nonsteroidal anti-inflammatory drug; SC, subcutaneous (self-injection); TNP, trigeminal neuropathic pain.
[b] Insurance approval hurdles; expensive.
[c] Controlled substance.

Trigeminal neuralgia (TN) presents as an acute disabling disorder commonly associated with vascular contact of the trigeminal nerve at the dorsal root entry zone (DREZ) where the nerve enters the brain stem. In 1773, the English physician John Fothergill detailed the clinical presentation of trigeminal neuralgia. He described attacks of TN as severe, electric-shock-like, stabbing pain lasting seconds to minutes. TN is frequently associated with a facial grimace, which resulted in the diagnostic term tic douloureux. Treatment of TN runs the gamut from pharmacotherapy to surgeries including microvascular decompression and gamma knife ablation. However, as classic as the clinical presentation of TN may be, the presentation can vary, and treatment depends on an accurate diagnosis.

Neuropathic pain is subdivided into neuropathy and neuralgia. Before using or prescribing topical medications, one must understand the difference between neuralgias and neuropathies. According to the IASP's Terminology web page, a neuropathy is "a disturbance of function or pathological change in a nerve." The IASP defines neuropathic pain as "pain caused by a lesion or disease of the somatosensory nervous system."

Neuropathy often follows trauma and disease, whereas central TN is spontaneous. Neuropathies present as a more continuous, chronic discomfort ranging from moderate to severe and are often associated with sensory changes. Surgeries for neuralgias that intentionally or unintentionally injure the trigeminal nerve can change a neuralgia into a neuropaty.

Treatment of neuropathic pain, whether neuralgia or neuropathy, typically includes systemic medications that carry a variety of unpleasant side effects. In addition, the use of medications for neuropathic pain may be contraindicated in medically complex or compromised patients or in patients taking other medications that prevent their use. Topical medications are an alternative route of administration of medications for neuropathic pain with minimal, if any, systemic uptake.

Topical medications are not new. Patients have used over-the-counter (OTC) medications, such as topical anti-inflammatory agents, for decades for a variety of maladies, mostly musculoskeletal pain. Custom compounded medications for neuropathic pain have been effective and indicated as an alternative route of administration for the treatment of neuropathic pain disorders.

Anatomy and Discussion. The brain stem is divided into three sections: the midbrain, pons, and medulla. Twelve pairs of cranial nerves, divided into groups of four, emanate from the brain stem. Their functions vary, comprising purely sensory, special sensory, and motor functions, as well as homeostatic regulation of bodily functions. The fifth cranial nerve, the trigeminal (CN-V), comes from the pons, the middle section of the brain stem. It is the largest of the 12 cranial nerves and is subdivided into three distinct divisions: ophthalmic (CN-V$_1$), maxillary (CN-V$_2$), and mandibular (CN-V$_3$). The trigeminal nerve is responsible for sensation to the face and the dura (brain covering), as well as for motor function of the masticatory musculature (chewing). Injury to, or dysfunction of, this nerve may result in a variety of clinical problems, the most disabling of which is TN. Most cases of TN are associated with a vascular contact at the DREZ. However, damage to the trigeminal system can also occur peripherally, meaning located outside the brain and spinal cord. Such peripheral injuries or diseases of the trigeminal system in any of its three divisions can result in other forms of neuropathic pain that are similar to, but do not meet the criteria of, TN. Care must be taken to distinguish a peripheral vs. a central cause of trigeminal neuropathic pain.

The trigeminal nerve is unique, being different from other nerves in several ways. First, the trigeminal nerve is programmed for denervation. For example, the primary teeth of childhood (baby teeth) are lost and replaced by the secondary or permanent teeth. One by one, the primary teeth innervated by the trigeminal nerve are lost. The denervation of the primary teeth does not affect the trigeminal nerve; no disease or trauma is related to the loss of primary teeth and their loss of innervation. Second, the trigeminal nerve is bidirectional. That is, signals can travel both toward (afferent) and away from (efferent) the central nervous system (CNS). This is an important feature of migraine, in which activation of the trigeminal system results in an efferent signal producing inflammatory mediators at the nerve endings. The signals form new blood vessels in the dura, resulting in sensitization of the trigeminal system and afferent noxious signals entering the trigeminal system. This sterile inflammation gives rise to an afferent signal along sensitized nociceptors, resulting in the throbbing pain of migraine. A similar response may occur secondary to peripheral inflammation of other branches of the trigeminal system, resulting in chronic neuropathic pain.

Nociceptors, or pain receptors, are free nerve endings located all over the body, including the skin, muscles, joints, bones, and internal organs. Under normal conditions, nociceptors do not report a noxious or potentially harmful signal to the CNS unless there is actual injury or trauma. The somatosensory system is the network of neural structures in the brain and body that produce the perception of pain, touch, temperature, and body position. If the peripheral somatosensory system is diseased or traumatized, non-noxious signals such as a gentle breeze or light touch may be interpreted as pain.

Neuralgia, such as central TN, is typically characterized by a sharp shock-like pain lasting seconds to minutes. Doctors call this paroxysmal pain. Paroxysmal means sudden, uncontrolled, or intense.

Neuropathy, such as that following a trauma to or disease of the sensory system, results in more continuous chronic pain, often associated with somatosensory distortions (e.g., perception of cold as hot) or loss of sensation.

Peripheral neuropathy is frequently misdiagnosed as trigeminal neuralgia even though the origin of the pain is peripheral rather than at the DREZ. Peripheral neuropathies are effectively treated using topical medications. Medications useful for neuropathic pain that are custom compounded with the active pharmaceutical ingredient or ingredients are absorbed at the site of pain with no systemic or transdermal (through-the-skin) effect. While topical medications have a role in peripheral neuropathies, they are ineffective in central TN.

How Trigeminal Nerve Injuries Affect the Body's Normal Functions and Structures (Pathophysiology). Afferent nerves are not just single fibers but a collection of thousands of different types of cells carrying a variety of signals, including mechanical, thermal, and chemical sensitivity ranging from light touch to pain and the discrimination of temperature.

Disruption of nerve conduction as a result of trauma or disease can result in altered perception and inappropriate signals that are interpreted by the brain as painful. The extent of injury and the prognosis for recovery depend on the degree of injury.

Editor's Note: The next paragraph is intended for clinicians.

The Seddon grading system describes three levels of severity of neuronal injury and subsequent dysfunction. The most innocuous form of peripheral nerve injury is referred to as neuropraxia. This does not represent permanent injury and is characterized by the temporary disruption of neuronal conduction. It is fully reversible. Next is axonotmesis, a sensory dysfunction of the nerve in which some fibers are damaged beyond recovery. Axonotmesis does not completely resolve and may result in paresthesia or the sensation of tingling, burning, and numbness along with pain. The most severe of the three levels is neurotmesis. Neurotmesis is a severe injury in which the nerve has been transected or cut through and will not recover. Despite the loss of innervation, stimulus-independent pain may persist as a result of spontaneous activity of the proximal portion of the transected nerve, which remains viable. Chronic neuropathic pain along the trigeminal system is characteristic of axonotmesis and neurotmesis. The quality of this type of neuropathic pain can range from chronic discomfort to sensory changes and paroxysmal episodes, often leading to the misdiagnosis of TN.

Editor's Note: Nonclinical readers should begin again here.

The experience of chronic pain following trauma to the trigeminal system is referred to as painful posttraumatic trigeminal neuropathic pain (PPTTNP). Many patients experiencing injury from a dental or intracranial procedure report pain along the trigeminal innervation; this is not trigeminal neuralgia. In such cases, a diagnosis of PPTTNP requires a known injury to a major branch of the trigeminal nerve with symptoms including sensory changes lasting more than three months. Traumatic injury may also result in the formation of a neuroma, a mass of nerve and connective tissue that forms at the proximal (close) end of a transected (cut) nerve. Neuromas form at the end of transected nerves that fail to regenerate or reconnect with the distal (far) portion of the severed nerve. Neuromas are structures that constantly produce inflammatory mediators (endogenous chemicals that promote inflammation around the injured nerve to facilitate its repair). This results in constant inflammatory activity and discomfort along sensitized injured nociceptors.

Editor's Note: The next paragraph is intended for clinicians.

How Topical Medications Work. There are four targets for topical medications: peripheral receptors, primary afferent neurons, the dorsal horn of the spinal cord, and the pain inhibitory system. Dampening of peripheral nociceptive input is thought to be the mechanism for pain reduction in the use of topical medications. An accurate diagnosis facilitates recognition of the potential target for the pharmacologic action of topical compounded medications. Targets of topically administered active pharmacological ingredients include abnormal sodium-channel expression, upregulated adrenergic receptors, and inefficient pain modulation. Effective systemic medications include tricyclic antidepressants, local and topical anesthetics, and antiseizure medications. Inflammation responds to nonsteroidal anti-inflammatory drugs (NSAIDs), which diminish peripheral receptor sensitization. Chronic centralized pain may be affected by N-methyl-d-aspartate (NMDA) and α-amino-3-hydroxy-5-methyl-4-isoxazole propionic acid (AMPA) antagonists. Agents affecting γ-aminobutyric acid (GABA), such as anticonvulsants, are useful and affect pain inhibition and modulation. With varying degrees of efficacy, these medications, when administered systemically, are associated with unpleasant side effects including sedation, disequilibrium, and bone marrow suppression.

Editor's Note: Nonclinical readers should begin again here.

As TN often affects patients 50 years of age and older, complications associated with medically compromised patients and interactions with other medications may present a risk. The benefit of topical medication is the minimal risk, if any, of side effects and interactions. Topical medications can be the route of choice for medically compromised individuals with neuropathic pain. The optimal drug concentration can be administered at the site of pain. Topical medications are easy for the patient to apply. There is no need to titrate, and side effects are negligible, if any. There is no risk of overuse or abuse. The only consideration is allergy to ingredients in the topical, which may result in a local skin rash.

Topical medications are typically custom compounded. They must be compounded by an experienced, knowledgeable pharmacist to ensure consistent quality. If compounded improperly, even if the ingredients are correct, the penetration, depth of penetration, and speed may be compromised.

Penetration of compounded medications requires that the medications be broken down to nearly a molecular level. A description of the equipment necessary to accomplish this is beyond the scope of this brief discussion. Compounding incorporates these molecules into micelles. A micelle is the product of milling the medication to a molecular level and incorporating it, through use of a surfactant, with an inactive vehicle or carrier that passes through either the mucosa (mucus membrane) or the dermis (skin). A micelle can be compared to a soap bubble composed of both hydrophilic and lipophilic molecules. The lipophilic action penetrates the dermis or mucosa and facilitates the penetration of the hydrophilic component. The most common inorganic vehicle is typically a soybean product or soybean oil. It has a standard rate of penetration that can be adjusted by adding additional inert vehicle modifiers such as propylene glycol or ethoxy glycol, which can adjust the depth and speed at which the medication is absorbed. Shallow penetration is advantageous when treating sensitized nerve endings in the dermal layer. However, if the penetration is too rapid, the patient may realize only a brief positive response. The importance of properly adjusting the penetration rate cannot be overstated. Once the penetration is complete through various partitions of the skin and mucosa including the stratum corneum, epidermis, and dermis, the micelle breaks down and disperses the medication subdermally or submucosally. Topical medications used alone or in combination with systemic medications have been shown to be highly effective in providing rapid pain relief when compared to systematic medications alone.

Practical Implications. The primary use for topical medications is in the treatment of neuropathic pain disorders. As discussed, the trigeminal nerve system supplies sensation to the face and oral cavity. A disturbance of or injury to this system can result in the perception of non-noxious stimuli as painful. Over time, when untreated, pain tends to spread over a wider field and become more intense. Frequently, untreated chronic pain becomes the disease rather than a symptom of an underlying condition. Topical medications have the advantage of targeting the receptors at the site of prior injury and have a calming effect on previously sensitized peripheral nociceptive receptors. Beyond this, it is assumed that the peripheral dampening effect extends to the trigeminal ganglion. This dampening effect seems, over time, to markedly diminish noxious input. In one study, a custom compounded topical neuropathic pain medication, with pregabalin as the primary ingredient, was compared with combined therapy with systemic medications alone or topical medications alone. (Heir 2008) Patients in the study reported pain levels on a visual analog scale (VAS) ranging from approximately 7.5/10 to 8.6/10. Pain scores diminished by approximately 50% in all groups. However, topical medications alone, applied four times daily to the affected area over 3 weeks, demonstrated the fastest reduction in pain compared to the other treatments, with no side effects or systemic uptake. Furthermore, a comparison of topical medications alone with combined systemic and topical medications revealed that the combination treatment provided the greatest pain relief. (Heir 2008, 2022) The formulation of these compounds is beyond the scope of this article; however, more detailed information regarding actions and applications as well as formulations is available in the cited reference.

The use of custom compounded topical medications is not limited to the treatment of neuropathic pain. For example, several medications involving guaifenesin-based compounds have been effectively used for musculoskeletal pain, and compounds containing misoprostol as the active pharmaceutical ingredient have been used for the treatment of intraoral ulcers often associated with viral or autoimmune disorders. In addition, viral infections such as herpes simplex can be treated topically with excellent benefit using 2-deoxy-d-glucose (2-DG). (Heir 2022)

Conclusion. Pain mediated by the trigeminal system is not necessarily trigeminal neuralgia. A detailed history of traumatic injuries to the area supplied by the trigeminal nerve, including dental procedures, may lead to a differential diagnosis of a peripheral neuropathy rather than classic TN. Differential diagnosis is key. When neuropathic pain is diagnosed excluding TN as the primary source, the clinician is faced with the risk factors and side effects of systemic medications. Topical medications used to treat numerous neuropathic and other peripheral pain disorders can incorporate analgesics, antivirals, antibiotics, topical anesthetics, antidepressants, and various oral rinses. The side effect profile, especially important in the treatment of elderly patients with comorbidities and potential interactions with other medications is minimal. Topical medications thus represent a viable alternative for treating neuropathic pain.

1.4
Ketamine Infusions for Pain Relief

Mohan S. Ravi, MD; Hannah K. Rasmussen, MD; QiLiang Chen, MD, PhD; and Xiang Qian, MD, PhD

Facial pain represents a group of conditions that involve chronic or recurrent pain in the face. A variety of factors, such as nerve damage, inflammation, and muscular tension, can cause these syndromes, which can range from mild discomfort to debilitating pain, highlighting the complexity and heterogeneity of facial pain. The treatment of facial pain can be challenging and often involves a multidisciplinary approach. Existing medications and surgical options for facial pain have limitations. Anti-inflammatories, antidepressants, and anticonvulsants often provide only partial relief and can lead to side effects including bleeding, ulcers, weight gain, and rare complications such as immunosuppression and electrolyte disorders (e.g., syndrome of inappropriate antidiuretic hormone secretion [SIADH] with low sodium levels). As such, there is a need to identify pharmacological alternatives to address facial pain.

Ketamine is a dissociative anesthetic acting as an NMDA receptor antagonist that has emerged as a potential treatment option for facial pain. Dissociative means that the medication separates the mind from the body, causing a kind of floating sensation. NMDA receptors are widely distributed in the trigeminal nerve and other facial nerve pathways. When activated, NMDA receptors play a crucial role in the amplification of pain signals and central sensitization, contributing to the perception of severe pain. Ketamine exerts its analgesic properties by blocking these receptors. By doing so, ketamine is thought to reduce the amplification of pain signals and mitigate central sensitization in conditions where the NMDA system is hyperactive. This unique mechanism of action makes ketamine a promising option for managing facial pain and other neuropathic pain conditions. Although the use of ketamine for the treatment of facial pain is still being explored, early research suggests that it may be a promising option for patients who have not responded to traditional treatments.

This section examines ketamine's unique analgesic properties, its risks, and the current evidence for its use in treating facial pain.

Ketamine Pharmacology. Ketamine was first synthesized in 1962 and was initially used as a general anesthetic. However, in the 1990s, ketamine began to be used as an analgesic medication because of its ability to relieve pain at subanesthetic doses. Today, ketamine is used in a variety of settings for the management of chronic pain, including neuropathic pain, complex regional pain syndrome (CRPS), and cancer pain. Ketamine is thought to modulate central pain processing through its NMDA antagonism. Ketamine also affects other neurotransmitter systems, such as serotonin, dopamine, and GABA, which may contribute to its analgesic properties. In addition to its analgesic properties, ketamine has been shown to have anti-inflammatory and antinociceptive (pain-relieving) effects, making it a promising option for the treatment of chronic pain.

The pharmacokinetics of ketamine are complex and depend on the route of administration. Upon intravenous (IV) administration, ketamine has a rapid onset of action, with peak effects occurring within 5–10 minutes. The duration of action is 30–60 minutes, with a half-life of effectiveness of approximately 2–3 hours. Upon intramuscular (IM) administration, ketamine has a slower onset of action, with peak effects occurring within 15–30 minutes. The duration of action is more extended than with IV administration, typically lasting 60–90 minutes. Ketamine's pharmacology and mechanism of action make it a unique and effective analgesic medication. The various routes of administration provide flexibility in dosing and allow for individualized treatment plans.

Use of Ketamine for Facial Pain Conditions: Migraine Headaches. Approximately 12% of the U.S. population experiences migraines, which are pulsating and throbbing headaches, often unilateral, associated with nausea and vomiting, dizziness, and sound or visual disturbances. Current treatment options for migraine headaches include abortive medications (i.e., those working to stop a migraine as it is happening, such as triptans and ubrogepant), as well as preventative medications (e.g., β-blockers, calcium-channel blockers, tricyclic antidepressants, and Botox injections). Despite these options, many individuals have migraines that are resistant or refractory to currently available treatments. The burden of disease disproportionately affects women of childbearing age, low-income households, and the elderly. Thus, the discovery of new therapy modalities remains an active area of research.

Ketamine is one agent that is being studied for the treatment of migraines. Some researchers have hypothesized a link between NMDA receptor activity and migraine attacks. Specifically, increased levels of glutamate in the blood and cerebrospinal fluid have been found to be associated with migraine attacks, as well as with the neurologic process called cortical spreading depolarization, which is thought to be involved in the generation of migraine auras. It has been postulated that NMDA antagonists, such as ketamine, which inhibit these excitatory glutaminergic receptors, may block the propagation of migraines and their associated auras. However, the use of ketamine for this indication is still under investigation, and there is a need for more high-quality studies in this area.

Of the studies that have been completed, most show conflicting evidence for the benefit of ketamine in the treatment of migraines. For example, one retrospective study found an approximately 3-point drop in pain scores after an average five-day ketamine infusion compared to lidocaine infusion in patients with intractable migraine. (Etchison 2018) However, another randomized controlled trial conducted at a single-center emergency department in the United States compared 0.2 mg/kg IV ketamine (N = 16) to a placebo of 0.9% normal saline infusion (N = 18) and found no statistically significant difference between ketamine and the placebo for acute migraine management. Intranasal ketamine use for migraines has also been studied, with one double-blinded randomized parallel group trial finding that 25 mg of intranasal ketamine was able to reduce the severity but not the duration of aura in migraine, compared to 2 mg of intranasal midazolam as control. (Afridi 2013) Finally, subcutaneous administration of ketamine for migraine has been studied as well, with one study based in Europe demonstrating that 80 μg subcutaneous ketamine administered three times per day for 3 weeks provided significant treatment and prophylactic pain relief compared to 0.9% normal saline injection. (Nicolodi 1995)

Ultimately, although these studies suggest the possibility that ketamine can benefit those who have migraine headaches, the current data are not yet definitive or replicable, and further studies are required to determine whether ketamine administration in migraine headaches should be pursued as a standard of care treatment option, at what phase of care ketamine should be selected for use by individuals with migraines, and whether certain subsets of patients with migraines would benefit from this treatment more than others.

Cluster Headaches. Cluster headaches are severe episodic headaches that are unilateral, usually in the trigeminal distribution, lasting about 15 minutes to several hours, and often associated with ipsilateral (same-sided) autonomic symptoms such as lacrimation, drooping eyelid, and congestion. They are estimated to impact roughly 0.1% of the worldwide population and predominantly affect males. Current treatments include high-flow oxygen, triptans, steroids, and greater occipital nerve block for management of an acute attack and calcium-channel blockers (e.g., verapamil), lithium, melatonin, and topiramate for prevention of an attack.

The underlying pathophysiology of cluster headaches is complex and not fully understood, involving multiple pathways including the trigeminovascular pathway, trigeminal autonomic reflex, and hypothalamus and pituitary axis. Several studies have implicated glutamate and NMDA receptor activation within the trigeminovascular pathway as a mechanism for the development of cluster headaches. The kynurenine pathway has also been implicated in cluster headaches, with certain metabolites of the pathway that naturally inhibit NMDA receptors found to be significantly reduced in patients with cluster headaches. These studies would suggest that antagonism of the NMDA receptor with agents such as ketamine may provide a treatment option for cluster headaches.

Studies have assessed the efficacy of IV and intranasal routes of administration of ketamine for this purpose. One group based in Switzerland treated 29 patients with refractory cluster headaches (both episodic and chronic) with IV ketamine infusions; the infusion treatments lasted 40–60 minutes each and were repeated every 2 weeks up to four times. This group saw "complete abortion of headaches in 100% of episodic cluster headache patients and 54% of chronic cluster headache patients for a period of 3–18 months". (Granata et al., 2016) Another group in France performed a study with 17 patients, each of whom received a single IV dose of ketamine (0.5 mg/kg) combined with magnesium (3 g) over 2 hours. The researchers found that the patients saw a decrease in number of daily cluster headache attacks from 4.3 ± 2.4 before treatment to 1.3 ± 1.0 after treatment. (Moisset et al., 2020) In contrast, intranasal ketamine seems to have a less significant benefit, with a study in Denmark finding no significant reduction in pain levels 15 minutes after the administration of 15 mg of intranasal ketamine spray (given every 6 minutes up to five times) in a population of 20 patients with chronic cluster headaches, although there was a significant reduction 30 minutes following treatment. (Peterson 2022) Thus, although there is some evidence to suggest a possible benefit of ketamine in the treatment of cluster headaches, the primary conclusion from most studies is that there is a need for further study and randomized controlled trials to obtain better data on this potential treatment.

Trigeminal Neuralgia and Persistent Idiopathic Facial Pain.
Trigeminal neuralgia (TN) is a debilitating condition marked by paroxysms of intense, electric-shock-like pain along the trigeminal nerve. These episodes are sudden, brief, and recurrent, commonly

triggered by routine facial movements or stimuli. Persistent idiopathic facial pain (PIFP), on the other hand, is characterized by chronic facial pain with no identifiable cause or structural abnormalities. The pain in PIFP is typically a continuous dull, aching, burning, or throbbing sensation. Both conditions are challenging to control with first-line medications because a significant minority of patients with these conditions either have only a partial response to these medications or are unable to tolerate their side effects, resulting in interruption or termination of these medications. For example, in a 2014 retrospective study of 200 patients with classic TN over a mean period of approximately 8 months from the initiation of treatment (first-line agents for TN), roughly 27% of those on carbamazepine and 18% of those on oxcarbazepine developed undesirable side effects that led to the interruption or complete cessation of treatment.

Frequently, for clinicians, this has resulted in escalation to non-first-line medication options including ketamine infusions, which have been more rigorously studied in recent years for TN and PIFP. One study at a single academic medical center included 12 patients with refractory facial pain who received continuous ketamine infusions. Patients with TN were more likely to respond to ketamine infusion than those with PIFP. The responders required a lower dose of ketamine to achieve adequate pain relief, and they reported a greater reduction in pain scores than the patients who received intermittent ketamine infusions. The results of this study suggest that continuous ketamine infusions may be an effective treatment option for patients with refractory facial pain from both TN and PIFP but especially the former.

In another single-center study involving 100 adults (aged 20–70 years) with refractory TN, patients were enrolled into ketamine bolus infusion sessions every 4 days for three sessions. The ketamine infusion group showed a statistically significant longer-lasting analgesic effect at 3 months post infusion compared to the control group. (Mogahed 2017)

Side Effects and Risks of Ketamine. There are few absolute contraindications to the use of ketamine. According to the American College of Emergency Physicians (ACEP), these include its use in infants younger than 3 months of age or in individuals known or suspected to have schizophrenia. Relative contraindications published by the ACEP include its use in individuals with porphyria or in those with thyroid disease who are taking thyroid medications because of the increased sympathomimetic activity induced by ketamine. In perioperative management, ketamine has long been thought to increase intracranial pressure (ICP), so it is also often avoided in patients with CNS masses, hydrocephalus, or other conditions for which increased ICP is detrimental. Similarly, ketamine can raise intraocular pressure (IOP) and is avoided when increased IOP is undesirable (such as in glaucoma). Other considerations in the use of ketamine include side effects such as depression of the CNS, elevation of blood pressure, and hepatobiliary dysfunction with repeated use or abuse. Chronic use of ketamine can also be associated with bladder dysfunction.

Additionally, ketamine has the potential to be highly addictive. Ketamine is currently considered a Schedule III controlled substance by the U.S. Drug Enforcement Agency because of its addictive potential. Given the rising interest in ketamine infusions as a treatment modality for intractable chronic pain disorders, including headaches, consideration of the addictive nature of the drug is perhaps of renewed importance.

Adverse effects of ketamine can be considered in categories including common side effects in therapeutic treatment, long-term effects of repeated ketamine use, and symptoms of ketamine toxicity and severe overdose. Short-term side effects commonly seen during ketamine treatment can include disorientation, dysarthria (slurred or difficulty in speech due to weakness of speech muscles), arrhythmia (irregular heartbeat), dizziness, muscle rigidity, increased blood pressure, increased heart rate, visual or auditory hallucinations, and dissociation (emotional detachment and/or lack of connection in thoughts, memories, and sense of identity). These effects typically resolve with cessation of use or treatment. More serious complications of repeated ketamine use include structural brain changes such as loss of gray and white matter integrity, as well as irreversible damage to the bladder (known as ketamine bladder syndrome), which manifests as persistent discomfort in the lower urinary tract. Finally, symptoms that are more suggestive of toxicity or overdose include nystagmus (involuntary eye movement), excessive salivation, abdominal pain, nausea/vomiting, oversedation or unconsciousness, respiratory depression or apnea, cardiac dysrhythmias (irregularities), and seizures. Management of ketamine toxicity generally consists of supportive care. If ketamine has been consumed orally in large amounts, activated charcoal may be considered for gastrointestinal decontamination. Hemodialysis is not regarded as effective for the clearance of ketamine because of its large volume of distribution.

Conclusion and Future Directions. In conclusion, this section provides a comprehensive overview of the versatile role of ketamine in the management of various facial pain syndromes. Ketamine's history as a general anesthetic, coupled with its subsequent repurposing as an analgesic, underscores its unique pharmacological properties. The exploration of ketamine's potential application in addressing migraine headaches, cluster headaches, TN, and PIFP highlights the ongoing pursuit of better pain management options. Although some studies present promising results, the variable design and quality of research to date call for further investigation and more robust clinical trials to establish ketamine's efficacy in these specific contexts. This section also emphasized the complex risk–benefit considerations associated with ketamine's clinical application, including its side effect profile, potential for addiction, and contraindications. Therefore, a prudent, evidence-based approach is essential for its incorporation into therapeutic protocols. The future in this evolving landscape of pain management beckons for focused, high-quality research, potentially exploring topics such as the long-term effects of ketamine administration, optimal dosing regimens, and patient selection criteria. This comprehensive examination underscores the intricate balance between ketamine's therapeutic potential and the need for responsible and informed clinical utilization, shedding light on the complexities of ketamine's role in the evolving landscape of pain management.

Overall, although there has been rising interest in ketamine infusions or administration for the treatment of chronic headaches, the reported studies are extremely variable in design and quality, and the overall evidence inconclusive regarding the efficacy of this drug in this space.

1.5
What To Do If Pain Takes You to the Emergency Department or Urgent Care Facility
Mark E. Linskey, MD

Trigeminal neuropathic pain (TNP) is divided into "typical" and "atypical" varieties. Typical neuropathic pain is sudden in onset and resolution; lasts seconds to minutes; is described as sharp, intense, stabbing, or electric-shock-like in character; and is not associated with pain between the episodes. In contrast, atypical neuropathic pain can be characterized as dull, aching, burning, throbbing, and/or pressured. It can be present some of the time, all of the time, or all of the time with intermittent flare-ups in severity. TNP falls on a continuous spectrum. The patient's position on that spectrum can change over time with syndrome evolution or as a result of therapeutic interventions (Figure 1-1).

On one end of the spectrum, classic TN consists of typical neuralgic pain only. There are two hybrid syndromes in which both types of neuralgic pain are present, but in different dominance ratios. TN1 is when typical pain is present more than half of the time, whereas TN2 is when atypical pain is present more than half of the time. Two other syndromes in which only atypical pain is present occupy the other end of the clinical spectrum. The first, when the atypical pain is

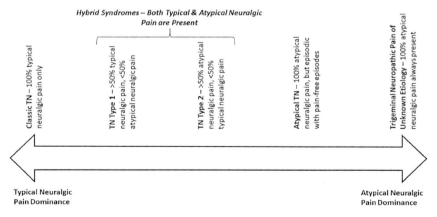

Figure 1-1. Clinical spectrum of trigeminal neuralgic pain syndrome.

intermittent, interspersed with pain-free episodes, is known as atypical TN. The second, in which some atypical pain is always present, is called trigeminal neuropathic pain of unknown (or obscure) etiology (TNPUE). The interventions described in this section focus on acute crises of typical trigeminal neuralgic pain. This means that the interventions will predictably work best for patients with classic TN and for the typical pain components for patients with hybrid syndrome TN1 or TN2. Although patients with atypical neuralgic pain also have severe acute pain flare-ups, the interventions described herein are less likely to help with this type of pain, which often requires standard pain pharmacological interventions such as narcotics and, more recently, ketamine.

Standard approaches for treating patients with general pain include acetaminophen (brand name: Tylenol), nonsteroidal anti-inflamatory drugs (NSAIDs), (such as ibuprofen or indomethacin) narcotics, ketamine, and other drugs that can be administered both orally and intravenously. These medications may prove useful for treating acute flare-ups of atypical trigeminal neuralgic pain. However, one of the unique characteristics of typical trigeminal neuralgic pain is that it generally does not respond well to these agents. One of the unique features of typical trigeminal neuralgic pain is that it characteristically responds best to anti-convulsive drug (ACD) treatment. These drugs generally include the first-line TN agents in the carbamazepine family (e.g., brand name: Tegretol) and oxcarbazepine (brand name: Trileptal), as well as agents in the GABA analogue family, which includes gabapentin (brand name: Neurontin) and pregabalin (brand name: Lyrica). Unfortunately, these agents suffer from several major drawbacks during an acute flare-up of typical TN pain:

- First, TN is characterized by tactile triggers in the trigeminal nerve distribution, and these agents can only be administered orally. If opening the mouth, taking pills, having liquid in the mouth, or swallowing are tactile triggers, an individual may not be able to take the medication orally.
- Second, these agents have pharmacokinetic half-lives that require several days of consistent oral dosing for drug levels to reach a steady state. If tactile-trigger concerns lead to missed oral doses, the circulating blood levels can decrease, resulting in

worsening acute pain flare-ups. This becomes an accelerating vicious circle over time.

- Third, even if an individual could somehow take the medication orally during an acute crisis, depending on how many doses had already been missed, the medication may take too long, or require too many doses over time, for an effective blood steady-state level to be re-achieved.

ACDs that can be administered intravenously (IV) in a loading dose that can immediately achieve a therapeutic drug level are needed to break the acute crisis of typical TNP. The mainstay and most proven IV agent for TN is phenytoin (brand name: Dilantin) and now its newer cousin fosphenytoin (brand name: Cerebyx). Phenytoin has a long history of use in TN, and in fact, it was the first ACD to be shown to be effective for TN. It can be loaded to a full therapeutic drug blood level if administered intravenously over 20–60 minutes, with telemetry monitoring for possible cardiac heart rhythm and hemodynamic blood pressure effects. Fosphenytoin is newer and safer to load and, along with phenytoin, has been effectively used for acute attacks of typical TNP. Once the pain cycle is broken with IV drugs, the patient can once again resume taking their better oral ACD medications and re-establish therapeutic blood levels of these drugs. If additional time is needed for several oral ACD doses to occur, the IV medication can be continued in a therapeutic maintenance dose regimen until the oral-dosing/blood-level goal is achieved, and the patient can be sent home on their oral drug regimen.

Patients in a typical TNP crisis in which they cannot open their mouth, take pills, and eat or drink may also be significantly dehydrated by the time they go to the emergency department (ED). In this case, IV hydration may be an important component of helping resuscitate them and helping them feel better.

Although no studies have been reported to date assessing their effects on an acute crisis of TN, new ACDs for epilepsy are constantly being developed. Two are of potential interest for the management of patients who are in typical TNP crisis because they not only can be administered intravenously but can also be fully loaded with the initial IV dose. These medications are levetiracetam (brand name: Keppra) and lacosamide (brand name: Vimpat). Although neither has been rigorously evaluated for treating TN, as ACDs have been, they retain

Note for Emergency Department or Urgent Care Physicians

Recommendations for Urgent/Emergent Care of Patients with an Acute Attack of Neuropathic Pain from Trigeminal Neuralgia

Patient Advice:
If you are experiencing an acute trigeminal neuralgic pain symptom attack, remember that narcotics usually will not work to relieve your pain. Furthermore, you may not be able to take your prescribed oral anticonvulsant drugs (opening or touching your mouth may be a tactile pain trigger). In addition, you may have missed one or more doses for this reason, and your blood stream drug levels may have dropped as a result. Finally, even resuming these drugs may not help in the short-term, as they enter your system too slowly. In an emergency, notify your treating physician and then seek medical attention at a local hospital that treats your condition.

To the Senior Emergency Room Physician:

The key drug to use is an anticonvulsant that can be loaded to full therapeutic blood levels intravenously (IV). Phenytoin (Dilantin) was the first anticonvulsant drug (ACD) shown to work for trigeminal neuralgia (TN). Deliver a 1 g load IV over 20–60 min with telemetry cardiac and blood pressure monitoring. This will break the acute pain cycle more than 90% of the time. Alternatively, fosphenytoin (Cerebyx) may be used (1 g phenytoin equivalent load) under the same monitoring conditions. Once the pain cycle has been broken, the patient can resume taking their better oral ACD medications, and they can even consider taking one or two extra doses, on a one-time basis, to catch up if they have previously missed a significant number of doses. If they are allergic to phenytoin or these medications do not work, two other ACDs (levetiracetam [Keppra] and lacosamide [Vimpat]) can be loaded IV and might help. These drugs have not been tested and proven for treating TN, but they are in the same therapeutic drug class and can be safely loaded IV.

Key points:

Neuropathic pain generally does not respond to standard analgesics, including opioids (narcotics).

It is usually managed with oral (per os [PO]) ACDs that can take days to achieve therapeutic drug levels.

The patient has come to you because they are in acute neuropathic pain crisis, they may have missed several PO ACD doses and may be unable to take PO ACDs in your ED because of oral tactile pain triggering, or they may not be on the right medication to start with (usually carbamazepine, oxcarbazepine, gabapentin, pregabalin, baclofen, or a combination).

Immediate Action Required:

Plan A: Administer a 1 g load of phenytoin IV over 20–60 min with telemetry cardiac and blood pressure monitoring (alternatively, fosphenytoin may be used [1 g phenytoin equivalent load]).

Plan B: Administer a 1000 mg load of levetiracetam IV over 5 min with telemetry cardiac and blood pressure monitoring.

Plan C: Administer a 200- to 400-mg load of lacosamide IV with telemetry cardiac and blood pressure monitoring.

Summary:

If the acute attack does not respond to an IV load of phenytoin or fosphenytoin, then it is reasonable to consider levetiracetam or lacosamide as alternatives in similar drug classes that can be safely loaded IV. Once the pain cycle has been broken, the better PO ACDs can be resumed.

For more information:

A. Zakrzewska, J. M.; Linskey, M. E. Trigeminal neuralgia. BMJ Clin Evid (online). 2014;2014(Oct 6),1207. https://www.ncbi.nlm.nih.gov/pmc/articles/PMC4191151/.

B. American College of Physicians. Trigeminal Neuralgia Module. ACP Smart Medicine. http://smartmedicine.acponline.org/content.aspx?gbosid=299. Must be a member to access.

C. Facial Pain Association Home Page. www.facepain.org.

D. American Association of Neurological Surgeons. Trigeminal Neuralgia – Causes, Symptoms and Treatments. https://www.aans.org/Patients/Neurosurgical-Conditions-and-Treatments/Trigeminal-Neuralgia.

Figure 1-2.   Single-page summary that individuals with trigeminal neuralgia can use to help in communicating with health care providers in crisis situations.

that theoretic potential, and as drugs that can be loaded rapidly intravenously. Thus, they may be worth trying for a TNP crisis. This may be particularly relevant for patients who are allergic to phenytoin or fosphenytoin. An empirical trial of IV loading of one of these two agents if phenytoin or fosphenytoin does not work or cannot be administered because of drug allergy would seem to be a reasonable (though unproven) empirical option.

For individuals with TN, we recommend that you carry with you, on your person (wallet, purse, or cell phone) at all times, a sheet of paper or card that you can show to a health care professional in the ED if you are in such an acute pain crisis that you cannot talk without triggering a pain attack. Figure 1-2 provides a single-page summary that you can/should also take with you to try and help in these crisis situations for communicating with your ED health care provider.

Editor's Note: Ideally, you should establish a relationship with a physician experienced in the care of TNP who agrees with this protocol and can be available to recommend to an ED physician their suggestions for its use. In an emergency, an ED physician may not have the time to review the references provided and come to independent conclusions on the safety of the recommendations in a timely manner. Ultimately, the ED physician must feel comfortable proceeding as they or a local consulting expert physician will be responsible doctor for your care. Physician-to-physician consultation remains the best option.

Disclaimer: This article discusses medical diagnoses and potential therapeutic interventions. It is intended for educational and background reference purposes only. It is not intended to prescribe any specific course of care or treatment. Actual care and/or treatment must always be prescribed by an appropriately licensed health professional in direct consultation with their patient in the setting of that specific patient–physician relationship considering their specific circumstances, as well as the risks and benefits of any intervention, which should be mutually reviewed and agreed upon onsite at that time.

Chapter 2
Types of Neuropathic Facial Pain

Anne B. Ciemnecki, MA

When we think about facial pain, most of us think about trigeminal neuralgia or trigeminal neuropathy. We think of pain in one or more of the three distributions of the trigeminal nerve. Put simply, the pain can occur near the eye, cheek, or jaw. It can be episodic, characterized by brief periods of lightning-like pain lasting for a few seconds to a few minutes, a refractory or rest period, another bolt from the blue, another refractory period, and so on. Or, it can be neuropathic, a lower level of aching, creepy, annoying pain that does not go away. Or it could be both.

Sadly, there are many more forms of neuropathic facial pain. In 2011, the Trigeminal Neuralgia Association (TNA) changed its name to the Facial Pain Association (FPA) to reflect this fact and to educate, support, and advocate for members the community who have different forms of neuropathic facial pain. Until recently, people with "other" forms of neuropathic facial pain mentioned that the FPA did not pay enough attention to their conditions. In this book, we are devoting the 10 sections of this chapter to other forms of neuropathic facial pain. To our brother and sister warriors with that pain, you are the rarest of the rare. We see you. We hear you.

This chapter covers the following topics:

- Glossopharyngeal neuralgia
- Geniculate neuralgia
- Occipital neuralgia
- Hemifacial spasm
- Burning mouth syndrome
- Anesthesia dolorosa
- Postherpetic neuralgia
- Autonomic effects of trigeminal nerve injury

- Bilateral facial pain
- Medical causes of facial pain

As an introduction to this chapter, we present a short anatomy lesson on cranial nerves. The names, functions, and locations of the 12 cranial nerves are presented in Figure 2-1.

There are 12 pairs of cranial nerves that emerge directly from the brain stem and carry information between the brain and parts of the body, especially the head and neck. The nerves are numbered with Roman numerals, I through XII, according to the order in which they emerge from the brain (from top to bottom). Note that some are solely sensory nerves, some are solely movement nerves, and some are both. Each nerve in the following list is labeled with an "S" for sensory, an "M" for movement, or a "B" for both.

i. Olfactory nerve: sense of smell (S)
ii. Optic nerve: ability to see (S)
iii. Oculomotor nerve: ability to move and blink your eyes (M)
iv. Trochlear nerve: ability to move your eyes up and down or back or forth (M)
v. Trigeminal nerve: sensations in your face and cheeks, taste, and jaw movements (B)

CRANIAL NERVES

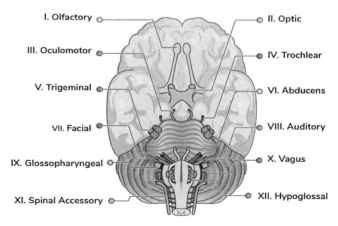

Figure 2-1.   Names, functions, and locations of the 12 cranial nerves.

   vi. Abducens nerve: ability to move your eyes (M)

  vii. Facial nerve: facial expressions and sense of taste (B)

 viii. Auditory/vestibular nerve: sense of hearing and balance (S)

   ix. Glossopharyngeal nerve: ability to taste and swallow (B)

    x. Vagus nerve: digestion and heart rate (B)

   xi. Accessory nerve (also called spinal accessory nerve): ability to move shoulder and neck muscles (M)

  xii. Hypoglossal nerve: ability to move your tongue (M)

If you are nerdy like me, you might want to remember the names of the 12 cranial nerves in order. I guarantee there will not be a test.

To remember nerve names, you can use the mnemonic

- On old Olympus's towering top, a Finn and a German viewed some hops.

Similarly, the nerve functions (sensory, movement, or both) can be remembered using the mnemonic

- Some say marry money but my brother says big brains matter more.

By the way, the occipital nerve, the culprit in occipital neuralgia, is NOT a cranial nerve. It originates from the upper cervical spine. I hope this brief anatomy lesson is useful as you read through Chapter 2.

2.1
Glossopharyngeal Neuralgia
Jeffrey A. Brown, MD, FACS, FAANS

Author's Note: The information contained in this section is not intended to provide individual medical advice, diagnosis, or treatment or to induce the reader to seek care with any specific physician. Always seek the advice of your physician or other qualified health care provider with any questions you may have regarding a medical condition or treatment and before undertaking a new health care treatment, and never disregard professional medical advice or delay in seeking it because of something you have read in this book.

Glossopharyngeal neuralgia (GPN) was first described by the one of the first modern neurosurgeons, Walter Dandy, as "paroxysmal pain frequently brought on by eating and swallowing with involvement of the root of the tongue and pharynx, with radiation to the throat and/or the deep ear structures". (Dandy 1932)

This description is still accurate.

What is the glossopharyngeal nerve?

It is the ninth of the 12 cranial nerves, meaning the nerves that directly enter or exit the brain, not the spinal cord, and it is anatomically closely related to the tenth cranial nerve, the vagus nerve. As the preceding definition notes, the glossopharyngeal nerve provides sensation to the throat and base of the tongue, the deep middle ear, and also the parotid gland. The parotid gland is at the base of the jaw. Injury to it will cause a dry mouth. The ninth cranial nerve provides taste sensation to the base of the tongue and some motor function to a swallowing muscle of the throat.

Dandy's definition was used by Peter Jannetta to select patients for whom he first performed vascular decompression of the vagoglossopharyngeal complex as the most appropriate treatment for this entity. (Resnick 1995) Note that Jannetta spoke of decompressing two nerves: the vagus and the glossopharyngeal. Why? The glossopharyngeal and vagus nerves compose a web of fascicles (slender bundles) such that a vessel in contact with the 9th nerve will also be in contact with the lower fibers of the 10th nerve. These also are sensory to the throat.

Distinguished trigeminal and glossopharyngeal neurosurgeons believe that glossopharyngeal neuralgia is an inaccurate description of this entity leading to neuropathic (stabbing) ear and throat pain. Glossopharyngeal neuralgia is more appropriately categorized as vagoglossopharyngeal neuralgia when caused by a vascular compression because of the close relationship of the fibrous web that enters the jugular foramen at the skull base. This is the opening in the skull that also allows exit from the brain of the large jugular vein, which drains blood from one side of the brain. For this reason, efforts to treat GPN by a rhizotomy, a heat injury to the nerve performed with a special needle, is a concern. The vein can be punctured. Surgeons who choose to section the glossopharyngeal nerve rather than decompress it have learned that they must also section the sensory fibers to achieve adequate pain relief. This leads to permanent, and sometimes uncomfortable, numbness in the throat. The controversy remains. Is GPN better treated by sectioning the glossopharyngeal nerve and adjacent sensory fibers of the vagus nerve or by attempting to decompress it?

What happens to the body with injury to the vagus nerve near the base of the skull? If the motor fibers of the nerve are injured, there can be weakness of the palate, giving the voice a nasal element. Trouble with swallowing follows weakness of the pharyngeal (throat) muscles. There may be weakness or even paralysis of the vocal cords, causing hoarseness. One of the lesser-known issues with vagoglossopharyngeal neuralgia is that, when the vagus nerve is involved, there can be speech difficulty, such as lowered volume of speech, hoarseness with ongoing effort, or perhaps a chronic cough.

The good news is that GPN is surgically treatable. In Jannetta's series, 79% of 39 patients treated over the course of 24 years had immediate pain relief, and 76% had continuing complete relief with follow-up of 6 months to 14 years, with a mean of 4 years. (Chen 2015, Zheng 2021) Many more series of patients by other centers have confirmed the benefits of glossopharyngeal nerve decompression for GPN. There has also been a small study of decompression surgery of the lower cranial nerves specific for dysphonia , that is, speech quality issues including chronic cough, breathing irregularity, and hoarseness. (Taylor 2015)

Finally, it may be possible for a person to have both trigeminal and glossopharyngeal neuralgia. When there is ear pain, it may not be clear whether it is from trigeminal or glossopharyngeal neuralgia.

Choose your physician with care to find one who understands the nuances of your care, and you should do well.

2.2
Geniculate Neuralgia

Alexander Ren; Christine Ryu; Araika Ramchandran; John Choi, MD; Lily H. Kim, MD; and Michael Lim, MD

Geniculate neuralgia (GN), also known as nervus intermedius neuralgia, is a rare facial pain syndrome characterized by sudden and intense pain felt deep in the ear canal. It typically affects one side but can also be bilateral. GN is a purely clinical diagnosis, meaning that there are no tests or imaging studies that can confirm GN. As ear pain can be attributed to various causes, a diagnosis of GN requires a thorough clinical assessment to rule out all other potential conditions. GN is challenging to identify because of its similarity with other facial pain syndromes, its location within the facial nerve, and the overall paucity of cases. To be diagnosed, you should consider consulting a neurologist; neurosurgeon; and an ear, nose, and throat (ENT) specialist.

Symptoms of GN range in severity, duration, and distribution. The most common symptoms are episodes of shock-like sharp or stabbing ear pain that last seconds to minutes. The pain can also feel dull and burning with occasional moments of sharp pain, and in some cases, the pain can spread to other areas of the face. The pain ranges from mild to debilitating. The episodes may last from a few days to weeks at a time with a gradual onset of persistent pain in the ear. Other symptoms of GN can include ringing in the ear, dizziness, migraines, and loss of balance. GN can be triggered by direct stimulation of the ear canal, such as touching or cleaning it. Because the pain can also spread to the palate and areas around the ear, GN can be triggered by swallowing, talking, chewing, and yawning. In some cases, cold wind or loud music can initiate an episode of ear pain.

GN is usually initially managed with medication, but if pain persists or medication side effects are intolerable, surgical treatment can be considered. Typical medications for GN are anticonvulsant drugs such as carbamazepine, and other treatment options include physical therapy, analgesic medications, radiation, and nerve block. Currently, surgical options include a transection or cutting of the nervus intermedius (NI) and/or a microvascular decompression (MVD) of the facial nerve. Overall, medications usually help the pain to subside up to a certain extent, but the efficacies of these nonsurgical treatments are still under review. Many studies have concluded that treatment options should depend on the condition of the patient experiencing GN.

Only a few case reports and series on GN exist in the medical literature, with less than 200 cases detailed in total. The scarcity of the literature speaks to not only the rarity of GN but also the limited evidence available to establish guidelines for treatment. As such, we recommend that you undergo a detailed analysis with a specialist.

Anatomy. Ear sensation involves a complicated sensory pathway that comprises the connection of many structures including the facial nerve, the geniculate ganglion, and the NI. Dysfunction along this sensory pathway causes the classic ear pain of GN; thus, it is important to be familiar with these structures, depicted in Figure 2-2.

- *Cranial nerve 7 (CN VII).* The facial nerve, also referred to as cranial nerve 7 or CN VII, supplies motor function to the muscles of the face controlling facial expression. There are also sensory fibers involved in taste, smell, hearing, and touch, as well as innervation of the glands that produce saliva and tears. The facial nerve splits from the brain stem into five distinct branches that carry out muscle functions to the face. The sensory information is collected back at the base of the cranial nerve and initially processed by the geniculate ganglion.

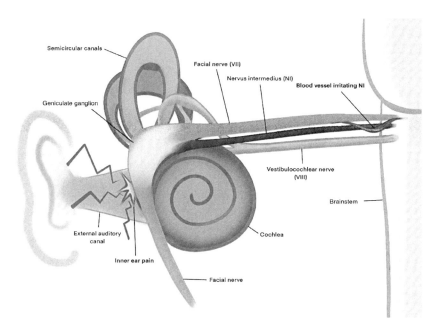

Figure 2-2. Graphical representation of the relevant anatomical structures in geniculate neuralgia.

- *Geniculate ganglion.* The geniculate ganglion is a sensory structure located along the course of the facial nerve in the facial canal within the petrous temporal bone. It is a collection of sensory nerve cell bodies that relay sensory stimulations from the fibers of nerve branches such as the nervus intermedius. It is responsible for transmitting sensory information involving taste, touch, and pain from the tongue and ear back to the brain.
- *Nervus intermedius (NI).* The primary structure believed to be involved in GN is the nervus intermedius, a small branch of the facial nerve. The geniculate ganglion contains the cell bodies of the nerve fibers from the NI, which are involved in transmitting a variety of sensations such as hearing, taste, and smell to the brain. The most relevant function of the NI is transmitting pain sensations from the ear canal, the eardrum, and the skin behind the ear. GN is believed to occur when the NI is damaged or compressed, resulting in pain felt deep in the ear. Abnormally large blood vessels have been associated with the compression of the NI.

It is important to note that the ear itself is innervated by three other cranial nerves, and the area covered by the facial nerve is also innervated by other sensory nerves such as the trigeminal, glossopharyngeal, and vagus nerves. There can be multiple or overlapping causes of nerve-related ear pain, and identifying the anatomy of the facial nerve may help to narrow down the possible conditions, as a diagnosis of GN can be established only when other types of ear pain have been ruled out.

Epidemiology. GN is a rare condition, and there is not much data on this facial disorder. Based on the existing literature, two-thirds of GN patients are women, and the onset of symptoms typically begins around 45 years of age. The prevalence of GN among different racial and ethnic groups is currently not known. Additionally, the geographical distribution of GN has not been well characterized, so it is unclear whether certain regions or populations experience higher rates of GN. GN is one of several similar facial pain disorders that differ in the location of the pain, the nerve(s) involved, and the triggers for pain. However, research on the more common facial pain disorders, such as trigeminal neuralgia (TN) and glossopharyngeal neuralgia (GPN), can be instructive in understanding and treating GN. For example, previous research on GPN also suggests that two-thirds of GPN patients are female. Furthermore, the average age when GPN symptoms begin is 50.7 years, with pain lasting about 5.7 years. Given these demographic similarities, physicians will often consider multiple facial pain disorders when evaluating ear pain.

Etiology. The cause of GN is not fully understood; however, it is known to involve the NI. One theory is that GN may be associated with a reactivated varicella zoster virus (VZV) infection, also known as shingles. When VZV infects the body, it can hide out in sensory nerves to avoid clearance by the immune system. After a period of dormancy, the virus can reemerge and create the classic symptoms of shingles, including light sensitivity, general discomfort, headaches, and a painful, itchy facial rash; the rash typically develops on areas of skin innervated by the infected nerve. When shingles involves the facial nerve, it is referred to as herpes zoster oticus or Ramsay Hunt syndrome, and this condition manifests as ear pain, facial weakening or paralysis, and hearing loss. Whereas shingles is known to commonly result in postherpetic neuralgia, or chronic pain in the area of a resolved shingles rash, there is little data to suggest that GN is a long-term complication of Ramsay Hunt syndrome.

Another theory as to the cause of GN is compression of the NI by a neighboring blood vessel, akin to the compression of the trigeminal nerve seen in TN. Mechanistically, the blood vessel may be enlarged or abnormally displaced to cause the compression, which would damage the nerve over time and generate a stabbing pain felt in the ear. It is important to note that vessel compression is not consistently observed during surgical exploration of the facial nerve. This suggests that, although compression may exacerbate GN symptoms, it is often not the primary causative factor in the majority of GN cases.

Clinical Presentation and Diagnosis. The clinical symptoms of GN can be challenging to identify because of its similarity to other facial pain disorders, such as TN, cluster headaches, and migraines. GN symptoms rarely affect both ears, but it is possible for both ears to be affected. Clinical symptoms of GN include a painful sensation in the afflicted ear; dizziness; loss of balance; sensitivity to light and sound; and tinnitus, which is a ringing sound in the afflicted ear. Some patients experience additional symptoms of excessive salivation or changes in taste. The ear pain can vary from persistent, burning pain to episodes of sharp, stabbing pain deep in the ear canal that patients often describe as an "ice-pick" sensation. Some patients experience both a constant burning pain and episodes of stabbing pain. GN ear pain can be triggered by cold sensations, such as a chilly wind, or loud noises. Additionally, actions that cause a patient's ears to pop, such as yawning, swallowing, sneezing, and touching the ear, as well as light exposure and high altitudes, can trigger GN pain. However, some patients undergo GN symptoms with no obvious triggers. Regardless of the different clinical presentations, GN significantly affects patients' quality of life (QOL).

The diagnosis for GN is a purely clinical decision, meaning that there are no specific tests or imaging findings that can definitively confirm GN. Notably, in the research literature, GN patients are often reported to have concurrent facial pain diagnoses such as TN, which can complicate the clinical picture. A thorough clinical history and physical examination are critical to elucidate symptoms and begin narrowing down the potential diagnoses. A physician will often perform a neurological exam to gauge the involvement of specific cranial nerves. To rule out structural causes of ear pain, such as tumors or vascular malformations, magnetic resonance imaging (MRI) scans are used to visualize the relevant nerves and any compressing bodies. Electromyography (EMG) and nerve conduction studies can provide insight into any abnormal excitability or sensitivity in the facial nerve sensory pathway.

Treatment. Once your physician makes a diagnosis of GN, they will typically recommend medications first, followed by surgery if pain persists. Regarding medications, the most common drugs used to address GN pain are anticonvulsant drugs (ACDs). These drugs inhibit the electrical activity of sensory nerves to reduce pain-related signaling. The most common first-line AED for GN and many other facial pain syndromes is carbamazepine. Despite the lack of large-scale studies of carbamazepine for GN, carbamazepine has been shown to be highly effective for TN. If patients experience no benefit or develop adverse effects (e.g., nausea, rash, dizziness) with carbamazepine use, alternative medications may be considered. Such alternatives include AEDs such as oxcarbazepine and gabapentin, the muscle relaxant baclofen, and the migraine and cluster headache drug methysergide maleate. Narcotic pain medications are not recommended for GN, as they have limited analgesic efficacy in facial pain disorders and carry a risk for addiction and abuse. Importantly, these medication recommendations are largely based on individual GN case reports and clinical studies conducted in TN, so the true efficacy of these medications for GN has not been rigorously tested.

If a patient's symptoms are not adequately controlled by medication, surgery is considered. All surgeries will involve a retrosigmoid approach, in which an opening is made behind the ear to access the cranial nerves. The definitive procedure to treat GN is sectioning of the NI. NI sectioning was among the earliest surgical procedures reported for GN. The most common complications observed are decreased hearing or hearing loss on the side of surgery, facial paralysis, dizziness, vertigo, loss of taste and smell, and a cerebrospinal fluid leak. When complications are present, they are typically transient. In the largest case series of NI sectioning available, 11 of 64 patients experienced a partial temporary facial paralysis that fully recovered. No patients experienced permanent hearing loss or a postoperative cerebrospinal fluid leak (Gupta 2022). Surgeons will usually avoid performing NI sectioning if there is significant concern that hearing function will be lost.

When vessel compression of the facial nerve is observed, the neurosurgeon may consider a MVD. This procedure is frequently used in TN, where the most common culprit is an artery pressing on the fifth cranial nerve. In an MVD, the surgeon will place a piece of cushioning, usually a pillow of cotton-like material, between the vessel and CN VII. Sometimes, the surgeon will both section the NI and decompress CN VII if vessel contact is present, but in general, MVD of CN VII is not widely accepted as an effective treatment for GN.

Often, patients will present with multiple facial pain syndromes in addition to GN. This again speaks to the difficulty of isolating a specific cause of neuralgic ear pain. As such, a procedure to treat GN may also include procedures targeting the trigeminal and glossopharyngeal nerves. NI sectioning is rarely performed as an isolated procedure; many of the GN surgeries recorded in the literature also involved a rhizotomy or decompression of cranial nerves other than the facial nerve. Although these accessory procedures may help to resolve GN-related ear pain, no reported research has suggested that targeting CN V, IX, or X can reliably reduce GN symptoms. Moreover, neuralgic ear pain is not always resolved by NI sectioning. This likely reflects the previous point that the inner ear is innervated by multiple nerve types, so if the culprit nerve is not the NI, then NI sectioning is unlikely to address the root cause of the ear pain.

Conclusion. Geniculate neuralgia is a rare diagnosis for neuralgic ear pain, and patients should receive a thorough neurological workup to rule out more common causes of ear pain. For patients with GN, pharmacologic and surgical options are available that can be effective in managing symptoms. GN patients will often initially trial medications that have been shown to be beneficial in similar facial pain syndromes. If surgery is required, sectioning of the NI is the most well-documented procedure for GN.

2.3
Occipital Neuralgia
Konstantin V. Slavin, MD, FAANS

It is common in a facial pain practice or headache clinic to hear from patients about pain in their face and head that originates, focuses or culminates in the back of the head, the region that is called occiput. A patient's description of the pain location may—and usually does—help in making correct diagnosis, as most nerves in the head and neck region cover extremely specific anatomical distributions. The trigeminal nerve, for example, is the main provider of sensation to the entire half of one's face. Similarly, the sensation in the region behind the ear and above the hairline in the back of one's head is supplied by a specific group of nerves: the occipital nerves. There are three occipital nerves on each side, namely, the greater, the lesser, and the third occipital nerves, and all of them originate from the upper cervical spinal nerve roots, mainly from the second and third cervical levels (C2 and C3). (See Figure 2-3.)

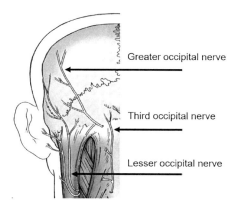

Greater occipital nerve

Third occipital nerve

Lesser occipital nerve

Figure 2-3. The occipital nerves.

As the sensory information from the occiput is carried by the occipital nerves to the central nervous system (CNS), it travels through sensory ganglia and nerve roots and then enters the spinal cord in the upper part of the neck. There, it is processed in the same area as is involved with sensation from the face and the rest of the head, the so-called trigeminocervical complex. These intricate connections explain the frequent overlap of occipital pain with various migraine and headache conditions, as well as some instances of occipital pain radiating into the forehead or being aggravated by facial pain.

It is important to notice, however, that, among many painful conditions that involve the occipital region, true occipital neuralgia (the subject of this section) presents a specific pain syndrome that can be successfully treated in most patients, as long as it is accurately diagnosed and addressed.

So, what is occipital neuralgia (ON)? It is a relatively rare condition that manifests itself with pain on one or both sides of the head (unilateral ON is seen in 85% of cases). The pain usually starts in the occiput and travels toward the parietal region all the way to the vertex.

Editor's Note: The parietal region of the scalp curves over the sides of the head, starting from the top and extending toward the ears. It contributes to the overall volume and shape of one's hairstyle. The vertex (or cranial vertex) is the highest point of the head, formed by four bones of the skull: the frontal bone, the two parietal bones, and the occipital bone. It is an area prone to hair loss.

ON is described as shooting, electric-shock-like, or stabbing in nature; in medical terminology, this is referred to as paroxysmal, lancinating pain. Very often, there is also a dull aching pain between the shooting attacks located in the same general area. The duration of attacks lasting from a few seconds to minutes, the severe intensity of pain, the presence of either tenderness over the course of the occipital nerves or trigger points within the occipital area, and pain or discomfort observed with innocuous stimulation of the scalp or hair are all characteristic features of ON. Another classical feature that assists in making a proper diagnosis is the improvement or disappearance of pain in response to numbing of the nerve with an injection of local anesthetic in the vicinity of the nerve in question (nerve block). Such blocks are used to both diagnose and treat ON, as the pain relief from a single injection may last for quite a long time. For an ON diagnosis to be made, the patient should be asked or tested for all of the mentioned features, keeping in mind that other conditions that present with pain in the occipital region (migraines, cluster headaches and hemicranias, tension headaches, cervicogenic headaches that arise from dysfunction of the joints within the spinal column and neighboring cervical muscles, etc.) must first be ruled out.

Very frequently, to rule out associated anatomical pathology, it is necessary to perform appropriate imaging of the head and neck; this would usually include MRI of the brain and the cervical spine. The imaging would allow detection of Chiari malformations, cervical spondylosis, and vascular and neoplastic conditions; in most ON cases, the MRI studies are read as normal or almost normal.

Interestingly enough, the exact source of pain in ON remains unknown; it is commonly accepted as a neuropathic pain condition, meaning that the underlying process is the malfunction of the nervous system. The occipital nerves, the culprit of ON, appear to be hyperactive and irritated, but the reason for this irritation is often unclear. Multiple existing theories postulate compression or entrapment of the nerve or nerves anywhere along their course in the patient's neck and head, but there is no consensus or universally accepted understanding of the underlying pathology.

As with all chronic pain syndromes, the treatment of ON is administered in systematic fashion, starting from conservative measures, medications, and interventions, perhaps ultimately leading to surgery. As the natural course of ON may be self-limiting and the pain may improve over time, it may be prudent to avoid risky interventions early in the course of the disease, but medically refractory cases are often considered for invasive treatments as the pain may become disabling, thus making risks of interventional or surgical treatment justified.

Common initial treatments include the application of cold and warm packs, massage, and physical therapy; rest may also frequently reduce the pain. Among available medications, initial preference is given to conventional anti-inflammatory drugs and muscle relaxants; the next level of treatment would include anticonvulsants and antidepressants commonly used for neuropathic pain conditions, including gabapentin, amitriptyline, pregabalin, carbamazepine, and nortriptyline. Although useful in relieving the pain, opioid medications are to be avoided in ON and other neuropathic pain conditions.

Nerve blocks are considered next, and here, one may use the block or blocks for both diagnostic and therapeutic purposes. Nerve blocks may include both short- and long-lasting local anesthetics; the medications are injected in the vicinity of each suspected nerve, and as a result of injection, the territory that the nerve supplies becomes temporarily numb. Along with numbness, patients experience improvement or complete relief of their ON pain, but the duration of this relief tends to be longer than the duration of the numbness, and sometimes, the pain relief may turn out to be long-lasting or even permanent. This course of events, however, is observed in only a small fraction of ON patients, and therefore, the nerve blocks have to be repeated, usually with the addition of corticosteroids to the local anesthetics, adding an anti-inflammatory effect to the anesthesia.

Other interventional (nonsurgical) ON treatment options include injections of botulinum toxin, pulsed radio-frequency treatments, and short-term electrical nerve stimulation (called percutaneous electrical nerve stimulation or PENS). Each of these interventional modalities is able to provide a significant reduction in pain intensity in a majority of ON patients, but the longevity of improvement varies from person to person and permanent pain relief is rarely seen.

Surgery is reserved for the most refractory patients who fail to respond to nonsurgical treatments and those with intolerable pain who experience pain recurrence after the use of less invasive approaches. Although many specific surgical procedures are available for individuals with ON, these treatments are divided into three main groups: decompression, neurodestruction, and neuromodulation.

Decompression surgery is based on the presumption that the pain arises from the compression of the occipital nerve(s) along their course through the muscles and fascial layers, with additional aggravation from neighboring arteries that are expected to travel next to the nerves. During surgery, the nerves are released at one or several points, usually by cutting the adjacent muscle and fascia, and the additional compression points from the vessels are protected by physical separation of neural and vascular structures. In case of unsuccessful decompression or the recurrence of pain due to scar formation, there is an option to interrupt the transmission of painful signals or remove the hyperactive neural structures. This is accomplished by destructive interventions including neurectomy or neurotomy, ganglionectomy, and rhizotomy, which are aimed at the nerves, spinal ganglia, and spinal nerve roots, respectively. All of these interventions are considered established treatment options for ON, but all patients are expected to discuss with their surgeons the associated risks of complications and possibility of improvement, as well as contingency plans in cases of insufficient pain relief or pain recurrence.

A quite different approach in the treatment of ON is based on pain suppression with electrical stimulation that is delivered by an implanted device. This technique, called occipital nerve stimulation (ONS), was developed in the 1970s and perfected to its current shape in the late 1990s. It is now considered a standard approach to the treatment of medically refractory ON pain. Several years ago, practice guidelines backed by a national neurosurgical society (the Congress of Neurological Surgeons) recommended ONS for ON patients based on evidence gathered through multiple peer-reviewed publications. Nevertheless, ONS remains one of those procedures that require a complicated approval process from most insurance companies.

The surgery for ONS includes implantation of one or two electrodes in the immediate vicinity of the nerve so that the electrical pulses can reach the nerve when the device is activated. During the initial testing period (the trial), the electrodes are connected to an external device to check for the degree of improvement and presence of any side effects; these temporary (externalized) electrodes are usually removed at the end of the trial. Later on, the implantation of the permanent device involves insertion of both the electrodes and an internal pulse generator that serves as the power source and "brain" of the ONS system. The devices available for ONS today allow patients to turn stimulation on and off, make it stronger and weaker, adjust settings, and switch between different programs based on the pattern and severity of their pain, and all of this is done with an external "remote control" that communicates with the implanted generator using telemetry. Among multiple generators and systems available for ONS today are some devices that are rechargeable and can last, with proper recharging, up to 15 years. Figure 2-4 presents an intraoperative anterior–posterior skull X-ray showing placement of a stimulating electrode across the occipital nerves at the base of the skull.

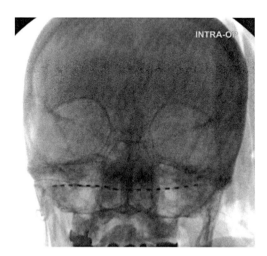

Figure 2-4. Intraoperative anterior–posterior skull X-ray showing placement of a stimulating electrode across the occipital nerves at the base of the skull.

No surgical treatment of ON is perfect—each modality has its own set of risks and limitations—but with proper diagnostic evaluation and clear expectations of treatment, it is possible to achieve lasting pain relief. Therefore, a diagnosis of ON should not be considered a lifelong burden but rather a treatable condition that can be improved and potentially cured as long as there is a well-informed patient and a team of experienced and enthusiastic physicians and surgeons.

> *Editor's Note: If a diagnostic block is consistent with ON and medications have either failed or initially succeeded but now cause intolerable side effects, then the least invasive surgical option is neuromodulation. Because it makes use of equipment that is approved for human implantation, but not specifically for ON, insurance companies are required to consider it "experimental" and deny coverage. Ideally, your neurosurgeon should provide a well-reasoned explanation during the appeal process for their proposed trial of its effectiveness to be followed by an evaluation of that trial's benefit and the need to proceed to a more permanent implantation. Depending on the insurance contract, there may be several layers of appeal, even to an independent entity. Success of the appeals process will need the involvement of you, the patient, to tell your story.*

2.4
Hemifacial Spasm
Jordan Dattero; Lilah Keating; and Raymond F. Sekula, Jr., MD

Hemifacial spasm (HFS) is characterized by irritating repeated spasms of the facial muscles in half of the face and a sense of fatigue when they occur. Individuals with HFS have described the sensation as feeling as if someone is pulling on half of their face. When asked, they have also described HFS as having constant pressure in their heads and feeling complete relief only post-surgery. Although the spasms are intermittent, over time, their duration can lengthen, and the spasms can become seemingly continuous. As for other neurological disorders, patients report that their spasms are sometimes triggered by anxiety, fatigue, or stress. The forceful spasms may cause involuntary, intermittent eye closure that leads to a loss of binocular vision. This becomes hazardous when actions such as driving can suddenly be impaired when unpredictable spasms occur, and half of the patient's vision is affected. It has been reported that sleeping and reading also become more difficult with the condition. HFS can also cause psychological distress, anxiety, and depression, as those experiencing the condition often isolate themselves from professional and social opportunities because of embarrassment from the uncontrollable spasms or concern that the spasms deem them unfit to perform certain tasks. When the spasms occur, the resulting facial asymmetry often elicits unwanted attention from observers. As the condition worsens over time, patients may experience partial closure of their eye and drawing up of the corner of their mouth. It is also common for patients to say that they hear new noises, a phenomenon likely caused by pulsations of the cochlear or facial nerve.

HFS is a rare condition that occurs in 9.8 per 100,000 people. An estimated 14.5 per 100,000 women and 7.4 per 100,000 males develop the disorder. Thus, women are twice as likely to be affected by HFS as are men. Asian populations are overrepresented among those with HFS. Onset occurs at an average age of 44 years. There have been a few reported cases of HFS as a genetic condition. However, in these cases, HFS exhibits autosomal dominant inheritance and low penetrance.

Diagnosis of HFS is based on clinical history and neurological examination. The spasms usually begin with the orbicularis oculi muscle (i.e., the eyelid muscles), but as HFS progresses, the spasms spread to the cheek and oral muscles. EMG helps distinguish this disorder from other similar disorders such as blepharospasm, tics, partial motor seizures, synkinesis, craniocervical dystonia (formerly known as Meige's syndrome), and neuromyotonia. For diagnosis and treatment, one must undergo a comprehensive medical evaluation and contact a medical professional who can discuss the treatment options.

HFS is caused by pulsatile vascular contact or compression of the facial nerve near the brain stem. Commonly, the anterior inferior cerebellar artery (AICA) or posteroinferior cerebellar artery is responsible. Compression from the artery, blood vessel, or tumor can also cause hyperactivity of a cluster of facial nerves within the brain stem, which further contributes to the facial spasms. In rare cases, compression of the nerve by a tumor or other problems can result in facial spasms. A high-resolution MRI scan of the brain performed using one of the special techniques known by the acronyms FIESTA and CISS and with gadolinium dye infusion will identify any vascular contact with the facial nerve or show a tumor or any other structural lesions.

Since the early 1980s, injections of botulinum neurotoxin (BoTN, also called Botox) have become the most common treatment for HFS. BoTN offers a nonsurgical treatment to provide some symptomatic relief in 92% of patients. BoTN provides relief from HFS by blocking the release of acetylcholine at the synaptic neuromuscular junction. In turn, without acetylcholine, the muscles cannot receive the nerve's impulses, and therefore, spasms are reduced. Effectively, BoTN injections reduce muscle activity by creating drug-induced muscle weakness.

BoTN injections have only a short-term relief period and have associated risks. After injection, the severity of spasms declines over a few weeks. However, symptoms tend to return within 4 months. Possible complications can include ptosis, blurred vision, and diplopia, all of which usually resolve within a few days or weeks. Repeated injections can lead to facial weakness and atrophy of the facial muscles. In this case, injection of the opposite side of the face may be used to achieve cosmetic effects. HFS tends to be a progressive disorder in which spasms become more frequent and intense over time. As minor contractions such as eyelid twitches may be effectively treated with BoTN, full-face contraction proves less effective to control with injections.

Once a blood vessel has been confirmed to be contacting or compressing the facial nerve by MRI, MVD surgery can be considered with a goal of removing the vascular contact.

MVD of the nerve can be performed by interposition or transposition of the nerve. At the time of this writing, neither technique has been shown to be superior to the other. Interposition can be used when perforators that supply blood to the brain stem are coming from the compressive blood vessel. To avoid injury to these perforators, polytetrafluoroethylene (PTFE) felt may be interposed between the blood vessel and the nerve, acting as a cushion that separates the blood vessel from the nerve and thus alleviating the pressure. Transposition is when the blood vessel is moved away from the nerve and affixed to a remote area. Neurosurgeons cannot assess whether they need to transpose or simply interpose a blood vessel until reaching the compression site during surgery and observing whether the blood vessel has perforators. In some instances, appendage slings are attached to the petrous dura to ensure that the problematic vessel is separated from the nerve; however, this is not always necessary.

A difficult component of the surgery is when the operative field is narrow for reasons such as a large flocculus (a normal brain structure) or an unideal location of the sigmoid sinus. In most MVD surgeries, the conventional retrosigmoid approach, in which the brain is entered from behind the ear, is used. However, when the operative field is narrow, alternative surgical approaches such as the extended retrosigmoid approach or the Retrolabyrinthine presigmoid approach can be used to gain better access to the site of compression. This just means that certain factors alter the best approach into the brain and provide sufficient access to the site of compression.

As with any surgery, there are some risks to MVD surgery, although they are low. The most common risks are facial weakness and partial hearing loss or deafness (1.5% of cases). Hearing loss may be lessened using brain-stem auditory evoked potential (BAEP) monitoring during the MVD operation to alert surgeons of cochlear nerve damage. An additional risk is leakage of the cerebrospinal fluid (CSF), which can lead to infection. CSF leaks can cause headaches, neck pain, ringing in the ears, loss of smell or taste, and meningitis. To avoid this complication, calcium phosphate cement can be used during the closure of the retromastoid craniectomy in surgery. A retrospective study using clinical data from 672 patients suggested that this decreases the rate of CSF complications, infection, or any other wound complications. Other low-probability complications include stroke, cerebellar hematoma, other cranial nerve injury, and death. Overall, serious complications in MVD surgery for HFS occur in less than 1% of cases, and recurrence can occur in 4% to 10% of patients. (Kaufmann 2023, Sekula 2013)

Despite a higher risk of complications, MVD is the only curative treatment. Additionally, patients who undergo this operation have exhibited a significant positive psychological impact. Many describe the success of surgery as the ability to regain confidence and restore engagement in daily interactions and relationships. This improved quality of life (QOL) was measured using a QOL questionnaire with unique questions related to the experiences of HFS patients. A retrospective study analyzed 242 patients who had undergone MVD surgery. The mean score improved from 22.78 ($\pm$ 9.83) down to 2.17 ($\pm$5.75) following the operation. (Lawrence 2018)

Why is MVD surgery so uncommon? A likely reason is that only 10% of individuals with HFS are referred to neurosurgeons. Most patients who wish to undergo MVD surgery are self-referred people who determined that MVD was a viable treatment option after doing their own research.

MVD surgery has proven to be successful in reducing long-term spasms in about 92% of cases, with low morbidity and mortality rates. Because of the rarity of this condition, the failure rate for the surgery is higher than it should be, perhaps because of the lack of specialized expertise in those who perform the surgery. Success rates of MVD for HFS are commonly derived from high-volume centers. The best course of action is to consult a surgeon who is an expert in this operation and performs many such surgeries each year.

Although it is up to the patient to determine which course of action they wish to pursue based on the severity of the condition and its impact on their QOL, the most sustainable and curative treatment option for most is MVD surgery. BoTN injections provide temporary relief and reduce the frequency and intensity of the spasms. This treatment would be most appropriate for individuals unwilling or unfit for surgery or a general anesthetic; yet, for most it is not a long-term solution. Additionally, when considering long-term costs, it is more cost-effective to opt for surgery than to continue with BoTN injections every few months indefinitely. See a neurosurgeon with experience. Ask questions. Listen to the answers. See Section 3.1 in the next chapter on what makes a neurosurgeon an expert for more advice.

2.5
Burning Mouth Syndrome
Gary D. Klasser, DMD, Certificate in Orofacial Pain

Burning mouth syndrome (BMS) is an enigmatic, idiopathic, chronic, often painful, clinical entity (condition). BMS does not have a well-established, universal, standardized, validated definition with field-tested classification systems or diagnostic criteria. It was first described by H. Fox in 1935. BMS has been called by various names depending on the quality and/or location of its intraoral pain presentation. Among the names are the following: glossodynia, glossopyrosis, glossalgia, stomatodynia, stomatopyrosis, sore tongue, burning tongue, scalded mouth syndrome, oral dysesthesia, burning mouth condition, and burning mouth syndrome. The use of multiple and heterogeneous labels shows the ambiguity and uncertainty that exists around BMS both within the scientific literature and in clinical practice. An unfortunate outcome of this approach is that it often produces a dilemma during the development and presentation of a definitive diagnosis while, at times, resulting in well-intentioned but misdirected interventions.

Because of the various definitions and multiple labels applied to BMS, it is easy to understand the frustration that people with BMS experience and the difficulties encountered by the clinician in evaluating and treating these individuals. This inauspicious situation exists because the patient is experiencing continuous burning intraoral pain that greatly affects their QOL while the clinician is struggling to identify any obvious clinical signs, even with the accompaniment of additional diagnostic testing or imaging.

There is debate among researchers and clinicians as to whether burning mouth is truly a *syndrome* or a *disorder*. A syndrome (a disease unto itself) is a collection of several simultaneous signs and symptoms of varying intensity, which, in the case of BMS, is a normal-appearing oral mucosa with a burning sensation, a feeling of oral dryness, and taste disturbances. In contrast, a disorder is a condition with symptoms of other diseases such as dry mouth being the cause of the burning sensation often reported by BMS patients. This debate regarding semantics is rather academic, as BMS is most likely more than a singular disease process with multiple causes and abnormal bodily functions. Clinicians diagnose BMS by ruling out other diseases or conditions. This is called a diagnosis of exclusion.

Epidemiology. According to international studies, the prevalence (proportion of a population affected by a medical condition at a specific time) of BMS is believed to range from 0.7% to 15% of the general population depending on the methodology used for assessment (self-report questionnaire or clinical examination) and the diagnostic criteria utilized (continuous or episodic burning pain, presence or not of clinical lesions). (Wu 2021) Most of the data have been obtained from cross-sectional studies and convenience samples with heterogeneous compositions, whereas population-based information originated mainly from national surveys. Because of these imperfections and deficiencies, it is difficult to establish an "absolute" for the prevalence of BMS. The condition is most reported in postmenopausal women, generally in their 50s and 60s, and rarely before the age of 30 years. Men may also develop BMS with a reported ratio between approximately 1:5 and 1:7 compared to women, depending on the study population. Prevalence appears to increase with age in both men and women. Gender differences may be explained by biological, psychological, and sociocultural factors; however, these factors are yet to be defined. It appears from these epidemiological studies that menopausal females have a particularly high incidence of burning mouth. Nevertheless, despite these findings, no significant differences have been found between women with and without BMS in any of the following factors: number of years since menopause, occurrence of surgical menopause, use of hormone replacement therapy (HRT), years of treatment with HRT, and years passed since the completion of HRT. Only one study has been conducted on the prevalence of BMS in relation to ethnicity, and no studies have reported the prevalence of BMS by social, educational, or occupational groups. (Adamo 2015)

Classification and Diagnostic Criteria. Several attempts have been made to develop an "ideal" classification system for BMS. It seems that the most practical approach in classifying cases of BMS is by dividing patients into either primary (essential or idiopathic) BMS (no other evident disease) or secondary BMS (oral burning from other clinical abnormalities). Because secondary BMS is associated with a preexisting condition or cause, it should be remembered that, once such a condition has been treated, the symptoms of BMS should either improve or disappear.

Over the years, several formal diagnostic criteria have been applied to BMS by individual researchers, clinicians, and various organizations. Unfortunately, despite similarities among some components of these criteria, there is no absolute consensus, nor has there been validation of any specific criteria. However, the most applied diagnostic criteria are as follows: intraoral burning pain or dysesthesia (an unpleasant abnormal sensation, whether spontaneous or evoked) recurring every day for more than two hours, for longer than 3 months, with no evident cause shown by clinical exams and/or investigations.

Clinical Signs and Symptoms. The clinical presentations of BMS are typically inconsistent and will vary from patient to patient. Patients often describe their oral symptoms with the following words: painful, burning, tender, tingling, hot, scalding and numbness; and sometimes the sensation is merely described as discomfort, raw and annoying. BMS is characterized by both positive (burning pain, altered taste, and uncomfortable sensation) and negative (taste loss and abnormal sensation) sensory symptoms. The burning is mainly located bilaterally (on both sides) and symmetrically in the front two-thirds of the tongue (71% to 78%), followed by the back and sides of the tongue (72%), the front of the bony roof of the mouth (25%), and the tissue lining the inside of the lips (24%), while often occurring in multiple sites. Other less commonly reported sites include the lining of the cheeks and back of the lips, the floor of the mouth, the hard and soft palates, and the throat (36%). Approximately 50% of BMS patients experience a spontaneous onset of symptoms without any identifiable triggering factor. However, about 17% to 33% of individuals with BMS attribute the onset of their symptoms to a previous illness such as an upper respiratory tract infection, previous dental procedure, or medication use (including antibiotic therapy), suggesting the possibility of neurologic alterations preceding the onset of burning in some patients. Other individuals claim that the onset of symptoms is related to traumatic life stressors. Typically, the symptoms occur continuously for months or years without periods of cessation or remission, with some reports suggesting an average duration of 2 to 3 years. There are reports of complete/partial remission (with or without intervention) in approximately 50% of patients and a complete spontaneous remission in approximately 20% of patients within 6 to 7 years of onset. (Tan 2020) The remission of symptoms, be it complete or partial, is often characterized by a change in pain pattern from a constant to an episodic form.

The pattern of daily symptoms is reportedly constant, with fluctuations in pain intensity and with approximately one-third of people with BMS experiencing symptoms during both wakefulness and sleep. Most individuals with BMS report minimal symptoms upon awakening, after which the symptoms gradually intensify during the day, becoming more aggravating toward the evening. About one-third of patients have difficulty with sleep onset, and some may awake during sleep as a result of the burning pain. The intensity of the burning pain has been described as moderate to severe, and in some cases, it is comparable to the intensity of toothache pain in regard to severity but not quality. In most individuals with BMS, the burning sensation intensifies in the presence of personal stressors; fatigue; and the intake of hot, spicy, and/or acidic foods. In about half of people with BMS, the intake of food or liquids and distraction seem to reduce or alleviate the symptoms. BMS patients have a significantly higher incidence of dry mouth, thirst, and taste disturbances, but they do not differ from healthy controls regarding changes in oral mucosa or dental problems. Those with BMS have more nonspecific health complaints (including sleep disturbances) and more severe menopausal symptoms as compared to healthy controls.

Etiology and Pathophysiology. Currently, the etiology (cause of a disease or condition) of BMS has remained largely unknown. The presumed etiology is best explained as the interaction between biological (neurophysiological mechanisms) and psychological and/or behavioral factors. Even though multiple local (physical, chemical, or biological), systemic, and psychological/behavioral factors have been found to be related to BMS, several of these factors should be considered as conditions important to the differential diagnosis

(diagnosis of exclusion) of oral burning, rather than as etiological factors implicated in BMS.

Furthermore, it has been suggested that, to establish a causal link between two factors, one must have good consistency of data, meaning that the association investigated must be present in all cases regardless of the number of ways in which it is studied. For a biologically plausible explanation to exist, there must be transparency regarding how the potential etiological factor causes the outcome, and the suggested association must be independently verified. It appears that the current literature regarding BMS does not consistently meet these criteria.

The pathophysiology (i.e., the disordered physiological processes associated with disease or injury) of BMS continues to be unclear, especially with the lack of any visible oral mucosal changes upon examination. The current suggested pathophysiology is multifactorial and encompasses changes in taste; changes in hormone levels; nerve damage, dysfunction, dysregulation, and/or alteration, CNS changes, autoimmune disorders, and psychological factors.

Diagnosis. BMS has for many years remained a diagnosis of exclusion. A thorough medical and dental history, as well a review of systems and listing of all current medications, are essential for developing a definitive diagnosis. The history should include the patient's description of their present concern, including a history of their symptom presentation, any associated symptoms, and a description of any previous and current treatments. The clinician should also elicit a measure of the intensity of the presenting pain using appropriate scales, as well as the character and distribution of the pain presentation. Factors that aggravate and lessen the pain should also be included in the history. Experiences regarding infections, diseases, and surgery should be ascertained. Questions should also be asked about dietary habits and the use of oral care products. An appropriate psychosocial history should also be considered as a component of the comprehensive history to determine the presence or status of any past or current psychosocial stressors.

Laboratory studies to rule out any local and systemic factors that may be responsible for the pain presentation will be guided by findings in the history and clinical examination. Testing for burning mouth pain may include studies of salivary flow and taste function, blood tests to rule out systemic factors, examinations of contact sensitivity and investigation for the presence of other biologic agents.

Adjunctive studies such as imaging should be considered if the pain presentation appears to be more complex, or atypical of the "normal" presentation. Such atypical presentations may include findings of sensory and/or motor disturbances, autonomic changes, or any other evidence suggestive of CNS pathology or neurodegenerative processes. Abnormalities or pathology of the salivary structures may also be identified through appropriate imaging studies. Measuring saliva flow may be used to determine if oral dryness is a key factor. Biopsy of the minor salivary glands may be a consideration if Sjögren's syndrome is suspected (see Section 2.10). Psychometric testing may be indicated to evaluate the influence of psychological and/or anxiety factors. In some cases, evaluation for gastroesophageal reflux disease (GERD) may also prove helpful.

Management Strategies. Definitive recommendations for the management of BMS are somewhat lacking in the literature. From a clinical perspective, the clinician must initially determine if the patient is experiencing signs and symptoms consistent with primary (essential, idiopathic) BMS or secondary BMS, in which symptoms are due to underlying local or systemic conditions. Secondary BMS requires appropriate diagnosis and treatment of the underlying condition(s). In primary BMS, the etiology is unclear, so management options are based on a patient's symptomatology.

Often, management involves a multidisciplinary team approach, often requiring multiple modifications of the management plan until an effective protocol is achieved. The importance of this approach cannot be overstated, as patients are often frustrated by a lack of understanding of this condition among clinicians. Currently, the clinician has a choice of three approaches or combinations thereof as considerations in management.

1. *Behavioral Strategies.* Behavioral strategies to be considered consist of self-help measures such as the cessation of parafunctional behaviors (clenching, bruxism, tongue protrusion) and/or the use of different oral care products, such as alcohol-free mouthwashes and

products without flavoring agents or irritating components (e.g., cinnamic aldehyde, sodium lauryl sulfate, tooth-whitening agents, anticalculus ingredients). Other products that could be discontinued include mints, gum, or other breath aids. Stress management approaches such as moderate exercise regimens, yoga, and tai chi may be attempted. Additionally, desensitizing appliances may be considered to reduce oral burning or as a habit-breaking appliance. Behavioral strategies utilizing professional assistance include cognitive behavioral approaches (which focus on how beliefs and thoughts influence behavior) used alone or in combination with other therapies and/or group psychotherapy have also shown efficacy in decreasing pain intensity.

2. *Topical Therapies.* Many topical therapies (involving the application of medication directly to the skin or mucous membranes) have been trialed in the management of BMS. These range anywhere from anxiolytics and antidepressants to mucosal protectants, herbal supplements, and low-level laser therapy (photo biomodulation). Many of these therapies have reported variable success rates. However, few well-designed comparative studies have been performed, thus hampering recommendations developed from evidence-based decisions.

3. *Systemic Therapies.* Systemic approaches (in which medication travels through your blood to cells all over your body) to manage BMS have used a vast number of medications from various medication categories. Some of the treatments used include antianxiety drugs, antidepressants, anticonvulsants, and antioxidants all the way to acupuncture and transcranial magnetic stimulation. The spectrum of diversity of the various agents employed attests to the lack of definitive knowledge relating to the etiology and pathophysiology associated with BMS. Hence, there is very little consensus around the "gold standard" therapy of choice to guide the clinician in providing an evidence-based approach for the management of this difficult-to-manage condition.

Conclusion. Despite the current knowledge gained from the scientific literature, BMS continues to be a rather enigmatic, misunderstood, and underrecognized painful condition. Symptoms associated with BMS can be quite varied, thereby providing a challenge for clinicians while negatively impacting the patient. Management of this condition also continues to be a challenge, as it currently targets only symptom relief without a definitive cure. However, scientific inquiry and knowledge are advancing, and through more robust and rigorous scientific studies, the ability to uncover the mysteries associated with BMS will result in improved patient-tailored interventions.

Editor's Note: See the Section 2.9, "Bilateral Facial Pain." Because BMS is a diagnosis of exclusion, potential treatable causes of bilateral dysesthetic facial pain include bilateral vascular compression of the trigeminal nerve. Patients with a Chiari malformation are more likely to have bilateral trigeminal neuralgia/neuropathy. This is because the Chiari malformation is a consequence of a temporary developmental arrest during hindbrain development. When fetal development restarts the posterior fossa, which contains the hindbrain and brain stem end up being smaller than normal. This pushes major blood vessels closer to the trigeminal nerves on both sides, making bilateral vascular compressive trigeminal neuropathy more likely. People with multiple sclerosis are also more likely to have bilateral trigeminal neuropathic pain.

2.6
Postherpetic Neuralgia

Trish Elliott, BS; Maria Merlano Gomez; and Julie G. Pilitsis, MD, PhD, MBA

Author's Note: Dr. Pilitsis receives grant support from Medtronic, Boston Scientific, Abbott, and the National Institutes of Health (NIH 2R01CA166379, NIH R01EB030324, and NIH U44NS115111). She is the medical advisor for Aim Medical Robotics and has stock equity.

Remember that time in your childhood when you and your friends wore mittens and socks on your hands all day? Maybe because your parents brought you to a "Pox Party," and after sharing a lollipop or chocolate milk, you developed an itch that you couldn't help but scratch... all over your body... the chicken pox. Before the vaccine was launched in 1995, the chicken pox was a rampant and seemingly inevitable disease among children, with 95% of adults today reporting having had the virus. Although the chicken pox vaccine has decreased the likelihood of the disease, the varicella zoster virus remains dormant in the bodies of those who experienced those 4 to 7 days of itchy agony long ago. Now, the same virus that plagued your body as a child has the potential to reappear, but in a different guise.

Shingles is caused by the reactivation of the chicken pox virus that has been dormant or lying in wait. With it comes the reappearance of a rash. Excessive stress, a weakened immune system, and aging increase the likelihood of virus reactivation. The good news about shingles is that, in contrast to chicken pox, you cannot get it from other people. Postherpetic neuralgia describes the condition in which the nerve pain persists in the area of the shingles rash after the rash has resolved. This can occur in 10% to 20% of patients. There is a higher risk of postherpetic neuralgia in those who have more severe shingles, older folks, or individuals whose shingles occurs on the face. Patients describe the symptoms as stabbing, stinging, or burning. Often, people visibly grimace during pain exacerbations. Individuals with postherpetic neuralgia will avoid touching the sensitive area. If it involves the face, they will try to avoid being out in the wind or in cold weather, or in the summer, they try to avoid being near air-conditioning breezes. They don't wear scarves or anything that touches the face. Even the light touch of moisturizer, make-up application, or activities such as shaving and washing the face can aggravate the symptoms. A pillow used when sleeping can awaken people if it touches their face.

There is no doubt that QOL can be affected. Aging is, of course, inevitable, but you can decrease the likelihood of postherpetic neuralgia, and if it occurs, its pain intensity. Trust me, I want you to conquer the tennis courts, tend to your tomato garden, hit a hole-in-one on the golf course, or climb Kilimanjaro at your painless leisure. And, yes, staying in shape, being active, and exercising regularly are all parts of your ongoing strategy.

So, let's discuss this strategy.

The prevention of shingles and the timely identification and management of shingles and/or postherpetic neuralgia are crucial.

The absolute best thing you can do to head this off is to get *the shingles vaccine!* Do this regardless of whether you had chicken pox as a child or not. The vaccine is highly effective and can prevent chances of shingles and its aftereffects. Even if you already have another type of facial pain, this is a wise decision if you are 50 years of age or older. If you do contract shingles, seek immediate care. Antiviral medications can limit the impact and severity of the disease. This is not a time to "gut it out." Treatment can prevent the dreaded aftermath.

When postherpetic neuralgia does still strike, treatments that are available are similar to those for any other type of nerve pain. Medications include typical nerve pain agents such as gabapentin and pregabalin, anticonvulsants, and antidepressants. In the past, tricyclic antidepressants and opioids were used, and they may be employed in rare cases today. Topical creams with capsaicin, menthol, or lidocaine are other options. Most often, these topical treatments are used in combination with oral medications. Less commonly, nerve blocks of the area with steroids and numbing medicine such as lidocaine may be used.

Integrated care allows for many additive therapies. Diet, meditation, relaxation, and biofeedback are all options. Optimizing hormonal and vitamin status has little downside. Acupuncture-related treatments pose another option for pain relief with few adverse effects. Use of acupuncture with medications holds particular promise, and one study showed that electroacupuncture reduced postherpetic neuralgia-induced insomnia and depression. (Yu 2020) In cases where these methods do not work, spinal cord stimulation has been successful in a subset of patients. Implanting such a device high in the spine where signals can pass to the brain stem has relieved facial pain in some cases. The stimulation of the device is controlled by the patient using a remote, and the pain is replaced by a light tingling sensation in some cases or no sensation in others. In rare cases, stimulation of the brain regions that affect sensation to the face with deep brain stimulation, motor cortex stimulation, or peripheral stimulation if the pain is in the face may be used. Peripheral stimulation involves insertion of electrodes under the skin of the painful facial regions, specifically, above and below the eye and along the jawline. These work similarly to the electrodes used in spinal cord stimulation when connected to a pacemaker-like device that is also implanted, but usually beneath the collar bone in the chest.

In summary, get vaccinated to prevent getting shingles! See a doctor early if shingles or postherpetic neuralgia does occur. The chicken pox may have scarred your childhood, but do not let this virus affect you in your later years.

2.7
Anesthesia Dolorosa
Jesse McClure, MD, PhD, PharmD, and
Julie G. Pilitsis, MD, PhD, MBA

Author's Note: Dr. Pilitsis receives grant support from Medtronic, Boston Scientific, Abbott, and the National Institutes of Health (NIH 2R01CA166379, NIH R01EB030324, and NIH U44NS115111). She is the medical advisor for Aim Medical Robotics and has stock equity.

When I was asked to author this article on anesthesia dolorosa, my first thought was that I have seen far fewer people with this condition now than I did earlier in my career. My second thought was that I had a hard time thinking of one particular patient I had treated who had a "textbook" version of the condition. This is a bit unusual, because, after 25 years of practice, when I think of a diagnosis, in my mind's eye, a patient's face or name or computed tomography scan comes up.

Anesthesia dolorosa is a Latin term that describes nerve pain that comes after a trauma to the trigeminal nerve, usually within 6 months of a surgery or an injury. Most often, the trauma occurs after a surgery intended to treat trigeminal neuralgia (TN) such as MVD, balloon compression, radio-frequency ablation, or radiosurgery. The incidence after a single surgery has been reported to be 1:1000, but because anesthesia dolorosa is a rare disease, it is difficult to truly identify how common it is. (Giller 2002) It is, however, more common after multiple surgeries, each with the purpose of causing nerve injury. Sometimes, patients describe anesthesia dolorosa as the sensation of "bees stinging the entirety of my face," and sometimes, they say it is "the feeling that goes along with a brain freeze," a cold electric sensation. Others may say that it is a constant burning pain.

The problem with the term anesthesia dolorosa is that there is no ruler that can be used to identify when you have it. It is a condition relative to each individual with trigeminal nerve injury. So, really, it is a term that corresponds to a chronic sensation of what can be called a severe form of "dysesthesia," meaning a burning, freezing, tingling, stinging discomfort.

For many years, anesthesia dolorosa has been considered a dreaded complication. Many patients have reported that the sensation was worse than the TN for which they were originally treated. These patient reports led surgeons to be more cautious and to restrict the amount of energy, pressure, or tension delivered to a nerve during surgery. During MVD surgery, nerve monitoring can improve safety. Furthermore, a better understanding of how anesthesia or the blood pressure control with anesthesia can affect nerves has led to more controlled outcomes. Thus, fortunately, anesthesia dolorosa is now less common after surgical procedures. More often now, cases are seen after facial trauma or surgical neurectomies (cutting of the nerve). Patients should be keenly aware of this complication if any surgeon proposes to cut a nerve as a form of treatment for facial pain, as this is a procedure with a high risk of causing anesthesia dolorosa.

When anesthesia dolorosa does occur, it should be treated as what is called a neuropathic pain condition. This means that further typical TN treatments such as MVD, glycerol rhizotomy, radiofrequency rhizotomy, balloon compression, and radiosurgery should be avoided. Neurectomy should never be done. Anything that could cause more damage to the nerve should be avoided. One reason physicians do not quickly move from one procedure to another in patients experiencing TN without allowing time for the procedure to work and for side effects to manifest is because of the potential for the development of this complication. Of course, there are times when immediate repeat surgery is necessary, such as when a postoperative MRI scan shows persistent or additional compression of the nerve or there are issues that limit the therapy from reaching the target during percutaneous procedures. However, in most cases, it is best to give 3 to 6 months between procedures, especially in cases where pain has improved but not to the degree the patient was hoping.

Anesthesia dolorosa remains difficult to treat. Fortunately, over time, symptoms may improve. What are other good treatments for neuropathic pain? They run the gamut and include means of treating the sensory, affective, and cognitive aspects of pain that occur in all chronic pain conditions for all patients, although the degree varies. It is unlikely that treating just the sensory component will resolve the pain adequately; treatment will often combine therapies. For the sensory component of pain, medications known to treat neuropathic pain, including gabapentin, pregabalin, anticonvulsants, antidepressants, and antispasmodics, are used. Historically, monoamine oxidase inhibitors and opioids were used in some cases, and they may occasionally still be used. Compounds including capsaicin and other pain creams may have benefits. Care needs to be taken when using such agents by the eye. There have been occasional reports of varying success with medications being administered directly to the painful area using catheters that are inserted within the spinal fluid space.

In general, the first surgical option is a procedure called high cervical spinal cord stimulation. It is designed to alter the firing of the tract to the trigeminal nerve that loops down in the spine just below the brain stem. The concept of its use is like that of a spinal cord stimulator for back or leg pain. A medical device that looks like a pacemaker to the heart can be used to create a type of white noise that is pain-relieving for the nerve. Device technology has advanced in the past decade. Many devices allow handheld or app-based management. Coupled with rechargeable implanted batteries, the devices are hardly visible and can be used for many years without the need for replacing batteries. In rare cases, stimulation to the brain through either the motor cortex or deep brain stimulation may be offered. Prior to considering surgery, a transcutaneous electrical nerve stimulation (TENS) unit may be used.

Western medicine does not typically have sufficient treatments for this condition, so an integrated approach may be needed. Noninflammatory diets, where foods that irritate the gut and body are avoided, are now being used. Auricular acupuncture, in which different regions of the body are reflected on areas of the ear, offers promise for some types of neuropathic facial pain. Additionally, vitamin or hormone deficiencies, which are not typically recognized, can worsen pain. A functional medicine evaluation may be helpful, although such evaluations are often not covered by insurance.

Living with chronic pain is taxing. It affects your physical and emotional well-being. It can impact your relationships both personally and professionally. It can leave you feeling completely helpless. It is important to recognize this and know that others with this condition feel the same. Mindfulness meditation can help to reduce chronic pain, and indeed, brain scans even look better afterwards. Yoga, tai chi, and biofeedback may aid in improving an individual's reaction to and awareness of the pain. It is essential not to go through this alone. Having a community of peers to talk to who are experiencing chronic pain or other forms of facial pain can offer comfort. Remember, one size does not fit everyone regarding symptoms or treatments!

2.8
Autonomic Effects of Trigeminal Nerve Injury
Jeffrey A. Brown, MD, FACS, FAANS

Author's Note: The information contained in this section is not intended to provide individual medical advice, diagnosis, or treatment or to induce the reader to seek care with any specific physician. Always seek the advice of your physician or other qualified health care provider with any questions you may have regarding a medical condition or treatment and before undertaking a new health care treatment, and never disregard professional medical advice or delay in seeking it because of something you have read in this book.

Editor's Note: When you have trigeminal nerve pain (TNP), do you sometimes have a red, runny, swollen, teary, or droopy eye on the same side as your pain? How about a stuffy or runny nose, or fullness in your ear? I do. I even know someone who needed care in the Emergency Department because he experienced cardiac arrest during an especially severe TNP episode. These are some autonomic corollaries or consequences of TNP.

Although not everyone experiences these autonomic effects, it is important to know what they are and why they occur. In this chapter, Dr. Brown talks about the autonomic corollaries of TNP and why they occur.

In 1908, a physiologist first described something called the "oculocardiac reflex." Push on your eyeball and your heart rate drops. As it turns out, this is the first understanding of the role of the trigeminal system in the control of those elements of the body that we cannot consciously control. The eyeball is innervated by the trigeminal nerve. Irritate it, and things happen in your body, not just in your face. Irritate it enough, and your heart can even (briefly) stop beating.

This is an autonomic function, where autonomic refers to the involuntary functions of the nervous system, the functions that one cannot consciously control. It relates to the working elements of the internal organs of the body, the muscles of the heart, blood vessels, stomach, and intestines and the functions of the lungs and the sweat and salivary glands. The autonomic nervous system also aides in digestion, relaxation, and even "instinctual" emergency responses to injury or potential injury.

Any form of injury, even minor irritation, to the trigeminal peripheral branches in the face will have some autonomic consequence because the wiring of the trigeminal nerve is intimately intertwined with the autonomic nervous system within the brain stem. It is the brain stem that runs the unconscious activity of the body. Think of it as the body's operating system, analogous to that of your iPhone or computer. If it gets reprogrammed, your phone can work better, but if it is damaged, things can literally go haywire. (Haywire is the thin, too-flexible wire used to hold bales [or bundles] of hay in the fields. Left alone, the wires tend to get intolerably tangled.)

One principle: The more intense the injury to the trigeminal system, the more widespread the effects, even down to the control of your digestive system. Why? The trigeminal nerve nucleus in the brain stem has connections to other nuclei that connect to the vagus nerve. The vagus nerve is appropriately named because it has "vague" or diffuse (autonomic) effects throughout the body. These interconnections go through another nucleus called the nucleus solitarius. A nucleus is the energy center of each nerve and the cable that emerges and enters into it. The output of the vagus nerve can be parasympathetic or sympathetic. One excellent way of understanding the difference is to use the rhyming phrases "rest and digest" and "feed and breed" to describe the parasympathetic plethora of functions. Some examples of parasympathetic functions include the following: The heart rate is slowed, and airway muscles in the lungs are tightened, reducing the amount of work the lungs must do. Energy is diverted to the bowels to help with digestion. The parasympathetic system puts the body to rest.

In contrast, the sympathetic system puts your body on alert. When activated, it enlarges the pupils in your eyes so you can see better. It diverts energy away from the digestive system to provide needed muscle energy to run away, along with increasing the heart rate to provide more oxygen to those working muscles, and even activating energy stores in the liver.

Together, the systems keep the body in balance. It is a complex computer system, indeed.

The problem is that, with trigeminal injury, the response can be a mixture of the two types of responses. Depending on the severity of the induced injury, it can also be inhibitory, instead of stimulating, to the parasympathetic system.

The point remains, however, that injury to the trigeminal nerve can be either at the peripheral level (in the face) or at the ganglion level (inside the skull and closer to the brain stem), at the nerve root level (between the ganglion and the brain stem) or at the brain-stem level. The closer one gets to the brain stem, the greater the consequences of injury.

Think of the brain and the brain stem as a complex electrical system. Electrons in the wiring can be moved quickly (high frequency, high voltage, high current) or more slowly (low frequency, low voltage, low current). Voltage refers to the power or strength of the pushing force delivered to the electrons. Frequency refers to how often those pushes are delivered. Current refers to the consequence of those two forces working together, leading to the quantity (volume) of electrons running through a wire in a given time period. By varying any one of these forces, if electrical energy is delivered to the brain stem, there can be different effects on the body.

I first began to research this topic when studying the effects of balloon compression on the trigeminal nerve while trying to understand how the operation to treat TN really worked. One important effect I observed was that, when the nerve root is compressed during the operation by the balloon, the heart rate will briefly slow. Blood pressure will drop, and then there will be a brief rebound rapid heart rate and rise in blood pressure. Why? Research in an animal model shows that low-frequency stimulation (at less than 50 cycles/second) of the lower portions of the trigeminal complex in the brain stem and spinal cord leads to a decrease in heart rate, a drop in blood pressure, a reduced breathing rate, and an increase in the motility of the gastric digestive system. This appears to happen because the sympathetic system is inhibited rather than the parasympathetic system being activated. The sympathetic nerves are activated by epinephrine. The parasympathetic nerves are activated by a different chemical, acetylcholine.

These responses differ from those seen with other reflexes such as the oculocardiac reflex; the diving reflex, which is a consequence of submersion of the face in cold water; or the nasopharyngeal reflex that results from noxious irritation of the mucosa of the nose.

All these responses are complex mixtures of chemical outpourings from things that happen to the face, that is, the trigeminal nervous system. What happens if you squeeze the trigeminal nerve at its root, as happens with balloon compression rhizotomy? The nerve gives one big "ouch," and out pours a surge of electrical discharge that yields a mixture of cholinergic and anticholinergic mediated effects. What happens in the body then depends on the unpredictable mix of stimulating and inhibiting nerve channels that are turned on.

Disease can do this as well. One way it does so is by causing inflammation, or the release of irritating chemicals. The inflammatory response is the body's effort to bring more blood flow to injured tissue to jump-start the body's reparative mechanisms. In the short term, it is helpful. If it persists, it is not.

What can we take away from this discussion?

There is, for example, a disease entity called SUNCT, which is an acronym for short-lasting unilateral neuralgiform headache attacks with conjunctival injection and tearing. All of these descriptive parts of the name are signs of trigeminal nerve irritation. Is this really a different entity, or is it another in the confusing plethora of manifestations of trigeminal nerve injury? From the preceding discussion, one could understand it to be the latter. TN is that, too.

TN is better understood, in my opinion, as a single form of TNP, meaning trigeminal nerve injury. It can manifest itself with brief bursts of short circuits, stabbing pain; or it can be felt by constant pain, often burning; or it can be a mixture of the two. Usually intermixed with the neuropathic (electrical, nerve injury) pain, there can be a residual aching pain. Aching pain is not nerve pain. It is what is called nociceptive pain. This is the type of pain transmitted to the brain by nerve endings in response to injury of the body. The pain felt in the face from neuralgia attacks, through another pathway in the that nucleus solitarius, can evoke this different form of pain as a secondary response.

In summary, the trigeminal nerve is intimately intertwined with the autonomic system of the body, and as such, any disease or injury to the nerve will cause an autonomic response that can be something so seemingly innocuous as a red face or possibly something as devastating as a full cardiac arrest. The difference is in the severity.

2.9
Bilateral Facial Pain
Jeffrey A. Brown, MD, FACS, FAANS

Author's Note: The information contained in this section is not intended to provide individual medical advice, diagnosis, or treatment or to induce the reader to seek care with any specific physician. Always seek the advice of your physician or other qualified health care provider with any questions you may have regarding a medical condition or treatment and before undertaking a new health care treatment, and never disregard professional medical advice or delay in seeking it because of something you have read in this book.

Is it real? Yes, it is—rare but real. Bilateral comes from Latin bi meaning two, and lateral meaning side or flank. Bilateral facial pain refers to pain on both sides of the face. It can occur concurrently, meaning that both sides hurt at the same time, or sequentially, meaning that there is pain on one side and then on the other. Bilateral facial pain more often occurs in people who have multiple sclerosis (MS), Chiari malformations, and a few other rare conditions.

We begin by examining why people with MS can experience bilateral facial pain. The brain consists of a mixture of *gray matter* and *white matter*. *Ganglia* are clusters of nerve cells found throughout the body. They carry nerve signals to and from the central nervous system (CNS). Large congregations of ganglia are in so-called gray matter. White matter is found in the deepest brain tissues. It connects the different parts of the brain. A straightforward way to visualize this is to think of the brain as a computer. The gray matter is the hardware. White matter represents the cables that connect the network and transmit signals. MS is a disease of white matter in the brain and spinal cord. Most nerves are not "naked." They are covered in a fatty substance called *myelin* that improves their ability to conduct impulses rapidly. The white appearance of myelin gives white matter its name. In MS, the sclerotic plaques that form are in the white matter and disturb its function. Because the trigeminal nerve has a high concentration of white matter and the face is extremely sensitive to touch, the trigeminal nervous system is prone to injury in MS patients. It is not limited to one side of the body.

Why do these sclerotic plaques cause pain? They injure the myelin, so nerves can be naked. When electricity surges through them, there can be short circuits that we feel as stabbing or sometimes continuous electrical, burning pains.

Because there is primary injury to the nerve, the TNP of MS is hard to treat. It is unlike TNP resulting from a vascular contact or distortion of the trigeminal nerve. These vascular abnormalities can be dealt with primarily by decompressing the nerve, that is, moving the offending artery or vein and placing a tiny pillow between the nerve and artery or vein to avoid further contact. That is usually not possible in people with MS. Sometimes, however, people with MS can have TNP for a reason unrelated to their MS and can be treated by decompressing the nerve. This is especially true if the MS has been inactive for many years before the onset of TNP.

Are there other ways for pain to be bilateral? Yes. Some young people with Chiari malformations may be more prone to bilateral facial pain. The Chiari malformation is a consequence of a temporary developmental arrest in utero of the early developing hind portion of the skull. This is the back of the skull that contains the cerebellum, which is the balance control portion of the brain. During the brief period when the skull is not growing, the brain is still growing. When the skull growth starts up again, the hindbrain does not fit into its package, and space is tight, sometimes tight enough that the hindbrain slips down into the spinal canal to find room. You can understand that, in this situation, arteries and veins in tight quarters are more likely to be forced up against the trigeminal nerve, which enters the brain stem in this region of the skull, called the posterior or back fossa or cave. Individuals with this experience in utero may be more prone to developing trigeminal neuralgia and having bilateral TNP. They may even have a combination of trigeminal and vagoglossopharyngeal neuropathic pain, as both areas would be subject to the complications of tight quarters.

Does anyone else experience bilateral facial pain? There is another group of people who have pain, but not with a compressive cause. They may have an immunologic cause of their pain such as scleroderma, lupus, or Sjögren's syndrome. (See the next section by Hossein Ansari, MD, on medical causes of facial pain.) These conditions can be diagnosed by laboratory studies and may be associated with other signs separate from the facial nerves, such as perennially cold hands, dry mouth, tight skin, or a butterfly rash on the face.

What about burning mouth syndrome? Because this syndrome is of unknown cause and unclear treatment, it should not be a diagnosis delivered lightly. Patients with venous contact on the trigeminal nerve are more likely to have continuous burning pain than those with arterial contact. If the pain is bilateral, vascular contact should be investigated before a diagnosis of burning mouth syndrome is issued. To make such a diagnosis, one has to undergo an MRI scan done with certain software adjustments that have the acronyms FIESTA, CISS, or VIBE. These techniques allow one to distinguish between spinal fluid, arteries, veins, and nerves. The MRI scan is done with thin cuts that provide the best possibility of seeing such vascular contact when the images are viewed in three different planes (axial, sagittal, and coronal) simultaneously. (See Figures 2-5 and 2-6.)

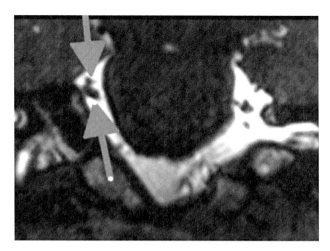

Figure 2-5. MRI image in the coronal (straight-ahead) view showing the right trigeminal nerve (lower arrow) in contact with an artery (upper arrow) in a patient with bilateral facial pain.

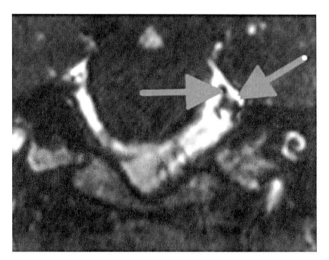

Figure 2-6. MRI image in the coronal (straight-ahead) view showing the left trigeminal nerve (left arrow) in the same patient in contact with loops of an artery (right arrow).

What happens when the diagnosis of bilateral TNP secondary to compressive neuropathy is made, and medication no longer provides relief? If surgery is needed, it should be done on the most painful side first. Surgery on the other side should be delayed for several months to allow time for recovery from the first operation. Bilateral injury to the brain from surgery in a single session is to be avoided, as it can inflict a devastating injury should it occur.

In summary, bilateral vascular compressive TNP is an unusual condition of an already unusual condition, so the diagnosis is best obtained from a physician well experienced in the treatment of TNP.

2.10
Medical Causes of Facial Pain
Hossein Ansari, MD, FAAN, FAHS

Facial pain is one of the most challenging entities for physicians to treat. This is due to the variety of its causes. These include neurological, dental (e.g., temporomandibular joint disorders, tooth and gum issues), and sinus- and nasal-related causes, as well as those related to rheumatologic and autoimmune disorders. This chapter discusses three autoimmune disorders that can cause facial pain: Sjögren's syndrome, scleroderma, and MS.

Nerve supply to the face comes from the trigeminal nerve, which is one of the 12 cranial nerves in the human body. A cranial nerve is one that directly enters or leaves the brain. The trigeminal is composed of three (prefix "tri-") main divisions. Each division has multiple branches that funnel down to the main sensory root before entry into the brain stem, as depicted in Figure 2-7.

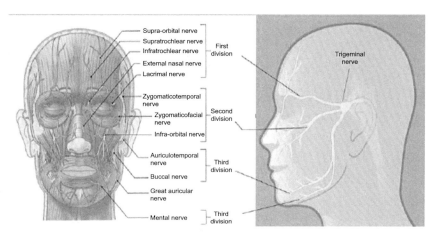

Figure 2-7.   Multiple small branches of the trigeminal nerve.

These branches supply the sensation to different parts of the face, mouth, tongue, nose, and sinuses. Any damage, injury, or disease that affects the trigeminal nerve anywhere from the smallest branches on the face to its origin in the brain can cause facial pain.

The evaluation of a person with facial pain includes both gathering a thorough history and examining the head, teeth, eyes, nose, throat, and even neck, because any of these structures can contribute to facial pain. Because of this heterogeneity of causes, individuals with facial pain often need to consult multiple practitioners to obtain a proper diagnosis and treatment.

Most of the time, facial pain is triggered by some form of trauma: a dental procedure, compression of nerves by blood vessels, or invasion by a tumor. Medical disorders that affect the trigeminal nerve can be a source of facial pain. In general, any pain that occurs as a result an injury to a nerve is referred to as a neuropathic pain. This definition is broad and covers more than 100 conditions. When the injury to the trigeminal nerve occurs in the brain due to compression by blood vessels, it is also known as trigeminal neuralgia (TN).

The most challenging cases of trigeminal neuropathic pain involve people with facial pain who do not have classical TN. Classical TN refers to intermittent facial stabbing pain with intervening pain-free periods. Other people are often labeled as having atypical facial pain or atypical TN. Some of these people may have a systemic medical disorder that also involves the trigeminal nerve, causing facial pain.

Among systemic medical causes, inflammatory and autoimmune diseases are the most common disorders that involve trigeminal nerves. Autoimmune diseases such as Sjögren's syndrome, scleroderma, lupus, and undifferentiated connective tissue disorder, can attack the trigeminal nerve and cause facial pain, sometimes similarly to TN. Individuals experiencing facial pain due to autoimmune diseases are said to have inflammatory trigeminal neuropathy or autoimmune trigeminal neuropathic pain. Surgery will not help these disorders.

Sjögren's syndrome is a chronic, systemic autoimmune disease that is more common in women. It is one of the more prevalent autoimmune disorders. Because its symptoms are sometimes mild, it might not be diagnosed. The main targets of Sjögren's syndrome are the exocrine glands, such as the parotid or salivary glands, which causes dryness of the mucosal surfaces. Dry eyes and dry mouth are the key features of this syndrome. If Sjögren's syndrome does not affect any other organs, it might not even be diagnosed solely on the basis of dry eyes or dry mouth because these symptoms are nonspecific and common in the general population. However, in Sjögren's syndrome, a variety of systemic manifestations may occur, including fatigue, musculoskeletal symptoms, cutaneous lesions, and internal organ and neurological involvement. According to some reports, up to 70% of Sjögren's patients may experience neurological manifestations.

Neuropathy is a classic neurological manifestation of Sjögren's syndrome; thus, trigeminal nerve involvement could occur in individuals with Sjögren's syndrome. In fact, the trigeminal nerve is the most common cranial nerve to be involved. As a result, in patients who have trigeminal neuropathy due to Sjögren's syndrome, with no other cranial nerve involvement, facial and trigeminal pain will be the only major symptoms of Sjögren's because the symptoms of dry eyes or dry mouth could be mild.

In patients with facial and trigeminal pain who do not have classic TN, the presence of some nonspecific symptoms could suggest the possibility of Sjögren's syndrome. These symptoms could include

- Unexplained fatigue or tiredness;
- Severe dry eyes that require treatment (Symptoms of dry eyes include stinging, burning, or itching; feeling of sand in the eyes; sore and swollen eyelids; discomfort when looking at light; and even blurry vision.);
- Severe dry mouth, which can present with the tongue sticking to the roof of mouth, feeling that food (specifically dry food) is stuck in the mouth or throat, and even changes in how food tastes;
- Frequent dental cavities despite good dental hygiene;
- Dry skin or vaginal dryness;
- Rashes (especially after being in the sun);
- History of multiple unexplained miscarriages; and
- Muscle and joint pain with stiffness and swelling.

These are symptoms that are usually not asked about by physicians if patients present with facial and trigeminal pain. Therefore, patients should be aware of this disease and pay attention to those nonspecific symptoms, particularly when they are diagnosed with atypical TN or atypical facial pain.

The diagnosis of Sjögren's syndrome is not always easy because the blood test for Sjögren's could be negative in up to 40% to 50% of patients with this syndrome. This is particularly true in people who are in the beginning of the disease process because their bodies have not made enough antibody to be detected. Therefore, in individuals with facial pain for whom there is a question of Sjögren's syndrome, consultation with a rheumatologist might help to obtain proper diagnosis and treatment.

Scleroderma is a chronic autoimmune disorder that is much less common than Sjögren's syndrome. However, because trigeminal nerve involvement is one of the most common manifestations of this autoimmune disease, it should be considered as a potential cause of facial pain. Scleroderma, similarly to Sjögren's syndrome, is more common in young to middle-aged women with peak onset at ages of 30 to 50 years.

Patients with scleroderma can have progressive skin tightness and induration, often preceded by swelling and puffiness. The other important symptom that can be suggestive of scleroderma is Raynaud's phenomenon. With Raynaud's phenomenon, there is a pale to blue to red sequence of color changes of the fingers or toes, most commonly after exposure to cold (Figure 2-8).

Raynaud's phenomenon is more characteristic of scleroderma, but it can be seen in other autoimmune disorders. Raynaud's phenomenon that is not associated with systemic sclerosis or other autoimmune diseases is known as primary Raynaud phenomenon. It occurs in 5% to 15% of the general population.

In addition to skin manifestation, scleroderma, similarly to Sjögren's syndrome, has many nonspecific symptoms, including

- Gastrointestinal symptoms, which can range from dyspepsia, bloating, and reflux to difficulty swallowing;
- Respiratory symptoms, such as progressive shortness of breath, chest pain, and dry persistent cough;

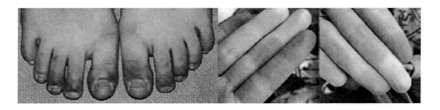

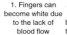

1. Fingers can become white due to the lack of blood flow   2. The fingers may turn blue as the blood vessels dilate to keep the blood in the tissues   3. Finally the fingers may turn red as the blood begins to return

Figure 2-8.   Color changes of the fingers and toes with Raynaud's phenomenon.

- Musculoskeletal symptoms, such as severe muscle pain, fatigue and weakness, and joint pain with loss in joint range of motion; and
- Kidney involvement, which typically presents as early-onset hypertension, which is usually resistant to regular treatment and can sometimes cause renal failure.

Bear in mind that the symptoms in Sjögren's syndrome and scleroderma, as well as other autoimmune disorders that can attack the trigeminal nerve, can be nonspecific. The entire clinical picture needs to be considered before suggesting these possibilities as the reason for facial pain. The most important factor is age of the onset of trigeminal pain. Because classical TN, which is the most well-known etiology for facial pain, is rare before the age of 40 years and unusual before the age of 50 years, individuals with facial pain in those age groups need to be aware of the possibility of an autoimmune disorder. This is particularly true because the most common age for the onset of autoimmune disorders is between 20 and 50 years.

Sjögren's syndrome and scleroderma are autoimmune disorders involving the trigeminal nerve outside the brain. In contrast, the third condition considered here affects the trigeminal nerve inside the brain, namely, MS.

MS is an autoimmune disorder in which the immune system attacks the myelin sheath around its own nerves. Recent research suggests that between four and six of every 100 people with MS experience TN. This is about 400 times more often than in the general population. The prevalence of TN in the MS population has been reported to be between 1% and 6.3%. TN is sometimes an early symptom in MS. In 10% of individuals with MS, the diagnosis of TN preceded the diagnosis of MS by an average of 5 years. (Houshi 2022)

Different people experience the pain of MS-related TN in different ways. It is most commonly felt in the cheek or in the upper or lower jaw, but some individuals experience pain up toward the eye, ear, and forehead or inside the mouth.

To understand why MS can cause TN, a short introduction of the nervous system will help. Nerve cells called neurons have two main components (Figure 2-9):

- *Axons* are a key component of a neuron. They conduct electrical signals between neurons.
- *Myelin* is the sheath or cover of an axon. Each axon is insulated by this sheath throughout its length to increase the velocity of the electrical signals it transmits, thus allowing signals to propagate quickly.

Demyelination occurs when the myelin sheath is damaged. Demyelinated nerves have spots, or plaques, with no myelin (Figure 2.10). When this damage occurs to the myelin sheath, electrical signals from the axons misfire when they are not supposed to fire.

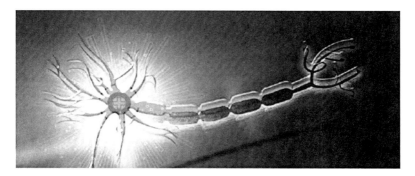

Figure 2-9.   Structure of a neuron with its axon surrounded by myelin.

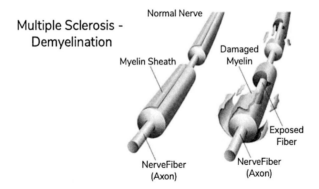

Multiple Sclerosis - Demyelination

Normal Nerve

Myelin Sheath

Damaged Myelin

Exposed Fiber

NerveFiber (Axon)

NerveFiber (Axon)

Figure 2-10.   Comparison between a normal neuron and a demyelinated neuron in multiple sclerosis.

This increased electrical activity presents as pain, which is classified as neuralgic pain.

Other than MS, myelin damage can be caused by any number of common and uncommon conditions. These include

- Infections,
- Inflammation,
- Metabolic disorders,
- Certain medications,
- Excessive alcohol use,
- Stroke, and
- Vitamin B_{12} deficiency.

Similar to classical TN, TN secondary to MS is characterized by a sudden, brief, jabbing, and electric-shock-like, recurrent pain with a distribution that is consistent with one or more branches of the trigeminal nerve. The paroxysmal attacks last from a fraction of a second to about 2 minutes and are typically provoked by simple stimulation of the skin or mucosa of the face and/or mouth. The pain can be triggered by everyday routine activities such as chewing, talking, or brushing teeth or even by being outside in a light breeze. However, characteristics that should raise the question of TN due to MS or other autoimmune conditions include the following:

- *Bilateral trigeminal neuralgia.* It is uncommon for classical TN to occur on both sides of the face, or bilaterally. In MS, an estimated 18% of patients have bilateral TN. Therefore, any patient presenting with bilateral facial pain requires a detailed work-up with particular attention to ruling out MS as its cause.

- *Pronounced sensory changes.* Patients who complain of significant sensory symptoms, either tingling or numbness on the face, are more likely to have an autoimmune condition, including MS. This is even more likely if patients have additional sensory symptoms in other parts of body, including feet and hands.
- *Continuous or constant pain from the onset of facial pain.* Patients with continuous face pain can misattribute the pain to dental causes. Bearing in mind that facial pain could be a symptom of MS-related TN, it is always helpful to keep this possibility in mind, especially before considering any major dental work. On the other hand, some patients with TN secondary to MS, such as patients with other types of TN, experience concomitant continuous, dull, or burning pain between attacks of electric-shock-like pain. The area of continuous pain is the same as the area of paroxysmal pain, and the intensity of the pain fluctuates between the episodes of those paroxysmal pain cycles. Therefore, a detailed history, in addition to a sensory exam and thorough work-up, is especially important to make a correct diagnosis.
- *Younger age of onset, particularly below 40 years of age.* It is rare for people under the age of 40 years to experience classical TN, so for those in this age range, it is particularly important to consider other causes of TN such as MS.

If, after a detailed history and exam, your physician suspects the possibility of MS as the potential reason for TN, a proper work-up needs to be initiated. Such a work-up should include the following components:

- *MRI scan.* An MRI scan of the brain, and in some cases, of the cervical spine, should be performed to look for changes caused by MS, such as signs of inflammation in the deep parts of the brain or spinal cord. Such changes are called MS plaques. TN secondary to MS is usually associated with a plaque in the area of brain called the pons, which is easily detectable by MRI. In most patients, MRI is enough to make the diagnosis. However, a normal MRI result does not rule out MS. In a small number of individuals with MS, it might not be possible to see the lesion(s) in an MRI scan, or it could simply be too early in the disease to detect the lesion(s). If TN is the only suspected symptom, further work-up is usually not recommended, but if there is a high suspicion of MS due to some other neurological symptoms, additional work-up might be indicated, as discussed further in the remainder of this list.

- *Spinal tap (lumbar puncture).* This test checks the fluid that runs through the spinal column. It is used to look for high levels of proteins and other substances that are signs of MS or a related demyelinating disorder.
- *Evoked potential tests.* These electrical nerve tests can help confirm whether MS has affected the parts of the brain that help with seeing, hearing, and feeling sensations. In these tests, some wires are placed on the scalp to test the brain's response as the patient watches a pattern on a video screen, hears a series of clicks, or receives electrical pulses on the arms or legs.
- *Blood tests.* There is no blood test to diagnose MS, but blood tests are used to look for substances in the blood that point to it. Most importantly, a blood test can help rule out conditions that look like MS.
- *Neurophysiological tests.* Results of trigeminal reflex testing, in particular, are abnormal in 89% of patients with TN secondary to MS, but they are abnormal in only 3% of patients with classical and idiopathic TN. This might be an extremely helpful test in patients unable to obtain MRI testing because of metal in their body such as a pacemaker.

According to international guidelines, there is insufficient evidence to support or refute the effectiveness of any medication in treating pain in TN secondary to MS. However, it is generally agreed that the first-line therapy for this pain is pharmacological and is based, as it is for classical and idiopathic TN, on the use of sodium-channel blockers such as oxcarbazepine or carbamazepine. It is critical that patients with MS treat their MS with medication that is specific for this condition. With advancements in medication for MS in the past decade, early and proper treatment of this condition might prevent the progression of disease and, as a result, also prevent the progression of TN. Surgical treatment, particularly MVD, is less successful in TN secondary to MS.

Chapter 3
Surgery for Neuropathic Facial Pain

Anne B. Ciemnecki, MA

As a peer mentor for the Facial Pain Association (FPA), the question I am asked most often is, "What should I do next?" My initial response does not include, "See a neurosurgeon." I have learned that, if I speak about neurosurgery initially, the person on the other end of the conversation shuts down. Having brain surgery is the last thing a person who is in excruciating pain wants to hear. Instead, I say that there are three things they need to do initially:

1. Do something to ease the pain. You need a break. You cannot explore your options or make a rational decision if you are in so much pain you cannot think.
2. Get a proper diagnosis. You cannot treat your pain if you do not know what is causing it.
3. Once you know what is causing the pain, consider all the available options (including medical, surgical, and integrative) and select the best one for you now and in the long term.

Part of the diagnostic process is getting a proper magnetic resonance imaging (MRI) scan. Orofacial pain specialists and neurosurgeons know the type of MRI to order and how to read them. If the scan shows a pulsation or vascular compression, I talk about the importance of considering microvascular decompression (MVD) surgery sooner rather than later.

There are two types of procedures to bring relief to people with trigeminal neuralgia. The first, an MVD, is the only procedure that is not intended to damage the nerve. Although technically brain surgery, an MVD is minimally invasive. It treats the cause of the problem by separating the blood vessel from the nerve that it is damaging. It offers the most long-lasting relief and minimizes the risk of postoperative numbness. Most people are eligible for this, even elderly people and people who have other medical conditions.

The other procedures are ablative, that is, destructive. They aim to eliminate pain by making a small cut (or a big one) to the nerve. Even radio-frequency procedures, such as gamma knife and CyberKnife surgeries, are ablative. Pain relief from ablative procedures is not always immediate. The relief does not last as long as relief from an MVD. Repeat ablative procedures are less effective than the initial ones. The numbness after an ablative procedure can be as uncomfortable as the initial pain. Although one can have an MVD after an ablative procedure, it may not be as effective as having an MVD initially if the ablative procedure left residual uncomfortable numbness.

Most people treat their pain with medications until the pain or the side effects of the medications become unbearable. Then, they move to surgical options. It is useful to see a neurosurgeon before you need surgery. A consultation with a neurosurgeon does not mean that you need to have surgery right away or at all. If you need surgery, you will be in pain and unable to make good decisions regarding selecting a surgeon or procedure. Knowing a neurosurgeon will be like having a security blanket, a connection with a doctor you trust. Experts can guide you and comment on the accuracy of your diagnosis, suggest different medications, and lead you to the best treatment.

In Section 3.1, Jeffrey A. Brown, MD, provides insight on how to tell if a neurosurgeon is an expert. In Sections 3.2 and 3.3, Richard Zimmerman, MD, discusses MVD surgery with and without Teflon. As you read these sections, remember that the objective of the surgery is to relieve the pain regardless of how the nerve is separated from the offending vessel. More research is needed on the long-term effects of Teflon MVDs versus non-Teflon MVDs. In Section 3.4, Margaret Tugend and Raymond F. Sekula, Jr., MD, show that, for individuals with classic trigeminal neuralgia, the chance of long-term pain relief increases for those who have an initial response to carbamazepine or oxcarbazepine and increased degrees of vascular compression of the trigeminal nerve. In Section 3.5, Navid Pourtaheri, MD, PhD, and Derek Steinbacher, MD, DMD, FACS, explain peripheral nerve decompression surgery for people with migraine headaches.

Editor's Note: If you are interested in surgery for neuropathic facial pain or the best type of magnetic resonance imaging, please read Facial Pain: A 21st Century Guide (2020).

3.1
What Makes a Neurosurgeon an Expert?
Jeffrey A. Brown, MD, FACS, FAANS

Author's Note: The information contained in this section is not intended to provide individual medical advice, diagnosis, or treatment or to induce the reader to seek care with any specific physician. Always seek the advice of your physician or other qualified health care provider with any questions you may have regarding a medical condition or treatment and before undertaking a new health care treatment, and never disregard professional medical advice or delay in seeking it because of something you have read in this book.

First, some basic requirements: There are a lot, but that is the point. Doctors educated in the United States are granted their MD degree upon completion of (most often) 4 years of study and clinical preparation after college graduation. They must pass a series of three examinations to be granted a license to practice in the state(s) of their choice. The first exam covers basic medical science. The second deals with the principles of clinical conditions. The last exam is taken during the first year of clinical training (internship or residency) and covers the application of medical knowledge to diagnosis and treatment. After completion, the MD degree is a general one and provides approval for the recipient to practice any field of medicine. Physicians who attended non-U.S. medical schools are granted their MD degrees from the country in which they studied. To be allowed to enter a U.S. clinical training program, they must take another version of this series of three exams that is specifically designed for foreign medical graduates. Osteopathic physicians (DOs) have a different degree program and different training programs, and they take different licensing examinations. Osteopathic medicine education is said to deal with patients "holistically." Becoming a board-certified neurosurgeon in the United States requires at least 5 to 6 years of training after medical school at one of about 100 carefully evaluated and approved programs and sometimes includes 1 or 2 years of elective, additional, focused (fellowship) training in a subspecialty of neurosurgery. These areas of training might include spine, pediatric, vascular, tumor, or pain neurosurgery. Fellowship training is not required. The final board certification occurs after several years of practice, submission of all operations performed during those years for independent review, and successful completion of an oral examination. In recent years, certification by the board must be renewed by further examination every decade. To maintain any state-granted medical license, physicians must complete 50 to 200 hours of approved continuing medical education biannually. More often now, some states are mandating reeducation in areas such as infection control. Finally, to maintain privileges to work at hospitals, neurosurgeons must complete annually scheduled education in hospital policies and practices.

So how does a neurosurgeon stand out among colleagues as an expert after all this education? Education is important. What comes next is what makes one an expert. Experience, dedication, passion, team development, personal contribution to the advancement of the field, the capacity for humanity, and empathy for others make the difference.

Let us take experience first: A seminal article reviewed data from a database representing one-fifth of nonfederal hospitals from 19 states for 1,590 MVD operations for trigeminal and glossopharyngeal neuralgias and hemifacial spasm. The authors learned that there were significantly fewer complications from MVD surgery by neurosurgeons who had performed at least 29 MVDs per year. Low-volume neurosurgeons' patients had a significantly higher incidence of brain hemorrhages after surgery and a need to drain spinal fluid after surgery (a sign of greater intraoperative bleeding). Twenty-nine percent (29%) of all MVDs at these hospitals were performed by a neurosurgeon doing only one MVD a year. (Kalkanis 2003) The hospital in which the surgery was performed was also an important consideration, especially for patients older than 65 years. Hospitals in which at least 20 MVDs were done yearly discharged significantly more patients to their homes than to another facility, such as a nursing home or rehabilitation center (5.1% vs 1.6%). For neurosurgeons, the corresponding percentages were 6.1% vs. 0.5% (only one of every 208 patients) for surgeons performing more than 29 MVDs a year. Complications were twice as frequent at low-volume hospitals and 12 times higher for low-volume neurosurgeons. (Kalkanis 2003) It is not just the neurosurgeon who needs the experience. It is also the team built around that physician in all aspects, including both the hospital and the team recruited by it.

What about those other aspects that make a physician stand out among other colleagues? The ability to communicate is essential. Does the doctor sit at your eye level when meeting with you, summarize the essentials of your health situation, and then elaborate, in understandable language, what they believe is your diagnosis and their recommendations for its treatment? Does the doctor then discuss the risks of any surgery recommended, the likelihood of each complication occurring, ideally the likelihood in their personal experience, and even the risk of not proceeding with surgery? This is the beginning of the informed-consent process. Note that it is an interactive process, not just a piece of paper slipped to you the morning of surgery. Does the doctor provide an opportunity for you to pose questions and then respond? All this takes time. Does the doctor allow for it? An expert technician must be matched by their expertise in the elements of being human, the essence of professionalism.

What does that mean? It means

- Integrity,
- Eye contact, and
- Use of power words—helping phrases.

Does the doctor exhibit the elements of compassion and personal engagement? These can be perceived in the doctor's "ESP":

- *Emotion:* The doctor reflects back their behavioral and emotional observation of you, the patient.
- *Stop:* The doctor stops to listen without interruption.
- *Plan:* The doctor provides a plan and summarizes.

And when leaving the room, do they ask an open-ended question, such as, "Is there anything we missed?"

A key to what makes an expert is how they handle an unexpected complication. Is the complication rapidly identified, and are all efforts made to limit the injury from it?

What if the physician believes that the best treatment is not something in their expertise? The ability to understand the limits of one's knowledge is also essential. Does the doctor help find another doctor and/or a facility with that expertise?

What is done after surgery can also be critical. There may be more to do. The problem may be ongoing.

An expert should not be an "expert" in only one thing. They should have other options to offer, other answers to the question, "What if this doesn't work?" We all hope that it does—but must be prepared if it does not.

3.2
Microvascular Decompression for Trigeminal Neuralgia
Richard Zimmerman, MD

When a person suffers from trigeminal neuralgia, many options exist that can help them manage or eliminate their pain. Both medical and surgical options exist to meet differing needs, but patients should understand that each option has risks, benefits, and relative rates of and durations of success. Choosing to have intracranial surgery is always serious, and a thorough explanation by healthcare professionals should precede any such decision. As one of the most common surgeries for treating trigeminal neuralgia, microvascular decompression (MVD) is the surgical option discussed in this section.

Introduction. An MVD is a surgical procedure used to treat trigeminal neuralgia (TN), both TN type 1 (attacks of pain) and TN type 2 (some constant pain along with attacks of pain). It is also effective in treating other related disorders such as glossopharyngeal neuralgia, geniculate neuralgia, and hemifacial spasm, but for this discussion, we will limit the topic to TN. Of the surgical and procedural options, MVD has the distinction of being the most effective treatment for TN. This holds for general success rates as well as longevity of success, and it allows for preserved nerve function (no numbness). Most neuro surgeons believe that this is a logical outcome, as MVD is the only treatment for TN that

- Corrects the anatomic problem causing the pain, namely, vascular compression of the trigeminal (fifth) nerve, and
- Does not include deliberate nerve damage as part of the procedure (all other procedures do, including radiation).

However, although the most effective, MVD is also the most invasive. Let us now take a closer look at the details behind TN and MVD surgery.

The trigeminal nerve is the fifth of 12 cranial nerves. Cranial nerves all emerge from or directly enter the brain or brain stem. The major function of the fifth nerve is to provide sensation from the face. A web of nerve endings comes together to flow through three openings in the skull: one above and one just below the eye and a large oval opening, the foramen ovale, at the base of the skull. These nerve endings converge on the ganglion, which is the energy center for each of the nerve fibers, in a small basin, Meckel's cave, and then narrow in a thicker nerve root (like the trunk of a tree) that is located in the spinal fluid space until it enters the part of the brain stem called the pons. The trigeminal nerve provides sensation from the eyes, teeth, tongue, and inside of the nose and mouth. The nearest named blood vessel above the trigeminal nerve root is the superior cerebellar artery (SCA). This artery (and sometimes other vessels) can elongate (common with aging) and form a loop that makes contact with the trigeminal nerve root. In some people, when a vascular loop pulsates against the trigeminal nerve at or near where it leaves the brain stem, it can cause pain. Not everyone with this anatomic variant gets TN, and it is unclear why it occurs in those who do.

The trigeminal nerve undergoes an interesting structural change as it enters the brain (as do all nerves as they enter the brain or spinal cord). Picture nerves as wires in a circuit. The long segments of nerves (axons) connect the body to the brain. And just like wires, all nerves have insulation for protection. This protective insulation is composed of a fatty compound called myelin, which helps conduct impulses rapidly. This is where we get to the fascinating (and potentially terrifying) part of the trigeminal nerve: the mysterious root entry zone (REZ).

The REZ is the site where the nerve is just outside the brain. Here, the myelin that surrounds the axons transitions from a type made by one cell to a type made by another kind of cell. The myelin covering the trigeminal nerve in the central nervous system (inside the brain) is produced by oligodendroglia cells. These exist only in the brain itself. When the trigeminal nerve leaves the brain to become part of the peripheral nervous system, the myelin manufactured changes over to that produced by Schwann cells. These exist only outside the brain. You can understand that the brain is protected by the skull, so nerves inside it are well protected. However, outside the skull, the nerves are subject to injury. So, they have a thicker form of myelin, or insulation, around them. There is a transition zone as the nerve enters the brain in which there is still some thin insulation. Something about that transition makes the nerve vulnerable to compression. This is why physicians who understand TN make a big deal about finding "a vascular loop at the root entry zone."

Although it is not known why the REZ is vulnerable, contact or compression of the nerve at this location can certainly create "abnormal conduction behavior"—that is, terrible face pain—even though, to appearances, there is nothing wrong with the face. Although the cause of the problem is pulsation near the trigeminal nerve REZ, few patients describe their TN pain in the character one would consider "pressure" or a "pressure sensation." The pain of TN is typically a sudden, sharp, electric, or stabbing pain. It is a short circuit of the nerve caused by the presence of unprotected nerve fibers stripped of their insulation from the constant arterial pounding.

Now that we have a basic understanding of the trigeminal nerve when it is not functioning correctly, we can explore the journey of having an MVD.

Discussing an MVD with a Surgeon. In most cases, the physician orders preoperative imaging with thin-cut MRI scans and three-dimensional studies performed using one of the techniques known by the acronyms FIESTA and CISS. These are acronyms for computer-programmed sequences that will show the nerves, arteries, brain, spinal fluid and their relationships. Three-dimensional means that the images are demonstrated in three different planes at once: straight ahead, from the side, and from the top or bottom. This gives the reviewer the best ability to determine whether there is a vein or artery in contact with the trigeminal nerve. Understand that, if the neuroradiologist reviewing your MRI images, is not familiar with the anatomy of TN, they may call the nerve "normal," which, to all appearances, it is. In addition to having an expert surgeon who knows what to do on "the inside," the experienced surgeon will be able to provide their personal interpretation of the images, which will help determine whether to offer you an MVD versus other choices based on the MRI results, as well as other considerations.

When selecting a surgeon, the best place to start is with a provider who has the time to speak to you and answer all your questions. Unfortunately, we do see MVDs that have not been done well, so do your homework and research your provider. Nearly all neurosurgeons complete their training with at least a little experience performing MVDs. However, finding someone who is an expert and focuses their practice on this condition and this specific operation will serve you well. (See the previous section, "What Makes a Neurosurgeon an Expert?") After surgical and nonsurgical options have been reviewed to your satisfaction and you feel that an MVD by an experienced surgeon is for you, it is time to prepare for surgery.

The Surgery. All MVDs are performed under general anesthesia. During MVD surgery, an opening is made in the bone behind the ear. Some spinal fluid is drained, and the space over the exposed brain (the cerebellum) is followed to the location where the nerve enters the pons and then on to the location of vascular compression. At this point, the magic occurs under the surgical microscope as the vascular compression is relieved (Figure 3-1). In the classical operation popularized by Dr. Jannetta, a tiny piece of Teflon felt was used to separate the blood vessel and nerve. In my particular practice, I try to avoid using Teflon, and instead, I employ a variation I call a microvascular transposition. Section 3.3 provides more information about this Teflon-free MVD. The risks of MVD surgery include the need for general anesthesia, the possibility of bleeding, and infection, as in all surgeries, as well as risks related to the patient's overall medical condition. Because the surgery takes place next to other cranial nerves, there is a small chance that hearing can be affected on the same side as surgery. To prevent this, monitoring of the nearby

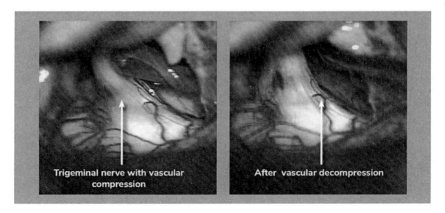

Trigeminal nerve with vascular compression

After vascular decompression

Figure 3-1. Intraoperative image of the trigeminal nerve with and without vascular compression.

nerves is routinely performed; this is known as intraoperative neuromonitoring or intraoperative electromyography (EMG) and brain-stem auditory evoked response (BAER).

After the decompression is complete, the covering (dura) of the brain is meticulously closed. The bone removed can be replaced and held in place with miniplates, screws, or cement, or an implant can be used instead. An inch of muscle at the base of the skull that was split is closed, and then the scalp above it is closed in layers.

The Recovery. Recovery from MVD surgery should focus on mobilization. I get my patients walking the night after their surgery. This helps reduce muscle spasms and prevents other problems such as pneumonia and blood clots in the legs and lungs. These latter two issues are risks after any surgery with a general anesthetic. Some patients have some nausea and dizziness after MVD surgery. These symptoms usually resolve in a few days and can be treated with medication, or a medication patch, worn behind the nonsurgical ear. Once the facial pain has stopped, patients can begin tapering their medications. The facial pain medications are not stopped "cold turkey," as this can cause significant side effects. Around 75% of MVD patients can leave the hospital the next day, possibly after two days. Postoperative pain medication is used for the discomfort at the surgical site behind the ear. Early mobilization and pain medication are the mainstay to support this recovery.

In conclusion, MVD is a successful surgery for TN. The first steps are obtaining a correct diagnosis; seeking good information prior to deciding; and of course, choosing an experienced surgeon.

Editor's Note: When should you seek the opinion of a neurosurgeon if you have been diagnosed with trigeminal neuropathic pain? As Dr. Zimmerman notes, you should seek out an "experienced" neurosurgeon. What makes one "experienced?" See the preceding section, "What Makes a Neurosurgeon an Expert?" And when should you seek out such a neurosurgeon? You should consult an expert in this field as soon as the diagnosis is made. This does not mean you need to have surgery right away. What it does mean is that, if you ever do have surgery, you have a connection to someone you trust. Also, neurosurgeons are the most knowledgeable physicians in the field and can help guide you to the best treatment, medical or surgical, and can comment on the accuracy of your diagnosis. Experts are identified as such because they combine the important elements of diagnostic acumen with empathy and surgical ability. Do not be afraid of them.

3.3
Teflon-Free Microvascular Decompression
Richard Zimmerman, MD

Editor's Note: In March 2021, the article "Microvascular Transposition Without Teflon: A Single Institution's 17-Year Experience Treating Trigeminal Neuralgia" was published in the peer-reviewed journal Operative Neurosurgery. The senior author and surgeon of the article is FPA Medical Advisory Board member Dr. Richard Zimmerman, of the Mayo Clinic in Phoenix, Arizona. The content of this section, provided by Dr. Zimmerman, shares some background behind the article, as well as a brief synopsis of the findings. Although copyright law prevents the FPA from providing copies of the paper, for those interested in reading the complete article as published, the citation is as follows: Operative Neurosurgery 2021 Mar 15;20(4):397–405.

Dr. Peter Jannetta championed MVD as a treatment for TN. Through his tireless support and work to help the facial pain community, Dr. Jannetta also made this procedure a part of mainstream neurosurgery. In the initial descriptions of this procedure, the technique used to elevate a blood vessel off the trigeminal nerve was to insert a small piece of sterile felt under or against the vessel such that the compression was eliminated. The use of Teflon felt has been effective, as demonstrated by the successful results that Dr. Jannetta and many neurosurgeons have achieved. As MRI quality became more sophisticated and detailed, it became apparent that re-imaging patients with post-surgical pain recurrance showed a mass of Teflon against the trigeminal nerve. Could it be that, in these cases, the surgery only replaced vascular compression with Teflon compression or that the Teflon against the nerve still transmitted vascular pulsations (Figure 3-2)? I decided that, in my surgical cases for TN, I would try to avoid using Teflon and instead simply relocate or transpose the position of the compressing blood vessel(s) away from the trigeminal nerve. To maintain the vessel in its transposed location, I used a biologic adhesive known as fibrin glue inside the brain that is commonly used in neurosurgery outside of the brain to aid in sealing off its covering, the dura. The goal of this technique was to completely

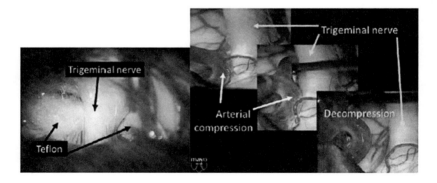

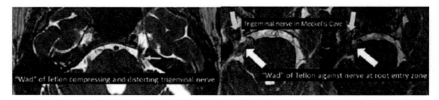

Figure 3-2.   MRI image showing Teflon compressing the trigeminal nerve.

remove anything whatsoever from touching the "sensitive" trigeminal nerve. Thus, I started performing "microvascular transpositions" (MVTs) or "Teflon-free MVDs." I did not invent this approach. Other neurosurgeons have published their series of TN surgeries employing a "noncompressive" technique. Variations on the use of Teflon have been described. These include the use of other types of sponges, sutures, slings, and aneurysm clips. This is not to say that there is anything wrong with the use of Teflon. However, the pattern that I observed in postsurgical recurrences of pain typically involved Teflon seen against the trigeminal nerve on imaging.

After almost 20 years of using this technique consistently, I wanted to evaluate and compare the long-term results of this strategy for treating TN. Thus, I adopted the method of patient-reported outcomes and sent a questionnaire to my patients who had a Teflon-free MVD to learn about their surgical outcomes. I contacted 102 patients and received 85 responses. The ages of those responding ranged from 20 to 89 years. The duration of time after surgery ranged from 9 months to more than 17 years. Long-term, pain-free results were achieved in 89.4% of patients with a mean follow-up duration of 6.9 years. This is a rate of success that compares with the reported outcomes in the literature. I was also able to examine the outcomes divided into the patients who provided a description of intermittent attacks of facial pain alone (TN type 1) versus attacks of facial pain with a background component of constant pain (TN type 2). Although both groups did well, I found that TN type 1 patients did better, with nearly 93% of TN type 1 patients pain-free at 10 years. This study has limits, and they are outlined in the full article. The conclusion, however, is that Teflon is not necessary for a successful TN surgery. Achieving a good decompression whether or not Teflon is used is the goal of MVD surgery.

Patients should always feel comfortable discussing any plans for an operation with their surgeon, including the option of having a Teflon-free MVD. However, given the widespread and classic teaching of using Teflon, it is not likely that many neurosurgeons will be experienced treating TN with vascular transposition. One therefore must decide whether they want to ask their surgeon to perform a procedure with a technique they do not routinely use or find a surgeon who is familiar with this technical nuance.

3.4
An Algorithm for the Surgical Treatment of Classical Trigeminal Neuralgia

Margaret Tugend, BA, and Raymond F. Sekula, Jr., MD

In the clinic, we are working to better understand which patients with TN can benefit from surgical intervention. We know that patients with classical trigeminal neuralgia (cTN) (also called TN1) fare better with most of the available surgical treatments than those with other types of TN. Information gleaned from a detailed history (i.e., a short conversation between patient and physician) allows the physician to make a diagnosis of cTN. Patients with cTN describe sharp, intermittent facial pain usually lasting for seconds or less and never for longer than 2 minutes or so. This pain does not encompass the posterior third of the scalp or the ear. Triggers include innocuous stimuli such as light touch, wind, or chewing. Attacks may occur numerous times each day with periods (from days to months) of remission. Sensory deficit (i.e., orofacial numbness) is not a related symptom. Most patients with cTN will wince (the so-called "tic douloureux" or painful spasm) with pain.

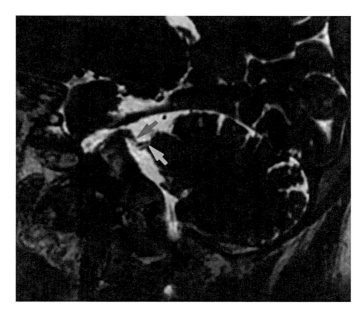

Figure 3-3.   High-resolution MRI image demonstrating trigeminal nerve deformation (purple arrow) by the superior cerebellar artery (orange arrow).

All patients with cTN will benefit from a neurosurgical consultation. Approximately 85% of patients with cTN will have evidence of vascular compression of the trigeminal nerve by high-resolution T2-weighted MRI images (which enhance the signal of water as opposed to fatty tissue). In our center, we perform high-resolution imaging (Figure 3-3) with a higher-power MRI magnet (i.e., 3 T) than found in community-hospital MRI machines.

Perhaps, more important than magnet strength is the "recipe" used to visualize the trigeminal nerve and adjacent vasculature. Too often, we review scans that do not allow a clinician to determine vascular compression of the trigeminal nerve. Why is this important? If a scan is interpreted as negative for vascular compression by a radiologist, the treating neurologist is led to believe that a referral to neurosurgery is unwarranted. We also know that the degree of vascular compression of the trigeminal nerve is important. Patients with more compression of the nerve do better with surgery. In some patients (as many as 15%) with cTN, there is no neurovascular compression. These patients do poorly with MVD. An analogy can be drawn to someone with tooth pain, but no structural problem of the tooth, who undergoes a root canal. The procedure just does not work and often worsens the pain. Those patients with cTN without evidence of neurovascular conflict or an inability to tolerate a general anesthetic may be best managed with a referral for an ablative procedure to the trigeminal nerve or ganglion or further medication management.

A patient's response to the antiseizure drug carbamazepine or oxcarbazepine provides helpful information for the clinician. Many patients report rapid relief of facial pain within just minutes of the first tablet or two of these drugs. Although we do not fully understand why the response to these drugs is an important predictor of response to neurosurgical intervention, we do know that it is important. A few years ago, we and another group developed a readily applicable, quantitative grading or scoring system to aid patients and referring clinicians in understanding whether MVD is the optimal choice (Tables 3-1 and 3-2). (Panczykowski DM 2020) Those with cTN whose pain responds to medication and who have arterial contact or an arterial deformity have a higher probability of achieving long-term pain relief from an MVD. For others, an MVD has a much lower probability of success and might do more damage than good.

One of the unique challenges for individuals with cTN is to *avoid* ablative procedures, if possible. Too often, neurologists and other clinicians relegate patients who are over the age of 65 years or in poor health to one of the ablative procedures rather than MVD. For a variety of reasons, this is a mistake. Although ablative procedures are useful in some circumstances, when patients have potentially fulfilling years ahead of them, these procedures are limited by a lack of durability (i.e., pain relief is short-lived) and increasing complications with repeat procedures. We and others have shown that individuals over 65 years of age and people with some medical conditions do as well as, or better than, others with a similar complication profile. Although the risk of stroke may be a bit higher for people over 65 years old, pooled data suggests that the risk of stroke is less than 1% in expert hands. (Sekula 2011) Consult with doctors treating all of your medical conditions to see if you are healthy enough for an MVD. In expert hands, an MVD is the gold standard regardless of age and even considering some medical conditions.

Table 3-1.   TN Scoring System[a]

Characteristic	Points Assigned for Characteristic
TN Symptom Type	
Nonclassical	0
Classical	1
Response to Medication	
No	0
Yes	1
Neurovascular Contact	
Absent or venous only	1
Arterial contact	2
Arterial deformity	3
Total TN System Score	1 to 5

[a]Abbreviation: TN, trigeminal neuralgia.

In summary, can the individual with cTN expect from a well-performed MVD? If you consider the scoring system in Table 3-2, you will notice that the chance of long-term pain relief increases with an initial response to ox/carbamazepine and increasing degrees of vascular compression of the trigeminal nerve. Although some individuals with cTN will experience a recurrence of trigeminal pain over time, the chance of pain recurrence is much lower with MVD than with any of the ablative procedures.

Table 3-2.   Probability of Long-Term Relief (Without Medication) from MVD Using TN Score

TN Scoring System Score	Probability of Long-Term Pain-Free Status (%)
1	4
2	16
3	44
4	76
5	93

3.5
Surgical Treatment of Migraine Headaches
Navid Pourtaheri, MD, PhD, and
Derek Steinbacher, MD, DMD, FACS

In 2007, the prevalence of migraine headaches in the United States was estimated to be 11.7%, or approximately 35 million people, with a greater proportion of women being affected (17.1% of women, compared to 5.6% of men). Migraine headaches also affect adolescents. The annual cost of treatment and medications for migraine headaches in the United States has been estimated as $13 to $17 billion, and the annual cost to companies in terms of workdays lost (112 million days per year) is in the range of $14 billion. Approximately 10 million Americans suffer from medically refractory migraine headaches.

Editor's Note: According to NIH, in August 2023, migraine headaches affected 12% of the population, up to 17% of women and 6% of men annually. This does not represent a change from the 2007 prevalence cited in the previous paragraph. An article written by Aylin Yucel, and Andrew Thach, published in the December 2020 in.the American Journal of Managed Care used a "Migraine Impact Model" to show that the burden of migraine headaches grew to 19.3 billion (inflated to 2019 dollars). Eighty-one percent of the burden is attributable to full days of productive workforce loss (absenteeism). The estimate does not include days worked with diminished productivity (presenteeism), which may add further indirect costs. One expects that burden will continue to grow. The increase calls for the surgical decompression solution that Pourtaheri and Steinbacher describe for carefully selected people with migraines who have persistent symptoms after medical management and those who cannot tolerate the side-effects of medical therapy.

The diagnosis of chronic migraine headaches should be performed first by a neurologist or other migraine headache specialist, based on the most up-to-date criteria from the International Headache Society. Next, a migraine headache journal, kept for at least 1 month, that documents the frequency, severity, and potential sites of the head and neck where the migraine headache pain may have originated is key to identifying surgical candidates. Frequent identification of specific site(s) of pain reveals "trigger sites" that may benefit from migraine surgery. Diagnostic procedures such as nerve blocks, injections of botulinum toxin (typically called Botox), and Doppler ultrasound may be useful in confirming trigger sites. At the time of a developing migraine headache, patients may be able to point to one or more sites of tenderness where the pain started, and if local nerve blocks performed at these site(s) improve symptoms, the patient would likely benefit from surgery at these site(s). Patients who present without a migraine attack are often able to recall and point to trigger sites based on memory. If injections of botulinum toxin into the muscles surrounding these specific site(s) lead to a significant improvement in symptoms over the next several months, the patient would likely benefit from surgery at these site(s). On the other hand, patients with vague, diffuse areas of pain at the start of a migraine attack or ocular migraine headaches are not surgical candidates.

The initial surgical treatment for migraine headaches involves thorough decompression of the affected nerves at the identified trigger site(s). Decompression primarily involves performing myectomies and/or fasciectomies (i.e., removing muscle and/or thin connective tissue surrounding the involved trigeminal or cervical nerve branch at the identified trigger site[s]). Doppler ultrasound at trigger sites is performed to help identify arterial branches that may be irritating a nerve, where arterectomy (or plaque removal, also called atherectomy) should be performed. Analysis of computed tomographic images is useful in identifying supraorbital foramen or notches, where osteotomies (bone removal) and fasciotomies, respectively, can be performed to release the nerve. After decompression, fat grafts are placed beneath or around the freed-up nerve at frontal and occipital trigger sites to pad the nerve from cicatricle changes and manage dead space after a myectomy. Neurectomy of a nerve branch is occasionally performed as a last resort during revision surgery in patients with persistent migraine headache symptoms after initial decompression; some improvement is obtained at the expense of temporary or permanent numbness in the dermatome for that nerve branch. Fat injection may be used as an adjunct either at the time of initial surgical decompression or at a later treatment date for patients with recalcitrant migraine headache symptoms following surgical decompression.

Traditionally, 73% of migraine headache patients treated with surgical decompression need multiple trigger sites (average of 2.6 sites) decompressed at the time of surgery. (Guyuron 2019) With fat injection, most patients (76%) need only one site to be injected (with a mean of 1.28 sites injected per patient). (Forootan 2017) Generally, these procedures are well tolerated with minimal morbidity. Incisions are small and placed in well-hidden areas to minimize the scar burden, seromas or hematomas are rare, and numbness following surgery is almost always temporary unless neurectomy is performed. The most common complaint is worsening of migraine headache symptoms in the acute postoperative inflammatory period, which generally improves after a few weeks.

Occasionally, successful migraine surgery may "unmask" secondary site(s) that patients describe as new sources of their migraine headaches. In these cases, patients should maintain a new headache journal and be evaluated for surgery at these secondary trigger sites. The success rate of migraine surgical decompression ranges from 79% to 90%. (Forootan 2015, Guyuron 2011, Kurlander 2016, Kurlander 2016, Ascha 2017) Factors associated with surgical failure are younger age of migraine onset, intraoperative complications, and two or fewer surgical sites. Factors associated with surgical success are surgery at a frontal or zygomaticotemporal (sensory nerve) site or at multiple trigger sites. Secondary fat injection has been shown to significantly improve or completely abate symptoms in 69% of patients with migraine headaches persisting after surgical decompression. (Guyuron 2019) These procedures likely improve symptoms because of the fact that trigeminal nerve branches in migraine patients are abnormal and surgical decompression or fat grafting reduces nerve irritation that may otherwise trigger a migraine headache. Successful migraine headache surgery requires working closely with neurologists or migraine headache specialists for appropriate patient diagnosis and medical management. The importance of careful patient selection and thorough analysis of long-term symptoms to determine an appropriate surgical candidate and operative plan cannot be understated.

Chapter 4
The Psychology of Pain

Anne B. Ciemnecki, MA

JoAnn Deak, PhD, authored a children's book in 2010 called *Your Fantastic Elastic Brain*. Check it out. There are multiple online videos of people reading it aloud. Deak tells readers that we are neurosculptors. We can shape our brains. We can stretch them by trying new things that build on things we already know. Just like lifting weights can build our bodies, exercising our brains can build them too.

Neurosurgeon Julie Pilitsis (Section 4.1) reminds us that chronic pain is a tridimensional experience that involves sensation, cognition, and emotion. *Neurosurgeons* address the sensation. As *neurosculptors*, we need to address the cognitive and emotional components. Lovette and Greenberg reinforce this idea in Section 4.3. They present a biopsychosocial model of living with chronic pain. Their suggestions describe ways that we can grow our brains to alleviate pain. None of these suggestions involve procedures or medication, just our brains growing and working for us.

Imagine Beth Darnall's Empowered Relief® (Section 4.6), a one-session, 2-hour class (not therapy) that teaches three core pain management skills rooted in mindfulness and cognitive behavioral therapy (CBT). Data from four published randomized controlled studies show that pain and symptom relief is effective 3 and 6 months after the class and that the 2-hour class is comparable to 16 hours of CBT.

Even more exciting is virtual reality (VR), which is revolutionizing the future of pain relief. VR is an immersive experience that transports people to new environments. VR diverts your brain's attention and emotions away from pain signals. In Section 4.7, the Collocas explain that the diversion creates a positive impact on various cognitive factors, ultimately influencing the way pain messages are transmitted through memory, emotions, and different sensory channels such as touch, sound, and sight. It sounds like magic to me.

If you want to try a more traditional pain management treatment, Section 4.4 discusses mindfulness meditation and presents three mindful exercises that people with chronic pain can do anywhere without the cost of trainers or equipment.

In Section 4.2, Leesa Scott-Morrow discusses four core temperament traits that she describes as the engine that drives our motivations. Everyone has some amount of these four traits. Working with a psychotherapist to determine how much of each trait you have can help you understand your reactions to chronic pain. She continues to explain that psychotherapy is not one-sided. Clients need to do some work to build a productive relationship with their therapist if they want to grow their minds.

Perhaps the easiest and most enjoyable way to alleviate pain is to join a support group (Section 4.5). Support group members share common experiences and concerns and provide each other with advice, comfort, and encouragement.

There are so many ways to sculpt your brain and alleviate your pain. Happy reading.

4.1
The Phil Mickelson Effect: A Holistic Approach to Chronic Pain Management
Julie G. Pilitsis, MD, PhD

"The only thing you can really control is how you react to things out of your control."

Better advice has probably never been given to any of us. It is relevant to the numerous roles I play in my life and something that I consider multiple times a day. As a surgeon, I often face an unexpected set of circumstances in the operating room such as a new team or a different piece of equipment. As a mother of former toddlers and now tween/teens, plans often do not go the way I had envisioned. As a patient, I often do not know how a new medication dispensed by my local pharmacy will affect my body.

Chronic pain affects people in many different ways, and there are many variables that may limit control over the condition. Physicians focus on the sensory experience and its treatment. They ask patients to evaluate their pain using the Numerical Rating Scale (NRS). "On a scale of 0 to 10, with 0 meaning 'no pain' and 10 meaning 'the worst pain imaginable,' what is your pain level?" Physicians use the reported pain level to assess response to treatment. Thus, the focus on sensation continues. Physicians and patients are less apt to consider other markers of success. More relevant questions perhaps are the following:

- Could you stand a minute longer than you did the day before?
- Were you able to do the dishes?
- Were you able to ride in a car?
- Were you able to sleep better?
- Did your mood improve?
- Were you able to enjoy time with family?

Why do we still use the NRS? Historically, its use goes back to the well-meaning idea of considering pain as the fifth vital sign, which, unfortunately, had the unintended consequence of contributing to the opioid epidemic. The NRS resonated with physicians by treating abnormal vital signs as something with which they were familiar. If blood pressure is high, providers give medications to reduce the value. The same is true for treating NRS values, and thus the focus on sensation continues. Although this approach may work for acute pain (e.g., a broken arm), for patients who have chronic pain, defined as more than three months of pain in the same area, it does not. Chronic pain goes beyond sensory changes alone as the brain's plasticity is altered.

In fact, chronic pain is a tridimensional experience that involves sensation, cognition, and emotion. However, there is a lack of guidance and adherence by both providers and physicians to treating components of pain that are not related to sensation. Why is this? For physicians not specializing in mental health, we often focus on fixing values like those reported using the NRS. We may advise our patients to limit their stress, but without concrete guidance on how to do that or integration of stress-reducing options into the formal treatment plan, patients rarely succeed on their own. Compounding the issue, patients with chronic pain have often been passed from physician to physician, and because of a lack of objective signs and/or a lack of response to treatments, they may have been told that the pain is just in their heads. This statement marginalizes what patients are experiencing. Further, it makes patients less accepting of any cognitive or emotional components of their pain and of future treatment strategies designed to treat those aspects of their disease. Indeed, chronic pain is a disease and something that people will have to learn to manage. That is not to say that people must suffer, and in fact, they should not. However, expecting to be pain-free for a lifetime is likewise an unreasonable expectation.

We need to consider how living in pain may affect our thoughts, our behaviors, and our moods. While we wait for our provider to aid in diagnosis and treatment, it is important to keep ourselves in the best physical and mental space possible to modulate our reactions and empower ourselves to keep moving forward. Much as we have to make good lifestyle choices when living with diabetes, we have to do the same with chronic pain. We may have to change certain behaviors. We may have to add meditation and yoga, a healthy diet that reduces inflammation, and good sleep hygiene to our lives. Changing our cognitive and emotional response to chronic pain is essential to our well-being. When working through the process of limiting pain, controlling our reactions is empowering.

In 2021, as I watched Phil Mickelson, a soon-to-be 51-year-old, win the PGA championship, I was struck by the fact that this man who suffers from psoriatic arthritis was able to achieve these goals. It was obvious that he was thinner and had worked on his swing. What was less obvious was what he had shared with interviewers: the role of meditation and yoga in his life over the previous few years. He truly had optimized his mind–body connection to accomplish the previously impossible. If we all did that, just think what we could do!

4.2
Harm Avoidance: The Role of One Inherited Temperament Trait in Chronic Facial Pain
Leesa Scott-Murrow, PhD, JD, LP

Editor's Note: The age-old "nature vs nurture" debate in psychology compares the relative importance of an individual's inherited qualities ("nature") versus their personal experiences ("nurture"). Although behavioral genetics enables researchers to quantify the relative contribution of nature to specific psychological traits, many are investigating how nature and nurture interact in complex, qualitative ways. In this section, Dr. Scott-Morrow focuses on a single temperament trait, harm avoidance. Although she recognizes the complex interaction of nature and nurture in harm avoidance, she clearly sits on the nature side of the fence. As you read this section, think about where you may fall along this continuum.

Every animal has a set of behaviors they use to defend themselves against danger. Perceived threats to survival require an urgent, immediate response, and it is for this reason that the brain mechanisms underlying the response to perceived threat have evolved to operate instinctually, in a wordless part of the brain. For all animals, humans included, defensive behaviors occur instantly in response to perceived threat; freezing in place, fleeing, or fighting, all occur automatically in response to danger. Securing survival is time-urgent; there is no time to think about taking defensive action.

For humans, the brain initiates a cascade of physiological changes that equip us to successfully respond to threats. Muscle tone increases to facilitate fleeing or fighting. Heart rate and blood pressure increase to ensure abundant blood supply to vital organs. Pupils dilate as the brain activates. These primal changes and many other associated changes initiate below awareness, outside the realm of choice. Most importantly, these physiological changes are involved in every kind of fearful response to some degree, even in those fearful experiences that do not involve threat to life or limb. Sudden painful experiences inevitably trigger the physiological threat response, even in instances when the pain is not life-threatening and even when the individual knows that the pain is not life-threatening. The cascade of physiological changes occurring in response to threats occurs even in response to threats that are purely emotional or imagined. The body cannot tell the difference between being exposed to a near-miss car accident and being suddenly surprised in a haunted house tour. For individuals with anxiety, the body can respond to a public speaking experience as if it were life-threatening.

For biologically complex animals, those with thinking brains, a lot of learning occurs in response to threatening experiences. We have the mental capacity to identify potential threats on the basis of tiny little signals in the environment and to adjust our behaviors accordingly. This blend of perception, cognitive interpretation, and behavioral response constitutes a kind of learning that is only partially conscious, however.

It is important to understand that, even though this kind of learning arises in response to the environment, it is ultimately biological. Newly learned information has to be stored in the brain in the form of a memory; this is a biological process. These memories have to wire themselves to other brain-based nuggets of knowledge in order to be useful; again, this a biological process. And the act of attaching meaning to these memory complexes is also ultimately biological. Learning at this last level is dynamic. What we know, and believe, can change, and when it does, our associated perceptions of threat also change. When our perceptions of threats change, our physical responses change. Change is possible, but because these stress-related processes occur instantly, largely below the threshold of awareness, change is difficult to achieve. Changing these responses requires becoming more self-aware in order to defeat, or override, the automaticity of the response.

Remember, the capacity to form fear–perception–action complexes evolved to protect animals (including humans) from the dangers of life-threatening injury. Because physical survival typically depends upon taking immediate action, the part of the neuroendocrine system that creates the stress response evolved to work very rapidly, too rapidly to include word-based cognition and analysis. The process of thinking about something that is happening and forming a problem-solving dialogue in our heads takes far too long to be effective under threatening circumstances; thus, the brain skips the problem-solving part to prioritize speed over everything else. Because nature has prioritized speed over all else, fear-based learning is error-prone. For example, if you have facial pain, the neuroendocrine system may fire a defensive reaction when you step outside on a windy day, without having actually felt any wind, or pain, simply because you have felt pain under windy conditions in the past. Indeed, the system may fire at the mere thought of going outside on a windy day, without your actually having stepped outside. As you can see, from a psychophysiological perspective, in the context of chronic pain, things can get complicated as unconscious learning compounds over time. Indeed, the more time an individual has struggled with pain, the more automatic defensive behaviors they will have learned, and the greater the likelihood this learning will involve error. This error will express itself in a set of beliefs, which, of course, the individual will resist changing unless they understand the necessity of doing so. Psychotherapists should approach this relearning process with compassion. Because fear-based behaviors and anxieties form automatically, they are difficult to identify. From the perspective of the person fearing pain, their beliefs feel correct and reasonable. Challenging the erroneous thinking that underlies pain-defensive behavior requires empathy, and it is crucial for the therapist to allow time for the patient to observe patterns in this behavior so that these patterns can be discussed in session. When it comes to automatic behaviors like fear responses, the methodology of change is technical and not particularly intuitive. If feeling anxious is a common part of your experience, it is a good idea to get professional help. Indeed, reading this section is a form of professional help, so let's keep going.

Let's dig a little deeper. As you can see, perception of threats and responses to perceived threats become extremely complicated because of our big brains. Because we have the ability to imagine things, we can worry about potential threats that will never happen. We call these apprehensive cognitions anxiety. It will not surprise you to learn that the tendency to feel anxious is biologically driven and that it powerfully affects personality structure. Some people see threats just about everywhere, whereas others easily shake off their worries. These two types of people will respond to facial pain in quite different ways. To illustrate these differences, consider fear of flying, a less provocative but more common situation. Imagine two people sitting next to one another on a plane that is flying through a turbulent storm. Because they are sitting side by side, their physical experience of turbulence is essentially identical. Yet, one person walks off the plane with little if any apprehension about their next flight, whereas the other person swears they will never get on another plane. These two people had the same objective experience during the turbulent flight, but their subjective experiences were quite different. They attached vastly different meanings to their experience based on the way they evaluate threats. Indeed, for human beings, the subjective experience of threat is an enormously powerful individualized force that shapes our beliefs and behavior.

Personality Structure. People are different from one another, but these differences are not random. The individual who will never fly again will likely respond fearfully to other scenarios they perceive to be dangerous, whereas their easy-going seatmate will not be as inclined to interpret situations fearfully. The difference between these two people is grounded in identity, or as we say in psychology, in personality structure. Their tendency to perceive a threat and evaluate it as potentially catastrophic, or not, is inherent in who they are. When I say inherent, I mean that this tendency is literally inherited.

For many decades, psychologists studying personality structure restricted their efforts to learning why certain people behave in ways that cause them interpersonal difficulty in most all settings. These psychologists were trying to better understand personality disorders. Yet, as a matter of logic, the existence of abnormal personalities in humans suggests there must be some human quality that constitutes a normal personality. Consequently, modern researchers have begun looking for the foundational aspects of personality, ones that define both normal and abnormal personality configurations. Their research tells us that personality has a structure, one that consists of identifiable traits, or factors, that are, for the most part, biologically determined. This research hinges on the assumption that these core traits are common to all humans and that, like other human qualities, these traits are coded in our genes. Eye color, a trait we all recognize as genetic, involves just a few genes. Certain dispositional behavioral traits are also genetic, but they are extraordinarily complex, involving the interaction of many genes. That makes the study of these traits difficult, but still possible.

Psychologists use true/false or multiple-choice tests that have been statistically designed to identify the traits that underlie personality. These tests query the individual about their self-perceptions, their beliefs about others, and their perceptions of the world at large. The most widely used of these tests have been translated into many languages, with data collected from people from many different cultures. After all, if something is truly biological at its foundation, it should be recognizable in all people, regardless of the individual's cultural or racial origins. Indeed, this research has identified a core set of personality traits that appear to be genetically based and universally human. Some research has identified four traits; other research has identified five.

C. Robert Cloninger, a Professor Emeritus in the Department of Psychiatry at Washington University in St. Louis, MO, is a leading researcher exploring heritable personality traits. I find his work fascinating, but more importantly, I find his research helpful in understanding my patients' experience of pain. I think a basic understanding of his research will be helpful to you, too, so let's take a look.

The Temperament and Character Inventory. Cloninger has identified four core personality traits, which he refers to as temperament traits, that appear to be genetic in nature. These traits are harm avoidance, reward dependence, novelty seeking, and persistence. (Cloninger 1993) The four temperament traits are best understood as the engine that drives our motivations. Harm avoidance is the degree to which we are motivated to avoid harm, just as it sounds. Reward dependence is the degree to which we are motivated by social rewards. These rewards can be as simple as a thank you or a hug, or as complex as the desire and effort to win an election or promotion. What all these things have in common is the need for positive interpersonal and social feedback to stay interested in something or someone. Novelty seeking is the degree to which we are motivated for new experiences. People who are high in novelty seeking tend to bore easily, and they are likely to be more impulsive than others who are lower in this trait. Persistence is the degree to which we are motivated to persevere toward a goal or task completion, despite frustration and fatigue.

Each of us has some amount of these four traits. People can be low, medium, or high on each trait, and their levels on each trait do not tend to change over the lifespan. Also, their level on one trait has nothing to do with their level on any of the other traits. For example, an individual might be high on harm avoidance and also high on reward dependence. Recalling the frightened person on the turbulent flight, maybe this person fears flying (high harm avoidance) but really wants to connect with family and friends over the holidays (high reward dependence). This person might board the plane in a near state of panic just to get home and see the family. The point is, even though these traits are independent of one another, they do interact to create the complex behaviors we identify as human.

Let's look at the interaction between harm avoidance and pain. From an emotional perspective, persons who are high in harm avoidance especially struggle when confronted with chronic pain. Research indicates that these individuals are more susceptible to depression and anxiety within the context of chronic pain than individuals who are low in harm avoidance. Most importantly, high harm-avoidant individuals are predisposed to fear-avoidant behavior and pain hypervigilance, which can cause a life-shrinking effect. Among my patients, there is a subgroup who pulled away from social activity with their families after the diagnosis of facial pain. These patients tend to be highly harm-avoidant individuals. Often, these patients tell me about experiences when they declined opportunities to go out for dinner with loved ones and friends, or they might have declined the opportunity to attend their child's dance recital, or they might have declined to attend an office party. The point is that they are pulling back from opportunities to interact with others all for fear they will suffer a facial pain attack during the interaction. They typically explain their social withdrawal in what seems to them to be rational terms. They might say that loud noises and busy environments cause them to experience pain. They might say that a young niece or nephew will want to be held, but they fear that, if they hold the child, the child might touch their face and cause a pain attack. It is not hard to imagine how harm-avoidant fears could cause devastating emotional losses in a marriage. Because of their high harm-avoidant nature, these individuals tend to imagine only negative outcomes. This is a behavior psychologists call catastrophizing.

Psychologists have developed successful ways of treating catastrophizing. Breaking the behavioral pattern that underlies catastrophic thinking can be done but doing so will probably require help. It is difficult to change this behavior without help, because, if you are highly avoidant, you understandably believe that you are doing the right thing by avoiding threats in as many ways, and in as many settings, as you can. But fear-avoidant behavior comes at a price. Constant fearful hypervigilance to pain is miserably distressing. It makes happiness impossible. Fearful social withdrawal inevitably negatively impacts relationships with family, friends, and colleagues, weakening these relationships and causing them to deteriorate.

It is crucial for the highly harm-avoidant person to recognize two things: (1) Their fears are a natural result of their temperament. It is certainly not the case that they are choosing to be fearful. Fear is an automatic response to pain for all people, but for the high-harm-avoidant individual, pain hypervigilance persists beyond the episodic experience of pain. These individuals become generally hypervigilant. (2) From the perspective of the highly harm-avoidant individual, hypervigilance is the only rational response to pain. This assumption involves cognitive error, but it does not feel like that to the highly harm-avoidant individual. A portion of the highly harm-avoidant individual's fear is directed toward low-probability events that are unlikely to occur, but it is difficult for the highly harm-avoidant individual to distinguish low-probability threats from high-probability events. All potential threats are regarded as highly, and equally, likely to occur. To harken back to an earlier example, most planes do not crash. But to the highly harm-avoidant individual, it feels like the plane they are in will be one of the few that does; this involves probabilistic error, but it certainly does not feel that way to the highly harm-avoidant individual. Consequently, they are overcome with fearful apprehension at the thought of flying, and they go to great pains to avoid doing so.

In the context of chronic pain, fear of low-probability pain-related outcomes inevitably develops in highly harm-avoidant individuals. Among my patients, I find that common fears include fear that all treatment will ultimately fail; fear that loved ones will abandon them because they are, at times, unable to participate in social activities; fear that, if they do participate in social activities, others will not take their pain seriously; fear that, if they do participate in social activities and choose to leave because of pain, it will anger those who are important to them; and fear that their relationships will fall apart, leaving them alone to confront overwhelming pain. In short, the list of catastrophic fears is extraordinarily long and highly personalized. Without learning to discern high-probability threats from low-probability threats, fear of pain will come to dominate one's experience. Indeed, over time, for highly harm-avoidant individuals, fears compound, and resulting anxiety becomes the dominant feature of their emotional experience. As this happens, these individuals avoid more and more activities, which causes their lives to progressively shrink to the confines of their homes, with little social interaction. Indeed, the interpersonal and experiential losses that come with persistent fear of pain and associated anxiety can be extreme.

In my experience, patients who struggle with high harm avoidance are relieved to have the support and guidance of a therapist once they make the decision to engage therapy. The therapist may be one of the few people who really understands what it is like for them to live with chronic pain. Certainly, the therapist knows how to technically address catastrophic thinking and help the patient unload unproductive worries. It should be said that the process of psychotherapy is not a one-sided effort. Successful treatment requires initiative on the part of both the therapist and the patient. Ideally, there should be a sense of compassion and understanding that is strong enough to support difficult work. This requires building a relationship, which will take time up front. Until that relationship solidifies, you should expect to be evaluating your therapist while feeling some degree of doubt about whether the relationship is what you want. That is normal. With time, however, if a good working relationship develops, doubt about your therapist will ease and largely disappear. I personally find my work with patients to be the most gratifying part of my life. These relationships matter to me, and I admire the effort my patients exert to feel better. I think of my patients as courageous people. I know how hard it is to leave behind hypervigilance to injury and pain. In the beginning, it is normal to feel extremely vulnerable, and it is during those moments that feeling trust for your therapist matters most. You should expect to have a warm and committed relationship with your therapist; anything less will not produce maximally successful results. But understand: you are part of building that relationship.

4.3
The Reality We Live With

Brenda C. Lovette, MS, and Jonathan Greenberg, PhD

Editor's Note: Portions of this article are reprinted from the following article: Lovette BC, Bannon SM, Spyropoulos DC, Vranceanu AM, Greenberg J. "I Still Suffer Every Second of Every Day": A Qualitative Analysis of the Challenges of Living with Chronic Orofacial Pain. Journal of Pain Research 2022;15:2139–2148. https://doi.org/10.2147/JPR.S372469. Originally published by and used with permission from Dove Medical Press Ltd.

Author's Note: We thank the Facial Pain Association for its contribution to data collection in this study.

Treatment of chronic orofacial pain is typically biomedical (e.g., focusing primarily on physiological factors). However, growing evidence suggests a connection between psychological factors such as stress, social considerations, and chronic orofacial pain symptoms and outcomes. The biopsychosocial model provides a useful framework for a more integrative assessment of the experiences, concerns, and priorities of people with orofacial pain. As implied by its name, the biopsychosocial model takes into consideration not just the biomedical aspects of living with a condition, (i.e., challenges relating to physical function and physiological aspects of injury), but also the psychological aspects (i.e., challenges relating to cognition, coping, emotion, and mental health or well-being) and social aspects (i.e., challenges relating to interpersonal, socioeconomic, community, and life participation factors). Identifying specific biomedical, psychological, and social challenges for individuals with orofacial pain is critical for improving care and working toward meeting their needs.

Listening to individuals with chronic orofacial pain as they share their lived experiences is the best way to learn about the challenges they face. Qualitative research methods (i.e., collecting and analyzing participants' experiences in their own words) can help shed light on people's own perspectives of living with chronic orofacial pain. For our study, we recruited 260 participants with chronic orofacial pain (e.g., trigeminal neuralgia, trigeminal neuropathic pain, persistent idiopathic

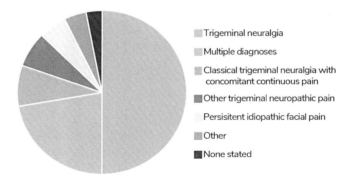

Trigeminal neuralgia

Multiple diagnoses

Classical trigeminal neuralgia with concomitant continuous pain

Other trigeminal neuropathic pain

Persisitent idiopathic facial pain

Other

None stated

Figure 4-1.   Distribution of orofacial pain diagnoses represented in the study.

facial pain, multiple co-occurring pain diagnoses, and others). See Figure 4-1 for a graphical representation of the distribution of diagnoses represented in the study. Participants were members of the Facial Pain Association (FPA). They responded to the question "What is the biggest challenge you face in managing your condition?" by typing their answer into a text box as part of an online survey. We compiled these responses and mapped them onto biomedical, psychological, and social themes. Figure 4-2 depicts the distinct and overlapping subthemes of participants' reported challenges across the biopsychosocial model.

Participants identified several biomedical challenges, including pain management, medication side effects, biological functions and related activities of daily living (e.g., sleep, eating, exercise), sensory triggers, and physical symptoms of stress and tension. Our findings illustrate how these biomedical elements impacted participants' overall health, wellness, and quality of life. We identified several recommendations to address these issues. For example, providers could discuss common medication side effects to empower individuals to make conscious choices about the cost–benefit balance of their medications. To address challenges with activities of daily living, providers should assess and treat sleep, communication, nutrition, and other aspects of self-care to boost people's health and function despite their pain. People with chronic orofacial pain may benefit from referrals including occupational therapy for modifications to activities of daily living, speech language pathology for treatment of communication and swallowing function, dietetics to address nutrition, counseling to

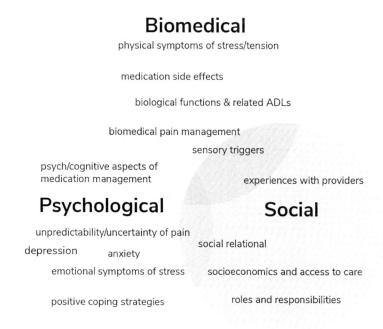

Biomedical
physical symptoms of stress/tension

medication side effects

biological functions & related ADLs

biomedical pain management

sensory triggers

psych/cognitive aspects of
medication management

experiences with providers

Psychological   Social

unpredictability/uncertainty of pain

social relational

depression   anxiety

emotional symptoms of stress   socioeconomics and access to care

positive coping strategies   roles and responsibilities

Figure 4-2.   Biopsychosocial model: Map of subthemes identified by participants in this study.

develop strategies to help manage sensory triggers, and pain–informed mind–body interventions to develop skills around stress and pain management.

Psychological challenges described by our participants included anxiety, depression, emotional symptoms of stress, unpredictability of pain, psychological and cognitive aspects of medication management, and positive coping strategies (e.g., resilience, mindfulness). Participants' psychological and emotional challenges were further reflected by the fact that 67% of them exhibited clinically meaningful symptoms of depression and 56% exhibited clinically meaningful symptoms of anxiety based on validated measures. Participants described the interplay of depression, anxiety, and general mental suffering with the severity of their pain condition. They additionally mentioned the unpredictability of their pain as a source of anxiety that impacted their ability or willingness to participate in social activities and work. Our results show the need for accessible and effective psychological programs to target these challenges. Such programs may include Cognitive Behavioral Therapy (CBT), mindfulness-based and relaxation interventions, and biofeedback.

Social challenges described by participants included changes to relationships, roles, and responsibilities; experiences with providers; and socioeconomics and access to care. Some described withdrawing from their communities and limiting their engagement in meaningful activities, which increased their sense of isolation and hopelessness. To address these social challenges, people with orofacial pain may benefit from treatment that involves spouses and family members. Clinicians may additionally provide individuals with chronic orofacial pain with resources such as orofacial pain support groups, online forums, and advocacy organizations (e.g., the FPA).

Participants described difficult experiences with medical providers and navigating care (e.g., distress around not being "believed" by their providers, difficulty obtaining a definitive diagnosis, and a sense that their providers were not knowledgeable enough). These findings suggest a need for more training and resources for providers who manage these cases and increased awareness of the prevalence of orofacial pain that does not have a known cause. Some participants described difficulty accessing care due to the cost of treatment and insurance coverage issues. This challenge may be particularly prominent for those who are uninsured, experiencing financial insecurity, or have fewer financial resources. To help with this issue, individuals with orofacial pain could benefit from the help of social workers to assist in navigating financial and social resources and work accommodations. Our findings also suggest a need for changes in policies such as reduced cost for effective pharmaceuticals and expansion of coverage to evidence-based complimentary therapies.

One unique aspect of this project was the inclusion of individuals with a variety of orofacial pain diagnoses. Although most previous research on orofacial pain "siloed" participants based on their different diagnoses, the current findings show more similarities than differences in challenges experienced among individuals with different diagnoses in our sample. These findings illustrate the wide range of challenges that individuals with chronic orofacial pain confront across the biopsychosocial continuum and suggest critical areas for consideration to improve future care.

4.4
Facing It: Mindfulness for Chronic Orofacial Pain – Mindfulness and Mindfulness-Based Interventions

Saige Fong, MS; Molly Becker, MS; and Jonathan Greenberg, PhD

The concept of mindfulness originates from early Eastern traditions and Buddhist philosophy. In its contemporary Westernized form, mindfulness is most commonly defined as "the awareness that emerges through paying attention on purpose, in the present moment, and nonjudgmentally." (Kabat-Zinn 1994) It is often described as having two main components: (1) regulating attention to whatever is happening in the present (e.g., whatever thoughts, feelings, and bodily sensations one is currently experiencing), coupled with (2) an intention of being open to and accepting of whatever arises. Thus, a person may be said to be mindful if they are attentive and aware of their current experience and try to be nonjudgmental and accepting toward it (e.g., noticing any resistance to one's experience and simply allowing it to be as it is). Mindfulness may be portrayed as a trait, a theoretical construct, and a psychological process, although it is most often described in the context of a meditative practice.

In the late 20th century, Jon Kabat-Zinn pioneered the incorporation of mindfulness practices into Western medicine through a secular intervention aimed at managing chronic pain and health-related stress (mindfulness-based stress reduction, MBSR). Since then, there has been an exponential growth in therapeutic interventions involving mindfulness. In the 1990s, Segal and colleagues combined mindfulness practice with traditional Cognitive Behavioral Therapy (CBT) in a treatment program intended to prevent depression relapse (mindfulness-based cognitive therapy, MBCT).

Other interventions such as acceptance and commitment therapy (ACT) and dialectical behavioral therapy (DBT) include mindfulness as a component in the treatment of various mental and physical health conditions. The utilization of mindfulness practices is continuously expanding in the treatment of a wide array of populations, as well as in nonclinical settings such as schools and businesses.

Mindfulness for Chronic Orofacial Pain. Pain is inherently unpleasant and aversive. It is natural for us to try to resist pain and have negative behavioral, cognitive, and emotional reactions to it. Although these reactions can help us avoid or minimize harm in acute pain (e.g., feeling startled and quickly moving our hand if we accidentally touch a hot stove), they are far less helpful in chronic pain, including chronic orofacial pain, when pain most often no longer signals that harm is currently being done to our body. Mindfulness encourages individuals to adopt a curious and nonjudgmental approach to the presence of pain and discomfort, which may decrease our behavioral, cognitive, and emotional reactions to it. A growing body of research suggests that mindfulness-based interventions constitute safe and effective approaches to chronic pain management. Reviews and meta-analyses of mindfulness-based interventions for chronic pain report that mindfulness decreases pain intensity, depression, and pain bothersomeness; improves quality of life; and reduces the interference of pain in activities of daily living.

Although research on mindfulness specifically for orofacial pain remains sparse, emerging evidence suggests that it is a promising means to aid individuals with chronic orofacial pain. A recent study suggested that specific facets of mindfulness, particularly adopting a nonjudgmental attitude, were associated with favorable pain and mental health outcomes such as decreased pain-related disability, depression, and anxiety among members of the FPA. (Greenberg 2022)

How May Mindfulness Help Individuals with Chronic Orofacial Pain? There are several ways in which mindfulness may potentially aid chronic orofacial pain. Some of these are as follows:

Reducing Anxiety and Depression. Living with chronic orofacial pain is stressful and may take a significant emotional toll. A recent survey of more than 300 members of the FPA living with chronic orofacial pain indicated that almost 75% of participants experienced clinically significant symptoms of depression or anxiety, and more than one-third reported taking antidepressants. (Greenberg 2022) Mindfulness-based interventions have been demonstrated to alleviate symptoms of anxiety and improve quality of life. (Ghahara 2020) Research further demonstrated that mindfulness-based interventions can reduce the length of major depressive episodes, heighten positive affect, and buffer against depressive relapse. These benefits have been partially attributed to increased awareness of calm, experience, and acceptance of their symptoms. (Burgess 2021) Mindfulness can also help reduce suicidal ideation and behavior, which are relatively prevalent among individuals with chronic orofacial pain. (Dibello 2022, Bertolo 2016)

Emotion Regulation. Emotion regulation refers to one's capacity to effectively manage and respond to an emotional experience. By observing emotions from a "detached" perspective (e.g., noticing phenomena arising and passing rather than identifying with them), individuals can avoid becoming overwhelmed by negative emotions surrounding their pain. Mindfulness practice also has the potential to open new avenues of thinking, including about pain, that can improve emotion regulation. Having an intense emotional reaction in response to pain, feeling victimized by the pain, and feeling overly critical of oneself or others are emotion-laden responses to pain that can become habitual and automatic. Research suggests that mindfulness may help change habitual patterns and increase the degree to which individuals can identify and implement novel, more helpful ways of responding than those they are used to. (Greenberg 2012) As mindfulness is characterized by curiously paying attention to things "as they are" (as opposed to our preconceptualized notions about them), it may increase one's capacity to respond in nonhabitual manners. Rather than ruminating on pain-related fears and engaging in harmful behaviors, new ways of responding to pain may become more accessible, thus improving emotion regulatory skills. This conclusion is in line with evidence suggesting that mindfulness can increase one's distress tolerance and capacity to be present with discomfort, further supporting one's capacity to effectively regulate their emotions. (Nila 2016)

Reducing Social Isolation. Chronic orofacial pain may have significant social implications, leading to social isolation and impaired quality of life. Many individuals with chronic orofacial pain face unique challenges with talking, eating, and making facial expressions, which are important for communicating effectively and creating social bonds. These challenges are particularly prominent for individuals with orofacial pain conditions such as type 1 trigeminal neuralgia (TN), who experience severe, spontaneous, and shock-like episodes of facial pain that last for varying intervals. The added uncertainty of spontaneous pain episodes causes many of these individuals to avoid social activities altogether, thus exacerbating their sense of isolation. Mindfulness has been shown to decrease feelings of isolation and bolster perceived connectedness with others. Mindfulness-Based Stress Reduction (MBSR) has been identified as an effective tool for managing loneliness, and participation in group-based mindfulness practices may also facilitate feelings of social connectedness. (Dreisoerner 2021) The impact of mindfulness on social isolation, particularly in the contexts of chronic orofacial pain and TN, warrants additional research.

Adaptive Coping. The "nonjudgmental" stance in response to pain promoted by mindfulness and its associated reduced reactivity can aid individuals in coping more adaptively with orofacial pain. A common nonadaptive response to pain, including orofacial pain, is pain catastrophizing—constantly thinking about how bad the pain is and its potential negative effects. Individuals with orofacial pain who tend to catastrophize their pain are more likely to experience higher rates of pain intensity and pain-related disability. Several studies have indicated that mindfulness is associated with decreased pain catastrophizing. (Rezaie 2019, Okvat 2022, Turner 2016) By observing and accepting such catastrophizing thoughts as passing events, one may stop "feeding the flame" of these thoughts and thereby reduce negative reactivity.

Mindfulness has further been shown to promote the use of other adaptive strategies of coping with pain and adversity. (Frostadottir 2019, Long 2021)

Many individuals with chronic orofacial pain tend to be harsh or critical toward themselves. Mindfulness has been shown to increase self-compassion, stave off self-blame, and foster treating oneself with kindness. Mindfulness has also been shown to increase qualities associated with adaptive coping such as expressing gratitude, exhibiting pain acceptance, displaying increased self-efficacy in managing pain, and leading a healthier and more active lifestyle.

Pain Awareness. Practicing mindfulness may benefit pain tolerance and awareness. Given that mindfulness commonly involves paying attention to one's body, individuals may begin to identify triggers for and patterns in their pain. Many people with chronic orofacial pain find that they tend to subconsciously clench their jaw or grind their teeth, particularly in stressful contexts. Increased attention toward these triggers can guide individuals to reduce unhelpful behaviors and thus reduce pain. Pain awareness also allows for curious, nonjudgmental observation of pain without resistance, including awareness of how pain naturally waxes and wanes over time, leading to a more accurate perception of pain (e.g., perceiving it as changing and dynamic rather than constantly severe). Some individuals with orofacial pain may experience pain hypervigilance, or overfixation on their current or next painful experience, as a result of constantly living on the precipice of another painful episode. Living in a state of constant worry may also prime them to magnify their pain experience, identifying unassociated bodily sensations as signs of an impending "attack." Indeed, a recent qualitative analysis of the experience of people with chronic orofacial pain found that the unpredictability/uncertainty of pain was a major stressor. (Lovette 2022) Mindfulness may ease this negative cognitive tendency and improve attention regulation, a mechanism that is vital for people with chronic orofacial pain given that pain and anxiety may distract from present experiences. Individuals may gently redirect their attention to neutral stimuli such as the sensations of their breath or sounds in their environment, and thus reduce hypervigilance toward uncomfortable sensations.

How Does One Practice Mindfulness? Listed here are several exercises that can be implemented anywhere. Note that, during each of these exercises, you will likely find that your attention wanders quickly to other topics and thoughts. This is natural, expected, and not a sign that you are doing anything wrong. Each time you notice that your mind has wandered, gently bring it back to the exercise.

With each return of your attention, you are training your mind to be more present.

- *Mindful breathing* is an exercise that encourages curiosity about breath as it is without trying to change it. First, get into a comfortable position for your practice, and then either close your eyes or lower your gaze, depending on your comfort levels. Begin to notice where you can feel your breath in your body, maybe in your chest, belly, or nostrils. Notice the sensation of your breaths in and your breaths out. Take a deep breath and exhale, placing your hand on your belly to feel the changes through expansion and deflation. Feel the warmth of an exhale and the cool air of an inhale in your nose. If your focus begins to drift, gently return to the sensation of your breath. Observe the quality of your breath with curiosity—whether it is jagged or smooth, rushed or slow, shallow or deep. Whatever you experience may simply exist without your trying to change it. Allow yourself to experience the sensations of breathing right here and right now.

- *Mindful body scans* allow for an increased, curious awareness toward bodily sensations that may have been previously avoided or feared, such as pain. Start by finding a comfortable position and then closing your eyes or lowering your gaze. Begin to direct your attention to your breath. What sensations do you notice? Perhaps the rise and fall of your chest or the coolness of your breath coming out of your nostrils. After several moments of attending to the sensations of breathing, focus on the soles of your feet. Notice any temperature, pressure, tingling, or lack of sensation here. Raise your attention up to your legs and any sensations that may live there. Should your mind naturally begin to wander, notice this without judgment and gently bring your attention back to the task at hand. Continue to allow your awareness to drift upward on your body, landing on your back. Maybe you can feel the sensation of your shirt against your skin or your back against a chair. What does it feel like? Guide your attention to your abdomen. Observe any tension you may hold there and release it with an exhale. Move up to your chest and feel the way it rises and falls with each breath. Bring your attention to your hands—you may experience buzzing or tingling here—and then to your arms and shoulders. Notice if you are holding any tension or stiffness there. Focus on any sensations present on your face and head. Once you have made it to the top of your head, see if you can experience your body as a whole. No need to change anything, but simply observe your body with curiosity and without judgment.

- *Informal mindfulness practice.* Although formal mindfulness practices are beneficial, people may find that they lack the ability to carve out time in their day for a recording or meditation. A key element of mindfulness is its properties as a tool that can be applied during any moment of the day: mindfulness in everyday life. There are numerous activities that one engages in over the course of a day that are often executed on "autopilot." You are encouraged to attend to sensory experiences that accompany such activities throughout the day with a mindful attitude. For example, when you brush your teeth, notice the sensory experience of the bristles against your teeth and the sound that it makes, perhaps the taste of mint. When you are outside, pay attention to the warmth of the sun on your face and the touch of a breeze. By applying a present and nonjudgmental awareness to basic daily tasks, individuals can become more grounded and appreciative of the small sensations, sights, and sounds that comprise the previously unnoticed moments of life. This allows individuals to manage their pain throughout the day. The benefits of mindfulness thus are available without the resources it may take to practice more formally.

Conclusion. Although research on the use of mindfulness for chronic orofacial pain remains limited to date, there is broad evidence indicating that mindfulness practice may help manage chronic pain and aid with specific challenges faced by individuals with chronic orofacial pain. The incorporation of mindfulness into the treatment of chronic orofacial pain can expand a growing movement toward viewing chronic orofacial pain through a biopsychosocial lens, accounting for the biological, psychological, and social factors affecting individuals with chronic orofacial pain, as well as the interactions among them. Given that mindfulness exercises are free and accessible, mindfulness may pose a safe, easy, affordable, and accessible means to help individuals cope with chronic orofacial pain.

4.5
Who Needs a Support Group Anyway?
Michele Cohen, LCSW, Fellow of the International Psychoanalytic Association

The topic of support groups is something close to my heart. When I was first diagnosed with facial pain, I recall feeling terribly alone and frightened. After I had searched on the term "trigeminal neuralgia" (TN) multiple times, Google led me to the FPA's website. From there, I joined multiple Facebook groups, which I found to be a mixed blessing. The groups were helpful in sharing information and dispelling some of the loneliness, but I wanted more. I had moderated support groups in the past for people dealing with medical challenges, and I felt that such a group would help fellow TN warriors deal with the emotional challenges of living with TN.

The TN groups that were active at that time were all in-person. I looked into the possibility of joining a group in my area but was not able to find one. It was my good fortune to meet Anne Ciemnecki online. Anne had been running a support group in New Jersey and was looking for participants. In 2017, we decided to offer a virtual support group, noting that it was difficult for people to attend in-person groups, particularly if they were in pain. This group, which has been extraordinarily successful, continues to meet weekly.

Of course, the world as we knew it, changed radically in March 2020. Suddenly, everyone was meeting virtually, in one way or another. The FPA also had to pivot immediately to working online, and at that time, I began to offer another weekly virtual support group. In 2023, I began a third group for people diagnosed with multiple sclerosis and TN. The nicest surprise about moderating these groups was how much they helped me deal with the emotional fall-out of trying to live with TN in a meaningful way. I no longer felt so alone, and because I was part of an active community of fellow warriors, I was able to spare my family the agony of listening to angry outbursts or sharp feelings of resentment, which only left me feeling frustrated and my family feeling guilty about how helpless and inadequate they were, seeing me in such terrible pain.

People feel helpless when they are in fierce and unrelenting pain and may be hesitant to join a support group. The helplessness we feel is related to a time long ago, when we depended on our parents to survive. As adults, we do have ways of soothing ourselves in the face of the normal dings and dents that come with being human, but for many, the stress and loneliness of TN causes a regression to feelings associated with an earlier time. These feelings are unwanted and difficult to manage, and people may become enraged or avoid them altogether, despite their wish to be helped. Getting rid of feelings, by either projecting them onto others or repressing them, may provide relief in the short run, but sooner or later, these unwanted feelings do return. If we fail to pay attention to them, we tend to develop emotional scar tissue, which is difficult to pierce. When scar tissue forms, people tend to become defensive and even more difficult to reach.

In addition, the uncertainty of never knowing how we will feel from one day to the next makes it difficult to make plans and sustain friendships and close relationships. Many people with TN are unable to work and miss the camaraderie of being part of a team. This leads to loneliness, anxiety, depression, and despair (among other feelings). As people with facial pain know, it is exceedingly difficult to survive the indignities of TN, but it is even harder to deal with them in isolation.

When I was first diagnosed with TN, I was too distraught to be interested in putting my feelings into words. Instead, I found myself inadvertently pushing people away. I felt as if no one understood me, and this led to my feeling even more hopeless. At the time, I simply did not know how to do anything but vent, scream, and close myself off from family and friends. Thankfully, the group was there for me, and the trust that had developed between participants helped me put words to what I was feeling, in a way in which I felt deeply understood. Finding words to describe our pain is difficult, but it can be done. We all wish to be validated and understood, but it isn't something that comes naturally. Looking at emotional pain is difficult. There are no guarantees ahead of time that paying attention to painful emotions will actually be helpful. It takes a leap of faith to join a support group.

People tend to be skeptical of looking closely at the emotional aspects of TN. This is understandable—who would want to willingly look at emotional pain when they are already in unbearable physical pain? It takes a certain amount of courage to move into, rather than away from, these kinds of feelings.

Support groups help people develop the ability to speak about facial pain, but we speak about much more than that. Before I became involved in a support group, I had accumulated a great deal of emotional scar tissue. I was angry, and it was difficult for me to keep my feelings in check. At the time, there were no words to describe how I felt, but with the help of the group, I was able to put my raw feelings into words. This helped me accept and own the feelings I had been avoiding.

Individuals with facial pain have few outlets to express themselves and need a safe space to talk with like-minded people. As a group develops, people begin to understand and respect the importance of attending meetings on a regular basis, which further deepens the group members' commitment to each other, and to the group as a whole.

You may be unsure about taking on a commitment to consistently attend support group meetings. This is understandable, as life often intervenes. Being in severe pain also makes it difficult, if not impossible, for people to consistently attend meetings, though using Zoom helps a lot.

I recall that, when my pain was especially vicious, I doubted my ability to moderate the group, but I did it anyway. To my surprise, being with my TN "family" was a welcome distraction for me. I have since encouraged others to try to attend, despite their pain. Group members also have each other's email addresses, so that we can share articles about facial pain and cheer each other on. Although I never "take attendance," group members do miss people and share concerns for them when they miss meetings. We are there for each other during times of difficulty, but we also enjoy celebrating the good times together.

When I begin working with a new support group, I emphasize the importance of creating a safe space, and I try my best to give people room to speak, if they like, or to listen without speaking. It is important to go slow and allow each member of the group to move at a pace that is comfortable. At first, much of the conversation tends to focus on treatments, physicians, and medications. People want to compare notes, and there is an audible sense of relief when they realize that others understand the challenges of living with TN. It is important to give group members as much time as they need to discuss the physiological aspects of TN. It is much easier to talk about the body than about the psyche, and it takes time to develop a language of the mind.

As group members become more comfortable with each other, the group feels safe enough for us to delve into distressful feelings such as anger, shame, and despair. As we become more comfortable owning some of these feelings, the group begins to feel less shame. This makes it safer to share even more with each other. Even though our pain may have felt out of control, changing how we dealt with it was something we could achieve. This made us all feel better. As many of us have said: as awful as it is to live in pain, there is some compensation in that we have been able to meet and get to know so many wonderful people who truly "get it." This has certainly been the case for me.

At this point, I would like to turn to my attention to the support group members. When I was asked to write a chapter for this book, I spoke to members of my support groups, asking them if they would consider sharing their experience of the group with you. After all, it is equally, if not more, important to hear their perspective, in addition to mine. I hope that the following vignettes give you a sense of what it feels like to be part of a support group. I think that you will gain as much from them as I did.

Vignette 1

In the past, I had belonged to support groups for issues with family members, but when I developed trigeminal neuralgia, I didn't have any idea of what I was dealing with and didn't even know anyone who had ever dealt with the condition. Like many of you, I went from pillar to post before even getting a correct diagnosis of my excruciating pain; an oral surgeon had given me a diagnosis of atypical burning tongue syndrome, which led to a dentist trying to alleviate my pain, to no avail. I continued to live in pain until my PCP [primary care physician] recommended an ENT [ear, nose, and throat doctor] who led me to a neurologist, who finally correctly diagnosed me.

And like many of you, I went online to see what I could find out about TN. At that time, there was little information except that it used to be called tic douloureux and was nicknamed "the suicide disease."

On one of my visits to my neurologist's office, I found the Trigeminal Neuralgia Association's (now the Facial Pain Association's) Quarterly newsletter and subscribed. It was through them that Anne C. found me and invited me to an in-person support group. This was the first time I had met people who were dealing with TN. Unfortunately, after a couple of years, I had to stop attending these evening meetings as I had trouble driving at night. And then I moved out of the area.

A few years—and several health issues later, I received word from Anne that she was part of a new support group that met through Zoom, and [she] invited me to join, which I was pleased to do.

I have now had a successful MVD and have been pain-free for 5 years. I still attend my support group meetings. Why? Hopefully, I can give back to those still in pain, not only with information and advice, but to be a friend and part of their support teams. And, who knows, with this invidious condition, I may once again need the support myself. (Jan S.)

Vignette 2

The support group members have become my best friends. The best meetings are gatherings when we do not talk about facial pain. It is wonderful to have conversations with people who have similar experiences. Once the group became cohesive, no topic was off limits. We discuss sex, life, death, travel, family, children, and current events. I look forward to the meetings every week. (Anne C.)

Vignette 3

I joined a support group after being diagnosed with trigeminal neuropathy from acute disseminated encephalomyelitis [ADEM].

ADEM is a neurological disorder characterized by brief, but widespread, attacks of inflammation of the brain and spinal cord that damages myelin. I was physically and emotionally drained. I started looking online and found the Facial Pain Association and the support groups. I still recall the first Zoom meeting as I tried to share my story and started crying intensely. It was a safe space and people understood my physical and emotional pain. My life has not gone back to "normal" or to pre-TN diagnosis but being part of this weekly support group has made me move forward and start enjoying the little things in life. (Nora C.)

Vignette 4

I am not sure if my life would have improved as it has if I were not part of this support group. Finding this group was like being reunited with long-lost family who put up with my quirks and my pain.

We share information, tips, and tricks, but probably the most valuable part of being in the group has been the emotional support we give each other. We laugh and cry, and then we laugh some more for good measure. But when you see a group member in pain, you have a good idea of how that feels. Who better to cheer you on than someone who has been there, done that?

Each group member brings a different personality and unique strengths and rounds out our group to make it just the right combination of receiving help and giving encouragement to others. What a blessing it is to be connected to my friends in the facial pain community through this group. (Kim F.)

It is my hope that we will continue to have the opportunity to support each other. TN is a tough disease to live with, and it is difficult for others to understand how debilitating it can be. This is further compounded by the fact that TN is invisible and rare. People who live with it need to know that they are not alone. It is too tough to weather the storms of TN without having people we care about share our journey. It helps to know that we are all in this together.

4.6
Empowered Relief®: An Evidence-Based One-Session Pain Relief Skills Intervention
Beth D. Darnall, PhD

The Problem of Pain. Chronic pain impacts more people than diabetes, cancer, and heart disease *combined*. Across health conditions, pain is the primary reason people seek medical care and costs the United States about $635 billion each year. (Committee on Advancing Pain Research 2011) Across disease conditions, chronic pain (>3 months) is the leading cause of work-related disability. Moreover, people often have more than one chronic pain condition (i.e., chronic overlapping pain conditions), which compounds suffering, disability, and treatment needs. Pain and disability rates are rising despite increased use of surgery and pharmaceuticals, which can have adverse effects. Minorities, women, older adults, and those of lower socioeconomic status are disproportionately not only impacted by ongoing pain but also experience the greatest barriers to effective pain care. Equitable access to effective pain treatment is an urgent national need.

Thinking Beyond Surgeries and Medications Only: The Need for an Integrated Pain Treatment Approach. The International Association for the Study of Pain (IASP) defines pain as "a negative sensory and emotional experience." (Taxonomy 1994) This is true for all pain conditions, including facial pain and specified conditions such as TN. The definition recognizes that, across varied medical diagnoses, all pain is processed in the central nervous system, where it is also influenced by many factors, including our thoughts, mood, behavior, history, and expectations for pain and treatment, to name just a few. Because pain is influenced by so many factors, it is important that pain treatment address these various factors and "dial down" the intensity of pain. Indeed, although we cannot control our medical diagnoses, we can address some of the factors that influence the severity of our pain, its impacts, and our suffering. This is the opportunity presented by treatments that are referred to as behavioral pain medicine, pain self-management, or pain psychology. With each of these approaches, the treatment focuses on helping people gain an understanding of what they can do to best control their pain and reduce its impacts. In so doing, people gain confidence in their ability to live with greater comfort and control, even within the context of an ongoing painful medical condition. It is important for people to have their pain addressed from an *integrated perspective*, one that does not rely on medications and surgeries alone but rather considers and targets various aspects of the person and their life (see Figure 4-3).

Behavioral Pain Treatments: Evidence and Access Barriers. Indeed, decades of clinical science show that evidence-based behavioral pain treatment can reduce chronic pain impacts, improve medical outcomes, and reduce the need for medical treatments for pain. Owing to the benefits and low risk profiles of behavioral treatments, multiple U.S. agencies have called for broad integration of such

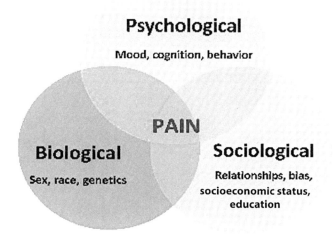

Figure 4-3.   Biopsychosocial model of pain.

treatments into national pain care pathways. Cognitive behavioral therapy (CBT) for chronic pain is the best studied behavioral treatment for chronic pain and is sometimes referred to as the "gold standard" behavioral pain treatment. Over the course of eight or more 2-hour individual or group sessions (16 hours of total treatment time), CBT attendees learn a variety of pain management skills and information. Attendees apply the information and skills by setting personal goals and creating daily action plans. Research suggests clinically meaningful benefits across a range of symptoms (pain intensity, physical function, pain-related distress, depression, sleep disturbance), with positive results lasting 6 months or more. (Cherkin 2016, Williams 2020, Darnall 2021) There are other evidence-based behavioral pain treatments, including acceptance and commitment therapy (ACT) (a variant of CBT), emotional awareness and expression therapy, and mindful-based stress reduction (MBSR). Although often effective and low to no risk, these treatments can be infeasible for many people because of time, costs, and lack of availability. In addition, some patients neither want, nor require, 16 or more hours of treatment time. As a clinical psychologist, I grew tired of seeing patients unable to conveniently access the care they needed and wanted. I created Empowered Relief® to provide broad patient access to effective, low-burden behavioral pain treatment.

Empowered Relief®: One-Session Pain Relief Skills Intervention Improves Patient Access. Empowered Relief® is a one-session pain relief skills intervention for people with acute and chronic pain of all types. The 2-hour intervention is delivered by certified clinicians to groups of patients either in person or online via Zoom or another conference platform. Empowered Relief® is not therapy; it is a class. Its content includes pain neuroscience education; participants acquire three core pain management skills and complete a personal plan for empowered relief (Table 4-1). These pain relief skills are rooted in mindfulness principles and CBT skills.

An NIH-funded randomized controlled trial of 263 adults with chronic low back pain revealed that single-session Empowered Relief® was of comparable benefit (i.e., not inferior) to 16 hours of CBT at 3- and 6-months posttreatment for reducing pain catastrophizing, pain intensity, pain interference, pain bothersomeness, depression, anxiety,

Table 4-1. What Is Empowered Relief?

- **One-session** pain relief skills class
- Delivered by a certified clinician
- **Can be received online or in person**
- 2 hours in duration
- Class content includes pain neuroscience education, experiential exercises, three core pain management techniques, development of a personalized plan for empowered relief, and a free binaural app for daily use
- Published data from four randomized controlled studies showed efficacy for pain and symptom relief 3 and 6 months after completion of the class (Darnall 2021, Ziadni 2021)

fatigue, physical function, and sleep disturbance. (Darnall 2021) A second study compared Empowered Relief® received online to usual care in 105 patients with chronic pain receiving care from a pain clinic. (Ziadni 2021) The results revealed high patient engagement and satisfaction, in addition to a similar pattern of reductions in pain intensity, pain interference, pain catastrophizing, pain bothersomeness, anxiety, and sleep disturbance at 3 months posttreatment.

Empowered Relief® for Surgery. Empowered Relief® has been studied in two surgical studies. (Darnall 2019, Ziadni 2022) For these studies, Empowered Relief® was tailored to the surgical context, and a digital version was created to allow patients to receive the intervention conveniently from home or in the hospital after surgery.

Empowered Relief® was first studied in women undergoing breast cancer surgery to compare the digital intervention (then called "My Surgical Success") to a health education control intervention that involved no active pain relief skills. (Darnall 2019) Women who engaged with My Surgical Success were found to require about one week less of opioids after breast cancer surgery relative to women in the control group, suggesting that Empowered Relief® helped speed the cessation of opioid use after surgery.

We next studied the Empowered Relief® digital intervention in 84 patients receiving orthopedic trauma surgery. (Ziadni 2022) The majority of patient participants received their assigned treatment on an iPad in the hospital on postoperative days 1 through 3. Patients who received the digital version of Empowered Relief® reported significantly less pain after surgery relative to controls, and the analgesic benefits lasted up to 3 months later, the last time point of the study. The results suggested that Empowered Relief® imparted clinically meaningful and sustained pain relief after surgery. Moreover, the results underscored the potential for low-cost, low-burden, brief education and pain self-regulatory skills to improve surgical recovery. We are partnering with health care organizations to embed digital and on-demand Empowered Relief® for Surgery into surgical pathways broadly.

Scaling Access to Empowered Relief®. Because its low-burden format requires only one session, Empowered Relief® can help many patients receive behavioral pain care, often conveniently from the comfort of their own home. Brief and home-based pain care can overcome many disparities that prevent people with the least means, and those in rural areas, from receiving the pain care they need.

Since the rollout of certifications in 2019, 1000 certified clinicians are delivering Empowered Relief® in 46 U.S. states, 26 countries, and 8 languages (Canadian French, French, Spanish, German, Dutch, Danish, Italian, and English), with expansions underway. Separate and tailored versions of Empowered Relief® exist across the continuum of care and across the lifespan (Table 4-2). Versions of Empowered Relief® exist for chronic pain and acute/surgical pain, and certification flexibly allows clinicians to deliver either or both versions.

Empowered Relief® is being delivered as "standard care" at multiple health care organizations, meaning that it is offered to every person who reports having ongoing pain. This addresses a common problem in the field: we tend to wait too long to provide behavioral

Table 4-2. Versions of Empowered Relief® and Availability Status

Tailored version	Status
Adult chronic pain	Available now
Acute and post-surgical pain	Available now
Adults with pain having challenges taking prescription opioids as prescribed	Available now
Active Service Members and Veterans with pain	Available now
Youth with chronic pain	In study; available in 2024

pain care. Now, rather than waiting until people suffer and offering behavioral pain treatment as a last resort when most treatments have failed, Empowered Relief® as standard pain care makes it possible for people to receive this class earlier in their pain journey. Thus, people will become equipped to best help themselves as they navigate the challenges of their diagnosis and the medical system. Organizations that have adopted Empowered Relief® as standard care include Cleveland Clinic Spine Surgery and the Cleveland Clinic Neurological Institute, multiple Veterans Administration medical centers, Cedars Sinai Health Care, Lehigh Valley Health Network, Allegheny Health Network, Brigham and Women's Hospital, Veterans Affairs Canada, the National Health Service in the United Kingdom, and Humana Neighborhood. Another benefit of the standard care approach is that it allows organizations and clinics to emphasize the applicability of this intervention to all patients, thereby destigmatizing it and boosting patient interest and engagement.

Research and New Directions. Various investigators are studying Empowered Relief® in different patient populations, such as individuals with chronic migraines and individuals who have experienced an acute back pain episode, to name just two. At Stanford, we are conducting a national comparative effectiveness trial of online-delivered one-session Empowered Relief® versus online-delivered eight-session CBT for individuals with chronic pain of any type (called the PROGRESS study). PROGRESS is a six-site national trial launched in January 2023 that is enrolling a total of 1650 adults from across the United States. (PCORI 2021) We aim to be able to say which behavioral treatment works best and for whom. The focus of this research is the inclusion of a diverse patient sample, including individuals from different areas of the country, of varied races and ethnicities, with varied pain conditions, and of different economic and educational levels. By including a patient sample that is representative of the U.S. population, we can best ensure that our study findings will be generalizable.

Other trends include an active study that is supported by the American Association of Pain Management Nursing. Principal Investigator Holly Watson and colleagues are conducting a national efficacy study of online nurse-delivered Empowered Relief® in people with chronic pain of all types. In addition, my group at Stanford

University is partnering with the Marfan Foundation to conduct a national online study of Empowered Relief® in individuals with Marfan syndrome and other Marfan-related rare diseases, with results available in 2024. Finally, we are partnering with the California prison system to provide Empowered Relief® to people who are incarcerated (Banerjee 2023).

How Can I Access Empowered Relief®?

- Check with your health organization to see if they offer Empowered Relief® within your clinic or at a nearby location. Many organizations offer it at no cost to you; others may bill your insurance company.
- Visit the Empowered Relief® website (https://empoweredrelief. stanford.edu) and check under the "Find a Provider" tab to see if there are certified clinicians in your area.
- Several certified clinicians offer Empowered Relief® online, and you can register for these class offerings regardless of your location. These national instructors are indicated on the Find a Provider page of the Empowered Relief® website.
- You may wish to join one of several active Empowered Relief® research studies. Chapter 7 of this book provides information about participation in research studies.
- If you are a clinician or health care leader who would like to adopt Empowered Relief® in your care setting, please visit the Empowered Relief® website (https://empoweredrelief.stanford. edu) and learn about the clinician certification process.

4.7
Virtual Reality for Orofacial Pain: Unlocking Its Potential in Pain Management

GianCarlo Colloca, MEd, MS, and Luana Colloca, MD, PhD, MS

Author's Note: The authors thank their temporomandibular disorder (TMD) patients for their inspiring role and continuous support. Some of the research described in this section was supported by the National Center for Complementary and Integrative Health (NCCIH): Grant R01AT01033 (Principal Investigator: L. Colloca).

Virtual reality (VR) is sparking interest as a pain management tool. Although its role in pain treatment is being explored, its potential in orofacial pain is still untapped. VR transports you beyond your surroundings, even embodying a new environment. This blend of technology and experience enhances pain tolerance and can notably reduce acute and chronic pain in real-world settings.

What is intriguing is that VR pain relief works at the bedside or at home, expanding its benefits. Custom VR rehabilitation aids movement-impaired individuals, while also enabling health care practitioners to gain hands-on training. The future holds the promise of more wide-ranging VR applications beyond medicine, and robust research is becoming increasingly available.

VR reveals a pain-managing future, offering a sneak peek. Through careful investigation and development, VR has the potential to revolutionize the experience, management, and treatment of pain.

People who experience jaw pain, known as temporomandibular disorders (TMDs), often have trouble finding the right help for their ongoing pain. TMDs affect about 5% to 12% of people in general, and it causes a great deal of difficulty for individuals and society. Sadly, it is not easy for individuals with TMD to find treatments that do not involve taking pills. In part, this is because there is no agreed-upon best care protocol for individuals with TMDs, nor is there much knowledge about how much therapies that consider both the body and the mind can help with TMDs and related issues. Moreover, to make the situation even tougher, there are not enough health care providers who know how to treat this condition.

VR could help with ongoing pain, whether it is lasting or just comes on suddenly. Although there is a great deal of detailed research about how exactly this works in acute and chronic pain, more research is needed especially for people with orofacial pain and TMDs.

Unlocking the Magic of Virtual Reality. VR is a computer-generated technology that creates immersive, three-dimensional environments or simulations. It is designed to simulate a user's physical presence in a digital or virtual world, allowing them to interact with the environment and objects within it. Recently, it has been proposed that VR offers a unique approach to alleviate pain in patients by redirecting the neural pathways typically associated with pain perception. In simpler terms, VR can be thought of as a technology that diverts the brain's attention and emotions away from pain signals. This diversion creates a positive impact on various cognitive factors, ultimately improving pain management and influencing the way pain-related messages are transmitted through memory, emotions, and different sensory channels such as touch, sound, and sight.

VR uses sights, sounds, and even feelings to create a different experience that might help reduce orofacial and other types of pain. For instance, imagine a person who has pain while walking. Through VR, they can virtually enter an environment in which they do not need to physically move their limbs, yet they can feel as if they are walking. This immersive experience can help distance patients from their current physical discomfort. Researchers are actively working to uncover the exact mechanisms underlying how VR benefits people in pain. Key aspects being explored are how VR operates through distraction, mood and emotions, and nerve system regulations, reshaping how we perceive the world around us.

Researchers such as Trost and co-workers have suggested four key features that make VR special: feeling present in a new world, becoming absorbed in this new world (like getting lost in a movie), interacting with the new world using your body, and feeling like your own "self" is there. This "embodiment" idea even helps in treating conditions such as phantom limb pain and spinal injuries.

Scientists such as L. Colloca and her team are studying how VR affects the body and mind. They are trying to understand how it can help with pain without using medicine or can be used as an adjuvant to typical treatments. VR creates "magic" but realistic places, and this can be part of a plan to manage pain naturally through a multisensory experience. Understanding exactly how VR changes how one experiences pain is particularly important for making best use of VR for this purpose. We have seen hints that VR can change the pain experience in many ways. It is not just what we see; it is also what we hear, feel, and even expect. There is still much more to learn. We need to figure out how our thoughts and feelings affect how VR helps with pain.

Understanding How Virtual Reality Helps with Pain. The Colloca research group performed a study to investigate how VR affects how we feel pain and whether we can increase the ability to tolerate pain through VR. (Colloca 2020) Study participants included healthy individuals, and the study investigated how their bodies and minds reacted to VR when they experienced a painful stimulus. Specifically, a painful stimulation was delivered through a thermode that became increasingly warm and that the study participants were able to control with a remote. The VR headset was mounted and displayed some jellyfish, nature, music, and relaxing ocean scenes. This was one of the first studies of VR that included appropriate controls for VR contexts (immersive vs nonimmersive) and multiple objective and subjective outcomes.

We wanted to determine whether VR could change how much thermal pain individuals could handle in a laboratory setting. We also investigated whether the painful stimulus made them feel different emotions, such as being in a better or worse mood or feeling anxious, when they were in the VR world. We even measured how their bodies reacted by measuring how their skin responded to pain and how their body's vagal nervous system was working.

The study results indicated that, when people used VR, they tolerated a higher level of painful thermal stimulations, and yet their bodies showed that they were more relaxed, even if they could tolerate more pain under VR conditions. It was as if their bodies were saying, "I'm okay, even though I'm feeling pain." The VR environment might have created such a state of relaxation that it allowed study participants to handle more self-administered pain while relaxing and experiencing mood improvements. Some of these results are presented in Figure 4-4, which shows that VR users exhibited increases in pain tolerance, reductions in pain unpleasantness, improvements in mood, and reductions in anxiety.

We also tested different variables, such as having people do a memory task to contrast the effects on pain tolerance of distraction versus VR. This trial indicated that simply being distracted by VR did not fully explain why pain was experienced less intensely. Also, the memory

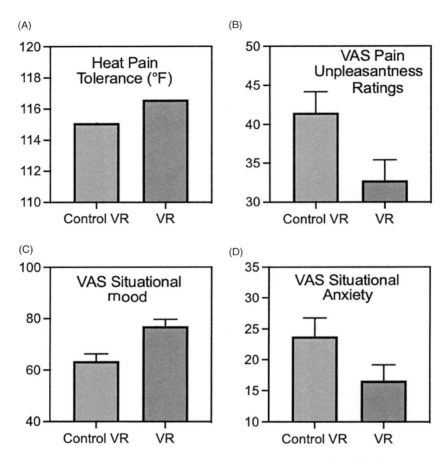

(A)

Heat Pain Tolerance (°F)

120 —
118 —
116 —
114 —
112 —
110 —

Control VR   VR

(B)

VAS Pain Unpleasantness Ratings

50 —
45 —
40 —
35 —
30 —

Control VR   VR

(C)

VAS Situational mood

100 —
80 —
60 —
40 —

Control VR   VR

(D)

VAS Situational Anxiety

35 —
30 —
25 —
20 —
15 —
10 —

Control VR   VR

Figure 4-4. VR-induced pain tolerance and psychological well-being, as shown by plots of (A) pain tolerance, (B) pain unpleasantness, (C) mood improvements, and (D) anxiety reduction for control VR versus immersive VR. These results collectively suggest that VR not only enhances pain tolerance but also promotes a state of relaxation, improved mood, and reduced anxiety. These findings are statistically significant.

Abbreviations: VAS, visual analog scale; VR, virtual reality.

task did not help with relaxation. Instead, people became more nervous during the memory task. On the contrary, it seemed that feeling relaxed in the body played a significant part in how VR helped with pain.

In short, we found that VR can help people increase experimental pain tolerance and improve their mood and anxiety. We also saw that the type of VR world matters. For example, being in a VR ocean scene rather than an opera (*La clemenza di Tito*, Mozart), which we created ad hoc for the VR headset, seemed to help the most, allowing study participants to tolerate more pain and feel better overall. The VR world appeared to provide people with a break from painful stimulations and help them relax. Moreover, the more an individual liked a VR world (e.g., the ocean vs an opera), the better they felt emotionally, and the less their pain bothered them. This means that how much someone enjoys a VR world can change how much it helps with both the experience of pain and general mood. It is as if the VR created a sort of multisensory experience that made thermal painful stimulations feel less intense.

Potential Mechanisms of Virtual Reality. Researchers have been investigating how VR might help reduce pain. Imagine being in a computer-made world that feels so real that you feel like you are actually there. VR can use features such as what we see and hear and even how we are feeling emotionally to help reduce pain. It is more like a distraction that our brain pays attention to instead of the pain. Our thoughts and expectations might also play a role in how well VR works for our experience of pain.

Scientists are studying this question in detail to determine exactly how VR affects pain and whether it can provide a helpful means of managing pain as an adjunct to medications or in the place of high-dose medications. Researchers want to know if different aspects of VR, such as what we see and hear and even how much we enjoy it, can change how much pain we feel. It is like solving a puzzle to make VR work the best way possible for people who are in pain. This is all still being researched, so there is much more to learn about how VR can help with pain relief.

Real-World Benefits of Virtual Reality in Hospitals. Researchers have been investigating how VR can help with pain relief, for example, for those who are staying in the hospital. This is pretty exciting because it is a new way to help in-patients feel better when they are experiencing excruciating surgery- or trauma-related pain. We have seen how VR can actually make a difference for patients at the bedside in the hospital.

One study used VR in a special way to help in-patients manage their acute pain. (Speigel 2019) In this study, patients were given VR headsets with an assortment of different experiences to choose from, such as being underwater or in a peaceful garden. The researchers then compared the experiences of these patients with others who just watched a regular television program about health and wellness. What they found was that the patients who used VR reported less pain than those who watched television.

Another study considered in-patients with injuries, including head injuries. (Morris 2023) In this case, two types of VR experiences were tested, one of which was relaxing, while the other was neutral. The VR experiences were also compared with use of a tablet with no immersion in VR contexts. The patients who experienced the relaxing VR reported less pain compared than those who used a tablet. The VR experience also seemed to make the body relax, which is good for healing. Even though the difference in anxiety levels was minimal, the patients felt that the relaxing VR helped them the most. Interestingly, a reduction was observed in the need for opioid intake to relieve pain. This result seems to be extremely meaningful in the effort to reduce opioid side effects and, potentially, to minimize the burden of overuse, abuse, and addiction resulting from the opioid epidemic. Interestingly, it was found that in-patients who liked the relaxing VR used less pain-relieving medicine, such as opioids, after a VR session. This suggests that VR might help reduce the need for strong pain medications while still making in-patients feel better.

Both of these studies demonstrate that VR can be used in hospitals to help patients manage their pain and feel more comfortable when handling severe traumatic and surgery-related acute pain, thus opening up a new and exciting way to improve in-patients' experiences while in the hospital.

Advancements in Virtual Reality for Chronic Pain Relief.
Researchers have investigated how VR can make a difference for people dealing with long-lasting pain. The efficacy of VR in terms of clinical pain reduction has already been examined for a variety of clinical conditions, including burning wound care pain (Hoffman 2011, Smith 2020, Scapin 2018), dental examination (Joda 2019, Sullivan 2000, Huang 2018) , and vaccination (Althumairi 2021, (Vandeweerd 2022, Real 2017), as well as chronic pain (Darnall 2020, Garcia 2022, Garcia 2021). Individuals with chronic pain have also found relief

through VR. One study used VR for just 5 minutes and found that participants felt much less pain during the VR session (Jones 2016). In another study, participants used VR for 21 days at home, and after a couple of weeks, they reported starting to feel better and being able to manage their pain more effectively. (Darnall 2020) Also, exciting is that the U.S. Food and Drug Administration (FDA) has approved a prescription VR headset device for managing chronic lower back pain (https://www.fda.gov/news-events/press-announcements/fda-authorizes-marketing-virtual-reality-system-chronic-pain-reduction). This device, called RelieVRx, uses VR to teach skills such as relaxation, shifting focus, and cognitive skills to help reduce pain and its interference in daily life. It is a new way of approaching pain management without relying solely on medication.

Other studies have shown that immersive VR treatments, such as those provided by RelieVRx, can significantly reduce pain intensity and interference in people with chronic low back pain. Individuals who used these treatments reported better pain management and improved quality of life. (Maddox 2023, Maddox 2022, Maddox 2022)

In the United Kingdom, researchers explored using VR for chronic low back pain. They found that participants who used VR therapy reported reduced fear of movement and overall improvement in their condition. This shows that VR can offer relief and positive changes for those living with chronic pain. (Eccleston 2022)

These studies are paving the way for a new approach to managing chronic pain through VR. As technology continues to improve, we can expect even more innovative solutions for people dealing with persistent pain

The Patient's Voice. VR is not just for games anymore; it is actually being used to help individuals with chronic orofacial pain. At the University of Maryland School of Nursing in Baltimore, MD, patients with orofacial pain are allowed to use the EaseVRx, another FDA-approved prescription-use immersive virtual reality system, for several weeks in an ongoing trial. RelieVRx offers a VR program that incorporates cognitive behavioral therapy (CBT), relaxation response exercise, breathing training, mindfulness training, cognition and emotion regulation, and pain neuroscience education. We interviewed some users asking to share their experiences.

Grace B., female, aged 35 years, White

My name is Grace. I have TMD [temporomandibular disorder], and I participated in a virtual reality study. The pain that I experience generally is not very extreme. It's more of a dull, more consistent pain. I hold a lot of tension in my face and jaw. The virtual reality definitely helped me to relax a little bit. I even got some like sort of brain tingles for certain sessions. I would do it after work—in the afternoon or early evening. It helped me to sleep. I felt that it relaxed my brain a little bit, relaxed my face a little bit, and it helped me to sleep a little bit better. So, I do really believe in that for helping with pain and thank you very much.

Jonathan T., male, aged 38 years, Asian

I'm very grateful for this experience using the VR device. It really helped me to control and cut down my pain. I'm just very, very happy with the technology and all the different features I had. [I'm] very glad to have participated in this experience because it had many different sensory modalities and tools that I used to reduce and hopefully eliminate my pain. I'm just very grateful for the lab for this opportunity to use this emerging technology. It has helped me immensely. Thank you so much.

Willis P., male, aged 52 years, Black

Sometimes I would just be [awakened] and amazed at the pain actually went away. It shocked me because I didn't think it would work. I was so amazed that I wanted to inquire about buying one for myself, I'm still in the process of getting one. I mentioned it to my pain doctor. They were aware of the technique and that it was a great experience for me. This should be something that I should get. It worked better than the medication. So, it's definitely something that I would definitely want to get. I'm hoping that one day soon I will, but I definitely know that it really does work. For anybody that would want to try it, I would recommend it 100%. Not 90%, not 50%, but 100% because it really worked. I'm thankful that I was chosen to be part of this experiment and was able to experience something like this.

Accessing VR for Pain Management. Patients interested in utilizing VR for pain relief have a few options for obtaining this technology.

Some health care providers and pain management specialists may prescribe VR as part of a comprehensive pain management plan. One example is RelieVRx, a VR-based pain management program that can be prescribed by your health care provider. Patients can inquire with their health care team about the possibility of using VR as a part of their pain management strategy. Insurance coverage for VR-based pain management may vary. Although some insurance plans do cover the cost of VR therapy when prescribed by a health care professional, others may not. Patients should contact their insurance provider to understand their specific coverage and reimbursement options. Importantly, there are various affordable or free VR programs and apps available. These can be accessed through VR headsets or even smartphone-based VR experiences. Some of these apps are designed specifically for pain management and relaxation (i.e., mindfulness). Although they may not offer the same level of customization and medical supervision as prescription-based options, they can still provide valuable help for pain relief. Patients can explore app stores and online platforms to discover free or low-cost VR programs that suit their needs.

The Colloca group at the University of Maryland School of Nursing has now enrolled more than 150 individuals with TMDs in VR treatment, and we have not observed any adverse events related to VR use in patients experiencing orofacial pain. Although we acknowledge the potential for facial sensitivity, we also emphasize that, with proper adjustments, such as lighter devices, additional padding, strap loosening, and shorter initial sessions, many individuals with facial pain may find VR to be a valuable tool for relaxation and improvement of pain outcomes. We encourage open dialogue between patients and their health care providers to ensure a tailored and comfortable VR experience that complements their unique needs and preferences.

Uncharted Territories and Future Research. As technology rockets forward, new doors swing open for the potential use of VR in fields such as education and medicine. In the realm of mental health, VR is making group therapy more accessible and inclusive. In education, VR classrooms immerse students in a dynamic learning environment, keeping distractions at bay and engagement high. Researchers are pushing the boundaries even further. By combining VR with eye-tracking technology, they are delving into the intricacies of human behavior such as monitoring patients for nonverbal expressions of pain sensation. This combination allows for the study of behaviors such as attention to cues, providing a peek into how our minds work in real-life situations. VR is also stepping onto the stage of art and creativity. Virtual galleries and exhibitions are bringing vibrant experiences to the public, offering an entirely new way to interact with art and culture. In the world of health care, VR is taking solid steps toward becoming a tangible tool. Its applications in clinical settings are no longer just theoretical but are now being put to the test.

Researchers have been busy exploring VR's potential in various aspects of health care, from therapy to pain management. This surge of activity has brought forth a wave of new ideas, products, and scientific insights. As VR continues to grow, we can anticipate even more breakthroughs, pushing the boundaries of what we thought was possible. The journey has just begun, and the road ahead is full of exciting twists and turns.

Chapter 5
Living Your Best Life

Anne B. Ciemnecki, MA

What is a "life hack"? We know that hacking at things means cutting into them with swift, heavy strikes. Computer geeks use the term to describe the act of using technical skills and knowledge to gain access to a computer system or network. The term life hack is a transformation of the concept toward life solutions, stuff unrelated to computer keyboards, things computer geeks might have to face in a world away from their screens.

Who doesn't love a life hack? What are your favorites?

Do you

- Hold a nail with a clothespin so you do not hammer your fingers?
- Label your jumble of cables using tags from loaves of bread?
- Use binder clips to keep the wires from getting into a tangled mess in the first place?
- Put a piece of colored fabric around the handle on your luggage so you can identify it easily when it comes off the carousel?
- Use different colored nail polish to distinguish keys from one another?

My most useful life hacks involve my pets:

- I clip a key ring with my house key onto my dog's leash, so I do not lock myself out when I take her for a walk.
- I hang bags of IV fluids on clothes hangers so I can give my pets subcutaneous fluids when I am home alone with them. Otherwise, it takes two people to accomplish the task.

And have you heard about the hack for getting all of the Nutella from the jar?

- Add a scoop of ice cream to the jar and eat the ice cream and Nutella from the jar. (I swear I have not done this, but it is tempting. I would probably use coffee ice cream and microwave the jar first...)

You might consider Chapter 5 to be a compilation of successful life hacks for people with trigeminal neuropathic pain (TNP). In Section 5.1, Dennis R. Bailey, DDS, discusses the bidirectional relationship between pain and sleep. He provides much information about sleep and sleep disorders. His hack is to manage sleep and pain disorders together. If you do, both will improve.

In Section 5.2, Megan Tudor Donnelly, DO, affirms that, with understanding, patience, and adaptability, romantic intimacy can thrive despite the challenges of TNP. She offers many hacks from the dating stage to the deepening of loving long-term partnerships. Reimagining intimacy is not a compromise.

In Section 5.3, Kenneth Casey, MD, FACS, a dear friend of the facial pain community, addresses one of the most frustrating components of having chronic pain, namely, meeting Social Security Disability requirements. His hacks: applying with multiple medical impairments or showing that your disability stems from a related medical condition that is listed in the *Disability Evaluation Under Social Security* manual, also known as the Blue Book.

We end our hacks in Section 5.4, where Lindsey Wallace, Certified Pharmacy Technician and Facial Pain Association (FPA) Young Patients Committee (YPC) Co-Chair, offers many ways to afford otherwise unaffordable prescription medications. She explains what you can do if a medication is not covered by your insurance, how to afford brand-name medications, and how to afford generic medications, and she also directs those on Medicare to the Extra Help and Low-Income Subsidy (LIS) programs.

Use these hacks, think up your own, and share them with your pain pals. You know, I bet that Nutella hack works with peanut butter and chocolate ice cream!

5.1
The Relationship Between Pain and Sleep
Dennis R. Bailey, DDS

The association between pain and sleep is bidirectional. Having pain may impact sleep quality, and not sleeping well may impact pain levels. The key to understanding this relationship is to understand sleep and to recognize common sleep disorders that impact pain. Unfortunately, for many people with pain, paying attention to sleep quality and recognizing a sleep disorder may not always occur.

Sleep Overview. Sleep is one of the three pillars of life, along with diet and exercise. The amount and quality of sleep is significant when it comes to living a long healthy life. It is important for everyone to understand what constitutes good sleep, what sleep is, and the disorders of sleep that can impact your health as well as your pain.

Under optimum conditions, the amount of sleep an adult should get is between 7 and 9 hours each night, according to the American Academy of Sleep Medicine and the National Sleep Foundation. To achieve your best sleep, your bedtime, and the time you wake each morning should be relatively the same. It is not true that older people require or need less sleep. However, as they age, many people may not get the recommended amount of sleep because of health issues or medications that impact their sleep.

There are two major types of sleep: rapid eye movement (REM) sleep and non-rapid eye movement (NREM) sleep. One common misconception is that REM sleep is our best or deepest sleep. This is not true. REM sleep is often referred to as dream sleep because this is when we are most likely to experience dreams. NREM sleep is made up of three unique stages based solely on brain-wave activity during these stages (Table 5-1).

Throughout the night, people go in and out of REM sleep and the different stages of NREM sleep. Typically, as we fall asleep, we transition through NREM stages N1 and N2 into NREM stage N3 and

Table 5-1. Stages of Sleep

Sleep Type	Amount of Sleep	Characteristics
REM	20–25%	Dream sleep; for memory consolidation
NREM		
Stage N1	5%	Transitional sleep stage between REM and NREM stages; lightest stage of sleep
Stage N2	50%	Light stage of sleep
Stage N3	20–25%	Deepest stage of sleep; also known as restorative sleep

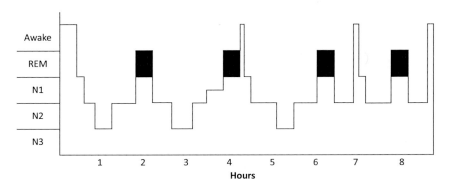

Figure 5-1. Stages of sleep during a typical night.

stay there for about 90 minutes. We then enter REM sleep for a brief period and typically go back to NREM stage N3. After another 90 minutes or so, we may go into NREM stage N2, or REM sleep, or both briefly, and then back to NREM stage N3 for a brief period. After approximately 4 hours of sleep, our deepest, restorative sleep is over. We then awaken, albeit briefly; we may or may not be aware of this awakening. For the balance of the night, we typically transition back and forth between REM sleep and NREM stage N2 with a possible awakening and longer REM periods (Figure 5-1).

When we experience sleep disruption, both the amounts of REM and NREM sleep and the stages of sleep may be altered. We may have more awakenings or disturbance in our sleep, referred to as sleep fragmentation, or more REM sleep or NREM stage N2. This occurs because of a variety of conditions, one of which is pain. These disturbances may result in our being tired during the day, having low energy, and having a reduced ability to concentrate. This can lead to other conditions such as anxiety and depression. Most importantly, sleep disturbances have the potential for increasing our pain and impacting our ability to respond to pain.

Two other significant factors are sleep quality (SQ) and sleep efficiency (SE). SQ is one's subjective perception of how well they slept and is often based on how rested they feel in the morning. In the case of pain, SQ may also be related to the perceived absence or reduction of pain. SE is typically reported as a percentage and is measurable during a sleep study by comparing the hours of sleep, which is determined by brain-wave activity, to the amount of time spent in bed. Having an SE of 85% or higher is the standard norm.

Sleep Disorders and Pain. Sleep and pain share a bidirectional relationship. Sleeping for fewer than the optimal number of hours may result in both increased pain and hyperalgesia, an increased response to painful stimuli. Alternatively, pain may lead to more sleep disturbance, as well as a deficient amount of sleep. Even people who do not suffer from a painful condition can understand the impact of a poor night's sleep. When a person has a disturbed night's sleep or a night of inadequate length or quality of sleep, they can feel more tired and less alert, and they may experience pain where pain is not typically present the following day.

Although sleep and pain have a bidirectional relationship, this relationship is not necessarily equal. Studies indicate that presleep pain does not necessarily predict subsequent sleep quality. Additionally, subjective sleep efficiency is the most reliable predictor of pain the next day. However, this applies mostly to pain on waking and for the first half of the day. It may not apply to pain later or in the second half of the day. A classic example of this is facial pain that involves the musculature. Many patients will awaken feeling minimal to no pain but experience an increase in their pain later in the day.

The deprivation of REM sleep leads to increased hyperalgesia the following day. A deprivation of REM sleep may also be associated with frequent disturbances in sleep, known as sleep fragmentation. In addition, REM sleep deprivation has been shown to impact and worsen nociception, that is, the perception or detection of pain.

Achieving a full understanding of how pain and sleep are related requires an understanding of the neurochemicals, also known as neurotransmitters, that transmit signals in the central nervous system and are involved with sleep, wakefulness, and pain. Many of these neurochemicals are interrelated, hence supporting the sleep–pain relationship physiologically.

Common Sleep Disorders That May Impact Pain. There are a wide variety of sleep disorders, some of which occur frequently. Many of these sleep disorders impact sleep quality and duration and, hence, can impact pain. Those with the greatest potential to impact both sleep and pain are as follows:

- *Insomnia* is the most common sleep disorder. It may be acute, for short periods of time, or chronic and ongoing. Insomnia can involve difficulty getting to sleep (sleep onset) or difficulty staying asleep (sleep maintenance.) Many people experience insomnia when they are stressed, mainly because stress comes with an elevation in cortisol levels, which promotes wakefulness. When pain is present, stress levels may be elevated, leading to more anxiety and thus increased difficulty with sleep.
- *Sleep apnea* is often associated with snoring and disruption in breathing during sleep. The most common type of apnea is obstructive, where the airway is blocked and the person struggles to breath, often observed as gasping during sleep. Sleep apnea is associated with daytime sleepiness, feelings of tiredness, mood swings, and memory issues. Eighty percent of people with sleep apnea have not been diagnosed. Of interest is a reciprocal situation. Many times, the bed partner of a person who snores or has apnea is impacted more than the person with the disorder because their sleep is disturbed; hence, they experience similar symptoms, feeling more pain and having poor sleep quality.
- *COMISA* stands for comorbid insomnia and sleep apnea, indicating that these two disorders co-occur. This comorbidity was first identified in 1973, and other studies since then have supported this relationship. Together, these two disorders lead to poor sleep quality and poor sleep efficiency, which potentially impacts pain.
- *Movement disorders* include restless leg syndrome (RLS), periodic limb movement disorder (PLMD), and sleep bruxism. RLS is typically found in the evening or during sleep initiation and is a clinical diagnosis based on the inability to sit still because of discomfort in the legs. PLMS involves the movement of mainly the legs during sleep and may disrupt sleep. It is diagnosed during a polysomnography, a multiparameter study of sleep that is a diagnostic tool in sleep medicine. Sleep bruxism

occurs predominately during stage N2 sleep and may disrupt sleep. An increase in N2 sleep is associated with an alteration in other stages of sleep. This disorder may also be associated with various orofacial pain complaints, as well as some types of headaches.

- *Narcolepsy* is the sudden onset of sleepiness. It may occur at any time and has been associated with an increased amount of daytime sleepiness or hypersomnia. When present, there may be an increased incidence of pain, especially chronic pain. Many times, people with daytime hypersomnolence are thought to have sleep apnea, so narcolepsy may be overlooked.

Orofacial Pain and Sleep. Orofacial pain encompasses a diverse group of disorders that involve the head, face, and neck, as well as the oral cavity (mouth) and related structures. Orofacial pain involves musculoskeletal, neuropathic, and mechanical disorders, all of which may involve pain and can impact sleep. Temporomandibular disorders (TMDs) are a component of orofacial pain that involve the head and neck musculature, as well as the temporomandibular joints. In one study, patients diagnosed with TMDs had a 36% likelihood of having insomnia and a 28% chance of having sleep apnea (Lavigne 2016).

Musculoskeletal pain is the most common of all orofacial pain complaints, often referred to as TMDs. Such pain involves the musculature of the head and neck area. Several of the muscles of the head, face, and neck all interact during the day, as well as at night. The muscles of the head and jaw function during chewing, speaking, and swallowing, and some are accessory muscles for respiration. The group of four muscles known as the masticatory muscles are the ones that most often are painful, especially when palpated. In addition, they have the potential to refer pain to distant locations. This was described several decades ago by Travel and Simons. What they described were areas in a muscle, termed trigger points, that, when provoked, would be felt as pain in another location. This is known as referred pain. As an example, pain in a muscle that moves the jaw may refer to a tooth or multiple teeth. These same muscles may refer to other areas such as over the eyes, the forehead, or the face and are

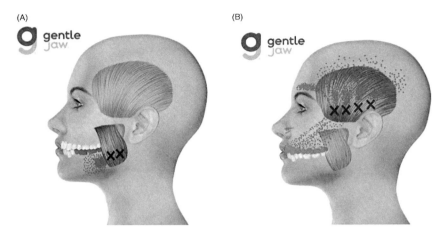

Figure 5-2. Based on the work of Travell and Simons, mapped trigger points (black X's) show possible areas (red) where pain may be felt: (A) masseter muscle and (B) temporalis muscle. Images courtesy of Dr. Rich Hirschinger, DDS, MBA, inventor of the gentle jaw.

potentially thought to reflect a headache or sinus problem. Travel and Simons mapped these trigger points, as well as the typical areas where the pain was felt (Figure 5-2).

The muscles of the neck are also important, as they help with posture and may also be involved as accessory muscles for respiration. The posture of the head is important and, when not correct, can also lead to pain that is experienced in a distant location, such as the face or jaw. The key factors that may impact head posture are previous trauma, such as a motor vehicle accident, working at a desk or computer with poor posture, or an airway that is compromised or restricted. Poor posture and head and neck support during sleep may precipitate pain that is experienced in the head, jaw, or face. The main nerve to the face and jaw, the trigeminal nerve, interacts with nerves from the cervical spine and is perceived as pain by the brain.

Neuropathic pain, and in particular trigeminal neuralgia (TN), is of particular interest in relation to sleep. Historically, TN was thought to be silent during sleep, indicating some type of protective mechanism so that it did not awaken the person. In 2008, however, it was found that this was not the case. Individuals with TN and their bed partners reported that awakenings were in fact present and common

(Devor 2008). Based on this finding and our understanding of how pain and sleep interact, it is evident that the disruption in sleep associated with TN may lead to symptoms of fatigue, including chronic tiredness and low energy during the day. There is a 20% chance that an individual with TN or neuropathy will have more awakenings during sleep or have poor-quality sleep.

Management of Orofacial Pain and Sleep. Managing any sleep disorder has the potential to impact pain positively. Therapies that may be most helpful include the following:

- *Cognitive behavioral therapy (CBT)* provides a series of lessons on how to calm the mind, relax, and improve sleep. Part of this therapy is termed sleep hygiene and is designed to eliminate distractions from the bedroom, thereby improving sleep onset, quality, and efficiency. CBT is offered by psychologists, and recently, online programs have become available. This program helps mainly with insomnia and is beneficial for pain management. Recently, an online prescription therapeutic program for chronic insomnia that is approved by the Food and Drug Administration (called Somryst) was acquired by Nox Health and should be available soon.
- *Mindfulness* is a form of meditation that can involve breathing exercises and guided imagery. The goal is to be able to achieve a feeling of relaxation in, and not overreact to, any situation.
- *Focusing on nasal breathing* as opposed to mouth breathing can be extremely helpful. Breathing through the nose increases oxygen uptake and improves oxygen levels in the bloodstream. There are aids to improve nasal breathing, called nasal dilators, that can be used at night. Aids to help prevent mouth breathing are available as well.
- If obstructive sleep apnea is suspected, consult a physician. The most common therapy is using a *continuous positive airway pressure (CPAP) device*. However, *oral appliances* are an option if the apnea is mild or moderate or if the issue is just snoring. An oral appliance moves the lower jaw forward and helps open and stabilize the airway, preventing the tongue from collapsing into the airway during sleep. These appliances may also address sleep bruxism, and this can lead to better pain control.

- Paying attention to a *good diet and adequate exercise* will help improve sleep and thus help manage the pain. Both diet and exercise are also important aspects of improved health.
- If medication has been prescribed for a sleep issue, seek an *alternate means* of addressing the sleep issue. For example, if medication has been prescribed to treat insomnia, use the medication for insomnia, but pursue CBT as well, as this may help reduce or eliminate the need for medication. Many medications have a negative impact on sleep. An exception is narcolepsy, for which medication is needed to address the physiologic cause.
- *Seek help from an orofacial pain specialist.* Recently, orofacial pain became a dental specialty. Dentists who have extensive training in this discipline are well versed in the management of orofacial pain conditions and can play a major role in helping people manage their pain. Orofacial pain specialists typically work in concert with all types of physicians, physical therapists, psychologists, and other health care providers to achieve an optimum outcome. Specialists in orofacial pain are also trained in sleep medicine, from both the diagnostic side and the management side. Most belong to the American Academy of Orofacial Pain.

Conclusion. The association between sleep dysfunction and pain is well documented. It has been reported that poor sleep is present in 50% to 80% of people with chronic pain (Ferini-Strambi 2017). However, the management of pain and sleep together may not always occur. In many cases, it may be necessary to prioritize either sleep or pain to adequately address the other. Regardless, paying attention to both will no doubt impact the priority issue as well. It is imperative that the sleep–pain bidirectional relationship be a consideration, so that optimum outcomes are the result. This will ultimately lead to more effective pain management and an improved quality of life.

5.2
Pain and Intimacy
Megan Tudor Donnelly, DO

Relationships are complex. They require time, honesty, patience, understanding, and emotional investment to succeed. Romantic intimacy is a fundamental aspect of human relationships, providing physical and emotional connection and fulfillment. However, trigeminal neuralgia (TN) pain can be triggered by even the slightest touch, such as a gentle kiss or caress. To approach the subject of romantic intimacy with TN, it is crucial to understand the condition's impact on the individual's life.

When one partner is living with a chronic pain condition such as TN, it can pose unique challenges to maintaining a healthy and satisfying romantic life. In this section, we explore how individuals with TN and their partners can approach romantic intimacy with care, empathy, and understanding.

Dating. There are certainly many people with TN who are single or dating. Having chronic facial pain can make finding the right partner challenging, but it is still possible. Even though TN can limit a person from doing activities that they might otherwise enjoy doing, such as staying out late, singing, dancing, going to loud places such as concerts, or doing activities in windy conditions, there are other activities and ways to meet a partner that do not involve these activities. Finding groups for new hobbies or interests, such as yoga, museums, acrylic painting, or a sci-fi book club, is a wonderful way to not only learn about new hobbies, but also make friends and perhaps meet a future partner.

Communication is Key. Open and honest communication is the foundation of any successful romantic relationship, especially when one partner is dealing with a chronic condition such as TN. Both partners should feel comfortable discussing their needs, concerns, and boundaries. If you meet someone new and are considering a relationship with them, I recommend being up-front with them about your medical condition and how it affects you. This is deeply personal information, and understandably, it is not the thing that you might want to tell a person on the first date, but if you foresee a future with them and want them in your life, they should know. You should use your discretion for when the timing feels right to discuss your health. As a blog post on facepain.org from April 15, 2021, states, "Romantic partners may eventually become caregivers, so it is important that they know the challenges you face. And if being in a relationship with someone who has facial pain is not something they can handle, then they are not the right person for you" (https://www.facepain.org/blog/helping-your-relationship-survive-despite-facial-pain/). If you are in a relationship, ongoing communication makes it easier for your partner to understand what you are going through, what your triggers are, and what you feel capable of doing at a given time. For example, you might have plans to go to the beach, but if it is too windy, you might need to change your plans. If your partner understands what you are going through, they will likely be more supportive and understanding of the need to change plans.

Remember that communication goes both ways, so your partner will need to have open communication with you in return. As discussed earlier, your partner may be your caregiver from time to time. They should have the opportunity to discuss how TN affects them, their needs, and their feelings. It is understandable if they may feel overwhelmed at times. That does not make them a bad partner, nor should you be made to feel like a burden for having your condition. Therapy or couples counseling can be beneficial to work through these complex emotions. As suggested on facepain.org, "make sure your partner has 'time off' every so often to take care of themselves, too. It is not just the person with facial pain who is going through this awful experience; partners, family, and devoted friends are along for the ride, too" (https://www.facepain.org/blog/helping-your-relationship-survive-despite-facial-pain/).

Educate Your Partner. If you have TN, take the time to educate your partner about the condition. Unless your partner has a background in health care, they might have extremely limited knowledge about TN. Share resources and information to help them understand what you are experiencing, both physically and emotionally. They will need to learn about the condition, triggers, treatment, and what to do (and what not to do) during an attack. You may want to invite your partner to attend doctor's appointments with you, as this is another way they can learn more about your condition, hear your physician's discussion and plan, and gain further perspective on how you are impacted by TN.

Regarding medications, it is helpful to educate your partner on potential side effects of your treatment. Many of the medications used for TN cause sedation, foggy thoughts (encephalopathy), mood change, or sexual side effects. Your partner also needs to understand that, although the goal of medication is for it to help with pain, it is not a cure-all. I have seen many partners who are trying to be supportive but have inappropriate expectations and overt frustration that a medication did not entirely eliminate pain and cure their partner. Pain relief can be incomplete, and breakthrough pain when medication wears off between doses can occur. More serious, but rare, side effects and risks also need to be discussed: What if a partner sees a new rash on you after you have started a new medication? They need to be educated about the risk of potentially life-threatening conditions such as Stevens–Johnson syndrome.

Timing Matters. TN pain can be unpredictable and vary in intensity. Be patient and flexible when it comes to intimate moments. Timing can make a significant difference in the comfort and enjoyment of both partners. For example, there is often a refractory period after a pain attack, in which the threshold to experience pain is greatly increased. In simpler terms, this means it is much more difficult to experience another pain attack during this refractory period that occurs right after an attack. One can harness the refractory period as a time to, for example, kiss their partner.

Likewise, when someone is going through a more painful time, whether it be a few minutes or even weeks, granting oneself emotional permission to avoid touches on that part of the face is quite reasonable. It is still always helpful for you to remind your partner that you still want them and appreciate their affection, but that you need to avoid ending up in worse pain. Your pain can fluctuate, and the unpredictability of TN pain can be a roller coaster for you and your partner.

On the other side, I recommend acting with spontaneity if you are having a good day. TN can steal so much, but when it is a better day, do not let it steal your joy. Take that opportunity to make last-minute plans with your partner. As recommended by facepain.org, "Suggest you see that movie your partner has wanted to see. Go for a walk because the weather is nice (and not windy). Show affection when you are willing and able to receive it. This can alleviate potential uncertainty on your partner's part" (https://www.facepain.org/blog/helping-your-relationship-survive-despite-facial-pain/).

Intimacy Reimagined. For many individuals with TN, certain sensory experiences can trigger pain. Work together with your partner to explore alternative ways to express affection. This may involve discovering nonpainful areas to touch or experimenting with several types of physical intimacy. Remember that romantic intimacy is not solely about physical affection. Intimacy quite literally means a close, familiar, and usually affectionate or loving personal relationship with another person or group. Emotional connection, verbal expressions of love, and quality time together are equally important components of a fulfilling romantic relationship. I spoke with one patient, who developed TN very shortly after her wedding, and she and her husband described how, as a result of TN and having to resort to other love languages, they have a very "flirty and cute" relationship, with a lot of hand holding, arms around each other's waists, and flirting banter, as a way to show their love and affection without focusing on what they do not have. This is reiterated by Jennifer and Dan Digmann (Jennifer and Dan both have multiple sclerosis, and Jennifer has comorbid TN) in a blog post on msfocusmagazine.org: "We no longer could kiss on the lips, but we soon found new ways to express intimate feelings for each other. Tighter and extended hugs, falling asleep while holding hands, and Dan's gentle kisses on Jennifer's forehead were the expressions of love that sustained us. These simple and meaningful acts actually pulled us closer together emotionally than we imagined was ever possible. Maybe it was because each act was rooted in the shared understanding that we are strongest when we're together" (https://msfocusmagazine.org/Magazine/Magazine-Items/Posted/Intimacy-and-MS-Make-It-Your-Own.aspx).

Emotional Support. Individuals with TN should prioritize self-care and coping strategies to manage pain and stress. Partners can play a role in helping their loved ones practice self-care, whether by assisting with relaxation techniques or simply being there to listen. It is best if your partner has patience, flexibility, and adaptability to accommodate your needs and expectations. Your partner can also help to encourage you to pursue hobbies and activities that bring you joy and fulfillment. Living with TN can be emotionally challenging. Chronic depression secondary to severe pain is common and should be actively addressed. Depression worsens pain, decreases libido, or both. Ensure that emotional support is readily available for both partners. Consider seeking the guidance of a psychotherapist or counselor who specializes in chronic pain and its effects on depression and relationships.

Your partner can be your advocate, particularly if you are not feeling heard by your physician. Partners can be your ally and another voice to speak for your needs and ensure that you receive appropriate medical attention, including seeking a second opinion if needed.

Caring Too Much. Although we all want an incredibly supportive partner, there are pitfalls when a romantic partner is overly enabling and if the focus of the relationship centers primarily on pain. This can encourage avoidant behavior, which can lead to stress and social isolation. This, in turn, can exacerbate limitations you place on yourself and create a dependent relationship. Dependency on your romantic partner is destructive to your self-esteem because it can reduce your sense of personal agency. Both you and your partner should encourage independence. Also, if conversations frequently focus on your pain to the exclusion of other topics, the relationship can falter because other relationship-maintenance issues are not being addressed. One way to avoid this pitfall is for your partner to not mention your pain and to avoid asking you if you are in pain if you have not brought it up. You need encouragement, not a constant reminder. Know that it is entirely acceptable to express when you experience intense pain. As advised by Leesa Scott-Morrow, PhD, on facepain.org, "As soon as you are able to authentically move away from focus upon your pain, do so. This will be reassuring for you and for your partner." She goes on to explain: "Understand that this experience is as terrifying for them as it is for you. Their experience of helplessness can be as great as yours" (https://www.facepain.org/blog/face-pain-relationships/). Your partner can also help to gently counter a spiral of negative or catastrophic thinking with reasoning (although psychotherapy is also often needed to unpackage catastrophic thinking). Staying active and motivated is incredibly important for your physical and psychological health if you have chronic pain. You need to maintain as much normalcy as you can, which includes staying involved in social activities and maintaining a routine, including keeping to a sleep–wake schedule, even if you are not presently working. Dr. Scott-Morrow states, "Work to retain activities that bring you pleasure and infuse your life with meaning" (https://www.facepain.org/blog/face-pain-relationships/). Make a point to actively try to participate in life, not just passively survive it. Avoid having your partner fall into the role of primary caregiver unless you need it. For example, after microvascular decompression surgery, try to limit the time of them in this role to what is needed and not to extend it further. If you can do something yourself, you should. Do not confuse caregiving with love or romance. Although there is overlap in the two concepts, they are separate things.

When To Move On. A partner who encourages and motivates but pushes you too far or feels that toxic positivity is the answer, or alternatively, a partner who enables pain behavior and encourages dependent behavior and panders to your pain—both are ultimately unhelpful and problematic. However, either of these partner behavior patterns can at least usually be remedied with education and couples psychotherapy because both come from the same place: care and concern. But what if a partner is overtly annoyed, unsupportive, belittling, and minimizes or disregards your experience? Or what if they make you feel guilty or unworthy of their love? These are massive red flags and reason to part ways and get out of that unhealthy relationship. You deserve better. Do not stay in a relationship with someone because you fear being alone or because you depend on them as your caregiver if they are otherwise not good to you. If they are not good to you, they are not good for you.

Better Together. The perception of pain is not just physiological but also psychological. Pain reception is mediated not only through the thalamus but also through higher cortical processes. Pain perception varies to some degree based on someone's state of mind. The best example of this is the experience that everything can hurt more—an example of allodynia—when someone is experiencing depression. But did you know that relationships can also affect pain perception? Research shows that patients in a relationship generally report less pain; they function better and are less likely to suffer from depression than patients who are single. Dr. Scott-Morrow explains, "Studies show that chronic pain patients experience lower levels of pain on days that begin with a sense of being happily connected to their partners; thus, relationship status can affect the patient's experience of pain on a day-to-day basis" (https://www.facepain.org/blog/face-pain-relationships/). However, the research suggests that the pain-related advantages of being in a relationship apply only to those in happy, satisfying relationships, "and even then, not in every case. When relationships are weak and distressed, pain patients tend to do poorly. They report more frequent and intense pain and show higher levels of disability." Patients in happy relationships with enabling partners also reported greater pain severity than patients in happy relationships with partners who were not enabling. This is another reason to aim for a happy, healthy, supportive relationship that fosters independence and brings out the best in each other.

Conclusion. Romantic intimacy can thrive despite the challenges of TN. It requires understanding, patience, and adaptability from both partners. By fostering open communication, seeking medical advice, exploring physical intimacy that does not exacerbate pain, and focusing on emotional connections, couples can maintain a loving and fulfilling romantic relationship while managing the impact of TN on their lives. Try to add levity to your day and encourage your partner to talk to you about non-pain-related topics, such as something funny they experienced that day. It is critically important that you continue to seek intimacy and emotional connection in ways that have nothing to do with pain. Aim to create a sense of normalcy in your life and in your relationship. A true partner will be there for you when you need it and when you need to talk about your pain experience and how it is affecting you. Such a person is along for the ride of both the good and the bad, in sickness and in health. But they also encourage independence and personal agency. And they should have permission without retribution to redirect you if you are in a spiral of catastrophic thinking. This is true for all relationships, but it is even more important when one's health is put to the test with TN.

Remember: Even though you have TN, it does not define you. You are capable and competent, and you have influence on your own life. You are still inherently the person you were before facial pain started. TN does not own you. You, being you, have something great to bring to any relationship.

Author's Note: When I was researching the topic of TN and intimacy, PubMed revealed zero relevant articles with any combination of the following search words: "intimacy," "romance," "sexual," "trigeminal neuralgia," and "facial pain." There are a couple of very insightful blog posts on the topic, as referenced in this section several times. But ultimately, this section could not have been written without the wisdom and insight of my many patients with TN who graciously shared their vulnerability and firsthand experiences in navigating romantic intimacy while living with TN.

5.3
Chronic Facial Pain and Social Security Disability
Kenneth Casey, MD, FACS

Editor's Note: There are two Social Security Administration programs that help people who meet disability requirements. The Social Security Disability Income (SSDI) program pays benefits to an individual and certain family members if that individual is "insured." This means that the individual worked long enough—and recently enough—and paid Social Security taxes on their earnings. The Supplemental Security Income (SSI) program pays benefits to adults and children who meet requirements for a qualifying disability and have limited income and resources. Although these two programs are different, the medical requirements are the same. For more information, see the website of the Social Security Administration at https://www.ssa.gov/benefits/disability.

The International Classification of Diseases, 11th edition (ICD-11), has a new code for chronic pain. This is good news for people with chronic facial pain. Previously, chronic pain had its own single designator in the ICD-10, namely, G89.4. G89.4 was labeled "chronic primary pain" and, unfortunately, included a hodgepodge of conditions lumped together, for example, neuropathic facial pain and chronic regional pain syndrome (which are not at all the same). In the new ICD classification, which became effective in January 2022, there are several subcategories for different types of chronic pain. Most importantly, there are now two new categories:

1. Chronic secondary headache or orofacial pain and
2. Chronic neuropathic pain

Either of these two categories can be used for patients with trigeminal neuralgia (TN), also called trigeminal neuropathic pain.

For the estimated 25 million Americans who are affected by chronic pain, this reorganized classification is good news, certainly on the medical and insurance front. The ICD is the coding system that insurance companies use to determine whether they will pay for medical services. In the past several years, ICD coding has devolved into somewhat of an adversarial relationship between insurance companies and physicians, hospitals, and even patients attempting to obtain reimbursement. This has led to increasing disparities in care.

Chronic pain interferes with daily functioning and is accompanied by stress. In the past, chronic pain was linked to psychogenic or mental health disorders. These are misclassifications. In 1986, Congress authorized an extensive review of this subject by doctors, lawyers, rehabilitation specialists, and representatives from the insurance industry. This was done because cases were being brought to court each year and individual judges were making decisions to clarify the definition of disability and the amount of disability that an applicant had incurred. In some different venues, and even among judges in the same venue, the results would vary widely. Congress recognized that this was not what they intended in setting up a pain section within the guidelines of the Social Security Administration (SSA).

The Blue Book, formally titled *Disability Evaluation Under Social Security*, lists impairments the SSA considers severe enough to prevent a person from working and lays out the medical criteria for determining if that person can receive disability benefits. Disability evaluation under Social Security starts with application of the concepts in the Blue Book, including the adult and pediatric listings of all currently accepted impairments in medicine and surgery. This is important because the presence of your impairment in the Blue Book simplifies the process. This is true for both adult listings and childhood listings. The evidentiary requirements include medical evidence, which is the cornerstone of the disability determination. It is up to the patient to obtain medical evidence demonstrating the impairment and the severity of the impairment. The SSA will try to help by obtaining hospital records (which may be otherwise difficult to get) and records from different physicians who may have seen you for this condition and treated you, even briefly (such as Emergency Department providers).

By law, specific medical evidence establishes that the claimant has an impairment and can show objective evidence based on acceptable medical science that covers the severity and the degree of impairment. The SSA may require that the applicant obtain additional consultative examinations to establish evidence related to the symptoms.

Evidence related to symptoms can include claimants' daily activities; the duration, frequency, and intensity of the pain symptoms; precipitating and aggravating factors; the type, dosage, and effectiveness of medications, along with their side effects; treatments other than medications that have been tried for relief, as well as other techniques such as massage or similar nonmedical approaches; and the impairment and limitations that the pain imposes on the claimant's day-to-day existence and lifestyle.

For individuals with TN, lack of appropriate codes makes accurate epidemiological investigations difficult and impedes health policy decisions regarding chronic pain and adequate financing of access to multimodal pain management. Chronic pain is usually defined as pain that persists or recurs for more than 3 months. However, in the Social Security lexicon, for pain to be considered chronic, it must have been present for a year, and it must be expected to last for at least one year. Chronic pain can be the sole or leading component, for example, in fibromyalgia or nonspecific low back pain. Under existing Social Security law, for pain to be considered in evaluating disability, there must be organic evidence of a physical or mental impairment that could be expected to produce that pain.

In summary, to be a candidate for Social Security Disability

1. You must have had the condition for one year and expect it to last for an additional year and
2. You must have supportive medical evidence, including:
   a. A medical evaluation that documents
      i. location of the pain;

  ii. duration of the pain;

  iii. frequency of the pain;

  iv. current medications used for the pain and their side effects; and

  v. other treatments and practices, including something as simple as rest or ice packs;

 b. Radiologic evidence of any anatomical abnormality.

Meeting these requirements will still not be enough to obtain approval for SSI or SSDI benefits. The SSA will want to review your residual functional capacity to evaluate how your symptoms affect your daily activities. This is a formal evaluation. Usually a neurologist, physiatrist (rehabilitation physician), or physical therapist conducts this evaluation.

Although individual claimants can certainly file for compensation, the number and widespread extent of court cases suggests that, all too often, legal help is necessary to pursue a claim to its conclusion. Most law offices operate under the premise that you, as a client, have obtained a good deal of the information for them; then they will seek more information from the individuals who you have identified as your primary physicians and other specialists consulted in the pain treatment process. Then, the law firm will proceed to file your claim. If necessary, the law firm will even proceed to court, all of which unfortunately comes at some expense to you. Your best chance for obtaining SSI or SSDI benefits for chronic pain syndrome is to apply with multiple medical impairments or show that your disability stems from a related medical condition that is listed in the Blue Book. Oftentimes, in a case involving this group of ailments that has been denied, a hearing before an administrative law judge takes place with or without legal representation. That judge is attempting to use the Blue Book, and in complex cases of chronic pain syndrome, the judge will need primary documentation of one of the conditions that you have claimed.

If we consider TN as an example, the codes could include both neuropathic pain and orofacial pain, which would be an example of multiple listings, thereby providing the appropriate legal status and legal weight to an argument for compensation. If you are denied disability status, counsel may facilitate your case.

Note from *Medical Editor Jeffrey Brown, MD, FACS, FAANS:* The SSA may require periodic reevaluation of your disability status. It can discontinue benefits if it believes that your condition no longer meets its criteria. It can reduce your benefits if you receive support from family for expenses or housing or if your income increases for any reason beyond its thresholds. There can thus be regrettable negative emotional consequences to what should only be a positive experience in your life.

5.4
Tips on Affording Your Prescription Medication

Lindsey Wallace, MBA, YPC Co-Chair, Certified Pharmacy Technician CPhT, Registered Technologist (Radiography) American Registry of Radiologic Technologists RT(R)(ARRT)

I was unprepared that the reality of having chronic health conditions would leave me in a state of financial insecurity. Over the past few years, I have learned to advocate not only for myself, but also for my patients. I want to share with you some of the most common questions we get at the pharmacy from patients who are struggling to afford their medication and what can be done to lower the cost.

Why did the insurance company reject a claim for medication, and what happens now?

Prior authorization: This is a term that nearly all of us have heard; however, many patients do not understand what it means or what the process is. If a medication requires a prior authorization, it could mean several things:

1. The medication is not covered by your insurance plan.
2. The medication is covered by your plan, but you must meet certain requirements for it to pay. When this happens, your doctor needs to submit information to the insurance company to prove that the medication is medically necessary.
3. The medication is covered by your plan, but it requires step therapy. This means that the insurance would rather pay for cheaper alternatives. If you have tried alternative medications and they were not a good fit for you, your doctor can submit this information to insurance to get the medication covered.

The next big question is what needs to be done about the rejected claim. When the rejection pops up at the pharmacy, the pharmacy will contact your doctor's office and inform them that a prior authorization needs to be completed. Your doctor's office will then contact your insurance company and provide them with the required information. Then, it is up to the insurance company to decide if it is going to cover the medication. Sometimes, an immediate response will be provided; however, it could take several days for the insurance company to decide if it will cover the medication. There is not much you can do during this process.

If the prior authorization is denied, there is still hope. Your doctor can appeal the denial of the prior authorization. If the appeal is also denied, they can file a second-level appeal. Finally, if that is denied, most insurance companies will let you ask for an external appeal through a third party.

What if a brand-name medication is not covered?

Patient assistance programs: The manufacturers want you to take their brand-name medications. They often have programs to help you get those medications. For example, if you are financially struggling or meet certain requirements, then you may be eligible for these programs. To see if you qualify, reach out to the manufacturer, and explain your situation. You will never know how they might be able to help you until you reach out.

Independent pharmacy programs: Some independent pharmacies are partnered with the manufacturers of brand-name medications. Through such a partnership, the pharmacy will sell the manufacturer's medication for an extremely discounted "cash price." This information should be listed on the medication's website.

If a brand-name medication is covered, how can I make it affordable?

Manufacturer savings: If you take a brand-name medication and have commercial insurance, manufacturer savings programs are your best friends. Nearly all brand-name medications have a coupon from the manufacturer. There are two ways to get manufacturer coupons: online and at your doctor's office. If you go online, search on "[drug name] savings," and click on the medication's website. There will be a quick form to fill out. Then, you download the savings card or receive it by email. Take the card to the pharmacy, so the pharmacy can apply the savings.

What if a generic medication is not covered?

Prescription savings cards: If a noncovered medication is not a name brand, prescription savings cards and programs can help you. There are websites where you can search for the name of your medication and find the prices of the medication with a coupon card at different local pharmacies. Not all pharmacies accept these discounts, however. Check with your pharmacy first.

Pharmacy savings programs: Grocery stores, wholesale clubs, and many retail pharmacies offer prescription savings programs. Grocery stores often have a list of medications that they sell for a discounted price for 30- and 90-day supplies. Wholesale stores typically offer a discount for those who pay for a membership to their club. The cost of the membership is well worth the savings. Many retail pharmacies are starting to offer similar programs. If you pay a yearly fee, you can receive huge discounts on your prescriptions.

What if I cannot afford my medication(s)?

State-run assistance programs: If you are having a hard time affording your medication(s), some states offer Medicaid programs that you can use as a supplement. Many states also have state pharmaceutical assistance programs (SPAPs) that may help pay for prescription drugs based on financial need, age, or medical conditions. Each state has different rules and requirements. Your State Health Insurance Assistance Program (SHIP) is a good source of information.

Assistance programs run by nonprofit groups: These programs will help pay for your prescriptions. There are several ways to find nonprofit assistance programs. If you are religious, check with your place of worship. Many will have assistance programs set up for their members that can sometimes even help people outside of the organization. Although I am unaware of a program for those with trigeminal neuropathic pain, there are some conditions with dedicated assistance programs that help with copays. If you have other conditions, it could be worth looking into this possibility. There are also programs online for those with low income or on disability benefits. If you need help, reach out to several programs and see what you qualify for. These programs exist to help.

Prescription savings cards and programs: Even if a medication is covered by your insurance, sometimes, you can get it for less by using savings cards and programs.

I am on Medicare. Are there programs for me?

If your income and resources fall below certain limits, you may be able to qualify for the Extra Help program to help pay for your drug costs and premiums. This program is also called the "low-income subsidy" or LIS. There are four ways to see if you qualify.

1. Check your Medicare and You handbook.
2. Call 1-800-MEDICARE (1-800-633-4227) (or TTY 1-877-486-2048), available toll-free 24 hours a day, 7 days a week.
3. Call the SSA Office (1-800-772-1213) or (TTY 1-800-325-0778) between 7 am and 7 pm, Monday through Friday.
4. Call your state Medicaid office.

If a drug you need is not initially covered, try these resources. You may get relief from pain and financial worries.

Edior's Note: Some U.S. residents purchase drugs from Canada at lower costs than U.S. pharmacies charge. While the Food and Drug Administration (FDA) prohibits such imports, it does not actively prosecute individuals who import up to a three month supply of drugs for their own use. Drugs purchased from Canada do not undergo rigorous U.S. FDA evaluation and regulation. Thus, there may be quality and safety concerns. ALWAYS consult with your doctor before purchasing drugs from a Canadian pharmacy.

Chapter 6
Our Stories

Anne B. Ciemnecki, MA

Storytelling is an art form that has been around for centuries. Storytelling transcends times and cultures. Storytellers entertain and inspire. They have the ability to transport listeners to another place and time. They make people laugh, cry, or think about the world in a new way. Storytellers have the power to change lives.

In Chapter 6, five brave souls who live with neuropathic facial pain and more tell their stories. We hear from a young person raised in a religious "cult," from a person whose pain was caused by compression from a tumor, from a person with multiple medical conditions including an amputation who says that facial pain was the worst of her afflictions, and from a young woman who managed her pain through two pregnancies and deliveries. These storytellers do not want your sympathy. They tell their stories to inspire you—perhaps to change your life.

My favorite artist these days is Brandi Carlisle. In her song "The Story," she sings:

> All of these lines across my face
>
> Tell you the story of who I am
>
> So many stories of where I've been
>
> And how I got to where I am
>
> But these stories don't mean anything
>
> When you've got no one to tell them to
>
> It's true, I was made for you.

Chapter 6 was made for you.

6.1
Telling Our Stories
Pari Shah, Rachel Chance, and Raymond F. Sekula Jr., MD

Editor's Note: Before we read five lived experiences of people with trigeminal neuropathic pain (TNP), Shah, Chance, and Sekula write about the real costs of TNP. To some extent, we all feel the challenges: pain, isolation, loss of a job, chronic fatigue, depression, lack of adequate health insurance, and the perceived or real burden on family and friends. The authors back this up with vignettes they found on social media, namely, on blogs such as "The Mighty" and "The Pain Corner" and on youtube. com. Despite these challenges, we are strong. We are not alone. We belong to a community through the Facial Pain Association (FPA) that advocates and educates. We have jobs, raise children, climb mountains, and make music. We are artists and grandparents. We are educators, judges, lawyers, doctors, writers, and business owners. Through conferences and support groups, we form strong friendships with others who have TNP. We are a force to be reckoned with within the public policy arena. In 2025, the FPA will launch a patient registry though the National Organization of Rare Disorders. We will pool data provided by members to advocate for ourselves. One of the first registry projects will be to demonstrate that our community needs and deserves government disability support. I tell my friends that I have turned pain into power. You can too.

"You can either let it defeat you, or you can rise up against it... If you're living with trigeminal neuralgia, you are one of the strongest people in the world"—*The Pain Corner*

Every year in the United States, 15,000 people are diagnosed with trigeminal neuralgia (TN), a diagnosis of extreme facial pain. They describe the pain in various ways, including "gnawing," "stabbing," and "electrical." TN is known for its insufferable episodes, which cause emotional and physical limitations to peoples' everyday lives, thereby diminishing their quality of life. TN may change the dynamic of families, trigger financial insecurity, and take years to diagnose, thereby significantly impacting one's mental health. Individuals battling TN are considered some of the "strongest people in the world." Many are advocating for themselves and others by telling their stories. Through background research and interviews with people with TN, we have tried to capture their experiences of battling TN.

This overwhelming, uncontrollable, falling-to-your-knees kind of pain can dominate one's life through repetitive attacks. Whether it's driving your child from school with an episode waiting for you around the corner or attempting to focus at work when the seemingly benign air conditioning triggers the trigeminal nerve, TN forces individuals to alter their lifestyle. Even though people with TN might prefer to stay within the comforts of their homes to avoid additional external stimuli, most have jobs to attend to, families to take care of, and a desire to return to normal life.

When interviewed, Kerri Salas, an individual with TN, stated, "I can't continue to have a work life… it's so hard with trigeminal neuralgia." Going to work is a routine that provides structure to many peoples' lives and imparts a sense of normalcy; however, work may be out of reach for people with chronic pain or intense episodes. A young woman who earned her doctorate in physical therapy took an extended break to undergo deep brain stimulation surgery for TN. Despite her original intention to return to work after 2 months, she has yet to do so because of her compromised abilities due to TN. An aspiring actor in New York City underwent microvascular decompression surgery, which was complicated by left-side paralysis in the face. This complication ended her career. Another woman, after working hard to develop an independent business, had to close down her company to fund her TN surgery; she ran through all of her savings. The economic instability of an unreliable income creates additional stress for people worrying about paying for surgery, medications, or fees for travel to TN specialists.

Individuals with TN who support their families feel incredible pressure to suppress their pain and carry on with their responsibilities. Although part of being an adult comes with balancing several factors such as work, family life, and self-care, adding a chronic pain shifts all those other factors to the periphery and demands central attention. As Samah Khan wrote in The Mighty blog, "when you've spent your whole day battling your own body along with trying to be civil to people you can't avoid, like family, you are too worn down and exhausted emotionally to partake in conversation" (Khan 2022). When researching TN and interviewing people with this condition, we noticed that TN often disrupts family dynamics and relationships. Salas explained, "I do think [TN] does [interfere with my relationship with my kids] because there are times I can't be as affectionate as I would like to, or I have to push their affection down because they don't understand it's hurting me—it's a struggle." TN pain and its effects may create a metaphysical barrier between people with TN and those around them. This isolation takes a toll on their mental health as they feel increasingly distanced from the people closest to them. A large part of the battle of TN is overcoming depression and learning to accept help from the community.

One patient said, "Just as I've learned to live with this disease, my husband and my kids [have] learned to live with it too; it's never just the person with TN." When one family member faces an issue, the entire family is affected. With any chronic illness, the family must make sacrifices to ensure the health of their loved one. With TN, the sacrifices can be financial, funneling all savings toward surgery and medication, or they can involve self-care, prioritizing responsibilities for the person in pain over oneself. With all that attention, patients often develop "self-perceived burden" syndrome, where they view themselves as a liability hindering their family's progress. They may perceive themselves as a chronic burden to their family and, therefore, try to minimize the appearance of their suffering. This feeling of burden is experienced across all age groups and medical morbidities. For example, the aspiring New York City actor mentioned previously had lost contact with close family during her TN process. She needed her eye sewn shut because of chronic infections resulting from TN surgery and treatments. Her sister refused to allow her son to see this, fearing that it would scare him, so she forced the actor to wear sunglasses around the family. When her nephew grew curious about the eye, she finally showed him. Her sister saw this interaction and forbade contact between the two. Currently, the actor runs her own online community called "Women in Pain," a support group recognizing women in similar situations. She has shown that a supportive community is of utmost importance. Being part of a community can improve morale and help tackle the complexities of

TN, many of which are not clearly appreciated by others. As another example, a study from the Iran School of Medical Science discovered that elderly people with chronic pain had been suppressing their pain to feel less like a burden towards their families. When researchers asked a group of individuals with chronic pain why they did not want to continue life support, 93% responded with comments such as the following: "I worry that my caregiver is helping me beyond their ability," "I worry that I will be considered a 'huge problem' for my caregiver," and "I am concerned that my caregiver's health will suffer as a result of my care" (McPherson 2007).

There is often a stigma associated with invisible disabilities—a psychological, physical, or neurological condition that is not easily recognized based on someone's external appearance. Examples include schizophrenia, diabetes, epilepsy, and TN. More than 42 million Americans have disabilities, and an overwhelming 96% of them are invisible. It is difficult to make anyone understand something they cannot see; therefore, the responses to encountering someone with these disabilities can range. Many people may respond by offering advice such as to take up meditation or to stop eating certain foods, despite not having any real expertise. Others may perceive people with these conditions as malingerers or weak individuals. Even families and doctors sometimes underestimate the intensity that their relative or patient is experiencing. The challenge of convincing others that you are experiencing this pain makes the diagnosis process frustrating—and often drawn out.

When first experiencing TN pain, often localized near the jaw or mouth, where a branch of the trigeminal nerve is, many people go to see a dentist for help. Dentists, sometimes unaware of this relatively uncommon condition, may perform unnecessary procedures in an attempt to alleviate the patient's pain. Salas recalls that she "had two root canals in [her] same front tooth that apparently never needed it." After much time and distress, a path of redirections and consultations will usually lead patients to specialists, such as neurologists and neurosurgeons. Meanwhile, all this time in between is filled with feelings of confusion, hopelessness, and pain. "I feel like I have been through the ringer, like I am actually 60 years old when I am 37," Salas describes. The frustration persists throughout misdiagnoses and doctors processing the subjective pain that the patient is enduring. This often leaves people in pain feeling confused and invalidated. One person shared, "before [my diagnosis], I was told 'well you have migraines, it's okay,' and it made me feel like I was weak and unable to deal with something that other people could." Another individual was even told that they needed to floss more, and others have been misdiagnosed with sinus infection, mononucleosis (often referred to as mono), fibromyalgia, and other conditions. These stories are all similar; they are filled with misdirection and confusion that leads the person in pain down a path of prolonged misery. Ultimately, reaching a TN diagnosis is based heavily on medical history, symptom descriptions, and physical examination. It also relies on ruling out the possibility of other diseases such as postherpetic neuralgia, cluster headaches, and temporomandibular joint disorders. Diagnostically, a magnetic resonance imaging (MRI) scan is often performed, but MRI does not always clarify the diagnosis. The time to diagnosis ranges for each patient: For Kerri Salas, it took two years, whereas for another patient, it took around two decades. Despite advances in medical technology and information, the path to a TN diagnosis remains delayed and complex.

Because of this delay of diagnosis and the stigma around invisible illnesses, acquiring disability insurance for TN can be extremely difficult. Many disability insurance services consider the doctor's assessment of a patient's pain much more seriously than a patient's description of their experience. Because TN patients often struggle to get a diagnosis or do not meet criteria for impairment, they cannot receive disability benefits. Even when they do receive a diagnosis of TN, the effects and pain of TN often do not meet the application's criteria. When Kiz, the author of *The Pain Corner*, a blog sharing her journey with TN, applied to the Personal Independence Payment (PIP) program, a service that financially assists people with long-term disabilities in the United Kingdom, she scored 0 points. She did not qualify for any services, as her TN diagnosis did not align with what the program defined as a disability. (The Pain Corner 2023) Disability across the world has many definitions, most related to employment. In the Netherlands, individuals qualify as having a disability if they are unable to earn as much as a "trained healthy" person in their community. In Germany, disability is defined by the country's social code as people earning less than a fixed income. (Nash Disability Law 2020) As seen through these definitions, disability is more of a social construct, and these national programs attempt to base their judgment of disability on how much or how little people contribute to society, rather than the hardship that the person is enduring. When asked about the Canadian Pension Plan (CPP), Cathryn Boadway, a TN patient, responded, "It all seems very much focused on whether or not I could be working, as opposed to whether my health and overall wellness is improved." (Boadway 2021) Many find disability applications daunting because of their time-consuming nature and long waiting process. When Salas was asked if she had signed up for the Social Security Disability Insurance (SSDI) program, she stated, "No I haven't [signed up] because I heard it was so difficult that it is not worth trying." Moreover, because TN is not listed as a disability on the SSDI website, it takes an extra step to prove to the program that you deserve the benefits.

A process that requires the stamina of TN changes one's perception of others. Patients report that having TN has given them empathy for others suffering from disabilities or chronic pain, saying, for example, "I know everyone suffers in some way, and I just keep hoping people do not have to deal with this pain." TN shapes a patient's life socially, economically, and psychologically, leading to a reflected view of the world. As Salas described, "Being strong is something we have to do; the world has to be strong, everybody has to, or we just get sucked up." Perseverance is key to battling TN. You advocate for yourself either in the doctor's office or through the disability benefits process, attempting to make others understand the extent of your pain. When asked how she continues to have hope through such a difficult process, Boadway explains, "I do not believe that we can really live ... without an underlying current of hope in our lives." She shared a quote from *Chronically Honest*, a popular Instagram account that illustrates the hardships of chronic illnesses, that she believes summarizes her view on hope while having TN: "It is so hard trying to balance remaining hopeful with not getting your hopes up too high due to the seemingly inevitable letdown" (Boadway 2021). This ability to continue to have an optimistic attitude toward the future, acknowledging that there is a part of your life you cannot control, is inspirational. If you look at the comments on the YouTube video *Life with Trigeminal Neuralgia - Cathryn's story*, a common sentiment is "I'm also going through this, thank you for sharing." As TN patients continue to share their stories through research, interviews, and social media, they realize that they are not alone. "When someone's willing to be vulnerable and let people in, it brings together this sense of community" (Boadway 2021). We thank all of the patients who are willing to tell their stories and appreciate this opportunity to share them with the world.

> Editor's Note: You just read about the challenges that people with Trigeminal Neuropathic Pain (TNP) experience. Now, read how five amazing people overcame these challenges. They are not unique. People with TNP confront and conquer challenges every day. You can too.

6.2
Facial Pain Will Never Steal My Smile
Laura Launderville

To my family, who has always believed my pain was real.

To my twin sister, who has always held my hand.

And to my partner, who has always seen me as just me, Laura.

I love you all so very dearly.

I come from a small rural town in the middle of nowhere, Virginia. Other small towns littered with farming fields surround me. Corn, cotton, peanuts, and soybean fields are close to my heart. When I see them, I instantly feel at home. I love watching the wind roll over the fields like ocean waves. Some of my fondest memories are walking down backroads and feeling the wind come off the fields and hit me, leaving my hair a windblown mess. I never expected to have those memories splattered with the worst pain I have ever experienced. I never thought the wind could hurt until it did.

Trigeminal neuralgia (TN) interrupted my life, making an unannounced, unnamed entrance when I was 17 years old. I had no idea then how painful life would become—and how much of an impact this pain would have.

I had dental work done—just a few fillings in my front teeth. A month or so later, a strange pain surfaced. I thought it was of dental origin, so I returned to my family dentist. He was confused but thought some of my teeth might be impacted. And so, the extractions started. The pain was beyond anything I can explain. The prescribed Vicodin did not even approach, let alone reduce, the pain. My dentist was utterly confused when I showed back up *after* the first extraction with the same pain. I knew something was wrong. That strange pain was *excruciating*. It was somewhere lodged in the back of my jaw and in the right side of my mouth. I could never fully pinpoint the pain for my dentist. So, when I showed up *again* in pain, he decided to pull another tooth, even though there was clearly nothing wrong with it.

Once again, the pain was there. It was stronger than the pain from a recent extraction. When I returned yet again, the dentist wanted to do another procedure, but he admitted that he did not know what was wrong. I knew deep down that this was not a dental issue. I stubbornly refused and decided to just deal with the pain.

Unfortunately, pain was not allowed to be shown in the world in which I grew up. Perfection was demanded; sickness was perceived as amoral and as a character failing. You could not really be "that sick" or in "that much pain." You couldn't be in pain at all. Being within this world taught me to hide my pain. I was forced to neglect my needs. Survival mode kicked in and thrust me forward.

I lived in survival mode for years, continuously slipping in and out of remissions. Terrified as my symptoms worsened, my facial pain spread until it took up residence in all three branches of the right side of my face. I was left at its mercy.

I finally found a bit of courage and reached out for help from my small-town primary care doctor. The doctor said to buy a night guard and the pain would go away. The doctor advised that I go to the dentist even though I shared my dental experiences. I was shamed for not going back. I was once again defeated, feeling unseen and unheard. I was brushed aside by doctors when it had taken so much courage for me to ask for help. I slipped back into survival mode.

My pain levels fluctuated, and I continued to adapt. I avoided things that would trigger my pain. I tried anything that would reduce the pain: soft and liquid diets, limited talking and laughing, staying out of the wind, and not touching my face. I even stopped wearing makeup.

I often wished that I would find what was ailing me, but whenever I reached out for answers, I was left feeling even more alone and scared. I continued to do what I could without the resources I needed.

I cannot grasp or put into words the fear, anxiety, and depression that accompany the experience of a rare condition such as TN. I would wake up to a new day and a new symptom. I have very emotional memories of the progression of my facial pain. TN slowly and steadily chipped away at my face and, with it, my life. My early 20s slipped away from me; each day was spent fighting the unnamed monster that had taken over my life.

The first breakthrough came from a library book. My twin sister had picked up a book about the human brain and was diving into it. Excitedly, she came over to me, book in hand, pointed to the diagram on the page, and said, "Laura, I think this is where your pain is!" I took a look and read the words "trigeminal nerve." The more I read, the more I became certain that this, indeed, was where my pain was located. That was the first time that I experienced hope. With that first breakthrough as a clue, I eagerly searched online for information. I finally stumbled across the term "trigeminal neuralgia." I was struck with fear with what I read. Then, I was reminded that I had survived this long; I deserved to name the pain that so negatively impacted my life. My next step was finding support groups online. The moment I read people's stories and symptoms, I knew this was what I had. I knew I had TN. And for the very first time, I knew I wasn't alone. It was through these support groups that I was pointed toward treatment and reassured that I was strong and supported.

Unfortunately, by the time I had found these answers, I was about to turn 26 years old and lose my medical insurance. I couldn't work. Medicaid was not available to me. I was in a rush to see a neurologist and get my diagnosis. I was desperate for some relief! My father pulled some strings, and I was able to make an appointment with his neurologist on the pretense of a migraine. I remember sitting on the exam table as I described my symptoms to the neurologist. His mouth dropped open, and as he pointed to my father, he said, "TN is a condition that people your age get, not a 17-year-old girl." He was in shock. I was not.

I knew that my pain was real, and I was determined to be heard, believed, and diagnosed. Two days before Christmas, I had an MRI scan. My neurologist thought there was a good chance that I had multiple sclerosis (MS) and told me to prepare for that or a brain tumor. This all terrified me, but I pushed through, knowing that, regardless of the diagnosis, I was close to getting answers. I remember going into the first MRI machine. The technician was kind and reassured me that I was in good hands. I waited over the Christmas and New Year's holidays until I got the results. With my twin sister holding my hand, the nurse told me I did not have MS and it was not a brain tumor. It was TN. The moment I got off the phone, my twin sister and I hugged each other, crying and jumping up and down excitedly. Not because of the diagnosis, but because *I had my diagnosis*. After nearly a decade, I had my official diagnosis. I cried tears of relief.

I would later find out that the radiologist who read my scans was the first person to fight for me. He argued with my neurologist, who still did not believe that I could have TN at my age. I will forever be grateful for that radiologist. He will never know how much getting an accurate diagnosis helped me or how much it meant to have someone advocate for me.

It took nearly 2 years before I found a treatment that helped. The world was shut down because of COVID, and that added to the extra wait time to get medical insurance and see a new neurologist. During that time, I experienced the worst flare-ups of my life. I remember barely being able to talk to the receptionist scheduling my appointment.

When she told me it would be a year's wait, I broke down on the phone, started to cry, and begged. I told her that I had TN and no medication. She found me an appointment within the next 2 months. I was lucky to find a neurology team that not only understood TN but also treated it. Once again, hope grew.

It took some trial and error, but at last, I found medication that relieved my pain. I had a 2-year remission. I had a few small flare-ups of pain, but adjusting the medication led me to a pain-free period. Could that change? Yes. I know that, any day, that could change. That is the reality of having something like TN. I try to live in the present. And I know that, whatever comes, I will get through it, because I already have.

TN took a lot from me; I won't lie about that. Honesty is important when sharing my TN journey. But I have gained from such a horrendous condition, too. TN brought not only pain, but also a community. I made wonderful friendships. I found an empathy for those in chronic pain. It is one thing for someone to say "I understand"; it's quite another when you know that the person saying those words really *does* understand. This condition has given me a passion to help others with facial pain and chronic illness. It has shown me a tenacity that I never knew I had. The truth is, TN has forever changed me as a person. And although I do not believe I needed to have something as painful and horrible as facial pain, with that pain has also come beautiful growth.

Fast forward to today and I never could have imagined I would be where I am now. For so long, all of life was about working through one episode of pain at a time. It was breathing through one attack and bracing for the next. It was bleakly looking at the future, and with it, the fear of never experiencing wonderful things because of my facial pain. Then, there was the fear of putting myself out there to experience wonderful things but being terrified of how to do so through the pain. I believed deeply that TN would steal joy from me. Steal happiness. Steal more time from me. Steal my very life. But I learned that pain and joy can coexist. Happiness is truly homemade. Facial pain did not have to be the deciding factor on whether I experienced wonderful things.

One of the things I genuinely wanted was a loving relationship despite TN. That took a lot of courage for me. And vulnerability. But it was worth it. I have experienced the vulnerability of putting myself in the dating world. And I have experienced love. I know the gentleness and compassion of a partner who still sees me as me and views my TN and health as just a part of me; not the whole of me. I am making a home with the love of my life and our two kitties, our little Luna and silly Charlotte, whose personalities are as different as their sizes. I love the life that I am building.

I love that, out of experiencing a unique pain, I have been able to give back to the empowering, wonderful, and strong community that welcomed me with open arms. This community breathed life into me when I so desperately needed it. It instilled in me the message that I was not as alone as I felt. It is a community filled with people who not only understand but genuinely care. I am honored that I belong to this community, I am honored to share my story, and I am honored to volunteer with the Facial Pain Association (FPA) and the Young Patients Committee (YPC).

I am grateful each day for my father, my twin sister, my other sisters, and my brother—the people who always believed that my pain was real. They have fought hard for me and have held me through TN episodes. My twin sister, especially, has been by my side on the darkest days. The darkness that comes with chronic pain often felt like it would swallow me up. I am grateful for my boyfriend, who has gently held me during the days when chronic illness overwhelmed me. He has reminded me of my strength and has walked hand-in-hand with me on my journey. My loved ones have been my rock; they have not only loved me, but also believed in me and championed me. I am blessed.

Over time, and with continuous healing, I am showing the 17-year-old me, who so desperately needed her pain to be seen and validated, that her pain was, indeed, real. And regardless of what others said, being bullied and not having been believed back then, she is seen now. And she is loved.

I have come a long way. And facial pain did not stop me. But most of all, it will never steal the smile within me.

> In memory of my friend and fellow warrior, Angel.
>
> She now flies with butterflies.
>
> August 18, 1993–May 2, 2022

6.3
Turning Pain into Hope
Vince Holtmann, MA, MS

June 11, 2008: I wake up, extremely nauseous, in an unfamiliar room. My head aches, as though gripped in a vice, and the room is spinning around me. And yet I know, without a doubt, that today marks a new beginning and is quite possibly the best day of my life.

The events leading up to that unforgettable day had begun about 3 years earlier. I started to experience sharp, yet brief shocks of pain on the left side of my face, above my teeth and just to the side of my nostril. I felt the pain when opening my mouth before taking a bite of food, and it would be gone before I had bitten down. I scheduled a dental appointment, but by the time of the visit, I was no longer having the pain episodes. The dentist took X-rays and said that everything looked normal.

On January 2, 2006, the pain episodes started again. Except now, they were lasting for several seconds and felt like jolts of electricity, considerably worse than the worst possible toothache. The only option for me to see a doctor that day was to see my allergist. Amazingly, he diagnosed something he had never diagnosed before in a patient: trigeminal neuralgia (TN), an extremely rare facial nerve pain. He informed me that TN is considered one of the most excruciatingly painful medical conditions and is often difficult to treat.

He prescribed Tegretol, which nearly eliminated the painful episodes, and referred me to a neurologist. The neurologist ordered an MRI scan, and a few days later, she called to reveal the news: "Mr. Holtmann, you have a mass in your brain." My heart started pounding. My thoughts immediately turned to brain cancer and how aggressive it can be. She was unsure whether the nearly 1-inch-diameter tumor was cancer. I would have to wait two exceedingly long weeks for more information from a neurosurgeon.

Although the neurosurgeon was fairly certain that the tumor was a noncancerous meningioma, its location was problematic. The tumor lay along my brain stem, pressing on five cranial nerves, including the fifth, or trigeminal, nerve. Exams also showed that I had hearing loss in my left ear and no gag reflex. I was deathly afraid of surgery and joked with family members to hide my fear. "Don't worry," I would tell them. "The surgeon says the operation is a real no-brainer." After consulting with three other local neurosurgeons, I was relieved to have CyberKnife radiation as an option to shrink the tumor. The neurosurgeon assured me that, if the radiation didn't work, I could always have surgery.

Within 6 months of the radiation treatments, the pain had nearly disappeared. But after about a year, it started coming back. After maxing out on Tegretol, I was now up to the maximum dose for Trileptal. That's when things began to snowball. My wife and I were eating dinner at a restaurant when I suddenly began laughing hysterically. My wife abruptly escorted me out as I staggered and laughed like someone who'd had too much to drink. On the way home, I developed double vision. We called the neurologist's exchange and were informed that I had a case of hyponatremia, or low sodium, and instructed me not to take any more Trileptal. The next day, the neurologist prescribed Keppra.

Gradually, my pain worsened. One morning, a steady barrage of lightning strikes of pain began shooting through my face every 15 minutes. I couldn't speak, eat, open my mouth, or clear my throat. The slightest movement of my face triggered excruciating pain. The attacks felt like someone had connected one electrode to my lip, another above the corner of my left eye, then pulled the switch to electrocute my face. These episodes were lasting for more than a minute instead of a few seconds, burning as if a hot frying pan were being held against my face. My eye and face turned bright red, the muscles around my eye spasmed, and tears streamed down my cheek. It was unbearable and unrelenting—every 15 minutes.

I called my neurologist's office that morning and again that afternoon, explaining that I was in severe pain. The Keppra clearly was not working. I needed to speak with the neurologist just as soon as she was available. The receptionist finally called back and informed me that the neurologist said she could talk with me at her next available opening in a week.

My wife decided to take me to the hospital emergency department (ED) instead of waiting for that appointment. Upon seeing a couple of my painful episodes, the doctors assured me that they were going to eliminate my pain. They promptly administered doses of two drugs I had never heard of before: Fentanyl and Dilaudid. For about 30 minutes, the pain level dropped considerably, until I became very nauseated and began vomiting. The vomiting immediately triggered the every-quarter-hour episodes of pain again. Against my wife's advice, my parents came to see me at the hospital. Soon realizing that they couldn't bear to watch me in such pain, they decided it would be best to go home and pray for me. It was a long, painful, sleepless night.

The next morning, another doctor suggested an intravenous (IV) drip of Cerebyx. Amazingly, by midafternoon, the pain episodes had stopped. I began to eat, talk, and feel good again. That's when my neurologist showed up with several medical students in tow. She was not happy that I had gone to the ED without her approval. "So, you think if you open your mouth to speak, you will have pain," she said to me. I nodded my head in agreement. "No," she said, "I want you to open your mouth and say it." When I said yes, she quickly replied, "Aha! If you would just open your mouth, you could speak." Then, she directed the nurse to remove the IV and discharge me. Horrified, I explained that I was only able to speak because of the IV medications and worried that, once those medications wore off, the pain would return. I will never forget her final words of advice to me: "It's pain. Learn to live with it!"

An hour or more passed as they readied the discharge papers. By now, the IV meds had begun to wear off, and I was in no shape to go home. I remember tightly gripping the bed rails as hospital staff threatened to have security remove me if I didn't leave. My nurse watched in disbelief as I cringed in pain. I finally gave in and left.

After another night of unrelenting painful episodes and sleeplessness, my wife took me back to the ED. The doctor insisted on calling my neurologist, who wouldn't allow them to admit me. I begged to see my neurosurgeon; I was more than ready for surgery now. In fact, I was more afraid of not having surgery than I had originally been of having surgery. Clearly, the radiation wasn't working. But my neurosurgeon sent a message stating that, as long as the tumor wasn't growing, he felt that there was no reason to consider surgery. I just needed to give the radiation more time—at least 10 years to try to shrink the tumor—and treat the pain in the meantime. I could hardly last 10 minutes, much less 10 years. I now faced the stark realization that the neurosurgeon wasn't interested in treating my TN, only the tumor. On top of that, my neurologist thought that the pain was "all in my head" and that only the fear of opening my mouth was both preventing me from speaking and causing my pain.

On September 13, 2007, at 3:15 pm, my wife and I were forced to walk out the doors of the ED for a second day in a row. Devastated and hopeless, I felt like my life had become a living hell. I found it hard to believe that such intense pain could exist. My only relief was to quickly attach several metal binder clips along my right cheek and around my right eye to try and match the painful side during each attack. I somehow felt that my newly discovered "pain matching" technique lessened the duration of the episodes.

By now, having come to fully understand why TN had once been described as the "suicide disease," I would have to begin choosing to live. It was a tough choice. In addition to the physical pain, I was tormented by painful thoughts: Would I ever work again, or would I just become a burden? How much life insurance did I have? Would it be enough to help my wife raise our three children on her own and help them make their way through college? Deep down, I knew I couldn't give up on my family. That was the one certainty.

The next few days were agonizing. As I would begin to fall asleep, my face would touch the pillow and trigger pain. I couldn't eat. By the fifth day, I had dropped 20 pounds on the "TN diet." I had been communicating for five days now by pen and paper. My wife had to go back to work the next day, and she feared what I might do when left alone. I asked her to let a church group of mine know that I was in a lot of pain and could use a few prayers. A doctor in the group called my wife within the hour, upset by the news. He said he would have the pain management doctor at his hospital call me. Then there was another call, from a neighbor who referred me to a pain website. There, I found a link to the website for the Trigeminal Neuralgia Association (TNA), now known as the Facial Pain Association (FPA). I noticed that a neurologist from my area was listed on the website, and I made an appointment to see him. As I continued to search the website, I found several interesting articles about Dr. Peter Jannetta in Pittsburgh, PA. The pain management doctor called and said that the Dilantin they sent me home with from the ED should start to take effect in a few days. Three days later, I began to feel some relief and steadily improve. Even though I was still in so much pain, I began to hope.

Eventually, I saw the neurologist from the association's website, and over the next several months, he closely monitored my blood levels for the Dilantin. I could accurately tell my doctor ahead of time just how high or low my blood levels were, based on how high or low my pain had been. Finally, I mentioned Dr. Jannetta's name during the visit. My neurologist said that he had previously been to one of Dr. Jannetta's seminars and that Dr. Jannetta likely knew more about the surgery of tumors causing TN than any other doctor. He suggested that I see if Dr. Jannetta agreed that I should wait for 10 years before considering surgery.

My medical records were sent to the offices of Dr. Jannetta. Dr. Jannetta called me a week later. After reviewing my records, he said he would not have recommended the radiation treatments. Although the radiation could shrink my tumor, it would likely never shrink enough to stop pressing on my trigeminal nerve. He suggested surgery as soon as possible. He believed there was an 85% chance of ending my pain. My response: "When can we start?"

That afternoon in June 2008, when I had woken up in an unfamiliar room, nauseous and my head aching, I had just undergone more than 6 hours of surgery. Dr. Jannetta had removed the tumor and performed his signature procedure, microvascular decompression (MVD). It was indeed the best day of my life. My facial pain was completely gone.

Unknown to me at the time, my church group had set up a prayer schedule with numerous people signed up to pray at church every half hour of my surgery. I googled my name years later and was stunned to see a website for a youth group at my church with an old post asking the group to pray for me during my surgery. Seeing the names of the kids, some I didn't even know, was humbling. To this day, I feel as though I've been given a do-over in life and often seek ways to give back, mostly through the FPA.

My first chance at giving back came just 3 months after my surgery. I decided to attend a national conference scheduled for the TNA (renamed FPA during the conference). I had never spoken with, met, or known anyone else with TN. I wasn't going there to look for answers, as were so many others. I was going as a sort of pilgrimage to finally meet "my people" and show them I care.

By chance, at the conference, I met Roger Levy, chair of the board for the association. When he learned that I was no longer experiencing pain, he asked if I would be willing to speak on the main stage during the following day's "Success Stories" session.

The next day, September 13, 2008, at approximately 3:15 pm, I stepped up to the podium to tell my story and share my message of hope. It was exactly one year to the day, to the hour, and nearly the minute, from when I had been thrown out of the ED for the second day in a row. Thanks to the care of doctors experienced with TN, the many association resources, and the love and prayers of faithful family and friends, I had come a long way in that one year.

6.4
Well, At Least I Won't Die From It
Stephen P. Fleming, MBA

Those words eased through my mind when I learned my diagnosis of trigeminal neuralgia (TN).

That was in 2009, and I was in my late 40s. In hindsight, there had been signs of what was to come. For example, one morning at the breakfast table I noticed a slight pain on the right side of my face, just above my teeth. This "twinge" only occurred as I was eating and eventually went away, only to return weeks later. After a few cycles of this, I reluctantly made an appointment with my dentist, thinking I must have a bad filling—*here comes the drill!*

If only.

At first, my dentist thought that maybe this was a lingering sinus infection, so she prescribed an antibiotic. But the twinge lingered— barely noticeable and only when I ate, and just during breakfast. Back to my dentist, where I made the self-fulfilling statement, "I still think it's this tooth with a bad filling," to which my dentist gladly agreed. Because the filling was extensive, this meant that the tooth required a root canal procedure by an endodontist. As root canals go, it proved rather easy.

Unfortunately, instead of this being the end of my story, it was just the beginning of my unexpected journey.

I'm a very blessed individual with overall good health. I have a loving and incredibly supportive spouse of 36 years and two beautiful daughters. They have helped me serve as an aging-services CEO for the past 25 years, and along with my work team, they have allowed me to lead in ways I could only imagine. And unlike so many who may be experiencing this disease, I have never been fully debilitated by TN. So, in so many ways, I have been blessed. Although I hesitate to "tell my story," I hope that it can lead to someone else's understanding of TN and how one can still lead a full and joyful life in spite of it.

Soon after my root canal, the "twinge" paid a return visit. Once again, the endodontist found no abnormalities. In time, the twinge became a pain far beyond a breakfast companion—it hurt even when the wind blew against my face, when I showered and water hit the right side of my face, and when I brushed my teeth. At this point, however, I turned to the internet, which revealed to me the condition known as trigeminal neuralgia (TN).

A few aging-services colleagues led me to a local neurologist who conducted a complete work-up. "This could be a brain tumor, or it could be multiple sclerosis, but it's most likely trigeminal neuralgia." Several subsequent MRI scans proved him right, and he prescribed the tried-and-true medication: carbamazepine (Tegretol).

Carbamazepine's side effects were significant: I had trouble staying awake at work, especially in the afternoons, and I had trouble with memory recall. Everything took just a little longer to get from my memory to my mouth; at times, this was very embarrassing, especially when I ran into someone whose name I should have easily recalled.

Worst of all, the initial dose of carbamazepine was not effective at alleviating the pain, so my neurologist threw in gabapentin, a medication used for nerve pain. Although ineffective, the side effects were unbearable, and this medication was stopped. On top of this, a brief steroid treatment made everything worse.

It hurt—sharp, knife-like pain—in the maxillary branch, referred to as V2, of my trigeminal nerve. This is the area above the upper lip, in my case, on the right side of the face, running diagonally up the cheek to the temporal area. Normally, this pain lasted only several seconds to maybe a minute, although it often felt longer. At its worst, the pain brought me to my knees and seemed to present more frequently, with the time between episodes decreasing—so much so that, after a day of multiple attacks, a dull ache ensued, only to be replaced by an episode of truly debilitating suffering.

Tweaks to my treatment regimen continued. As is common with TN pain management, my neurologist kept increasing the dosage of carbamazepine until I reached about 1100 mg/day. Eventually, the pain began to subside. Whether it was the correct dose of carbamazepine or simply my time for a pain-free "holiday," the pain became manageable to the point of being nonexistent.

After a few years on medication and the side effects that go along with it, I began contemplating a more invasive procedure to, perhaps, provide a longer-term solution. Again, through online sleuthing, I learned of a surgical procedure known as MVD, which I discussed with my neurologist. Here, he was cautious, spending more time on the risks than the benefits of going under the knife. He ultimately referred me to two neurosurgical specialty groups.

My wife, Anne, accompanied me on these consultative visits, and in addition to helping me "hear" what the surgeons were saying, she was and continues to be a supporting, understanding, and patient counselor. Relationships are vitally important when living with TN. They must be purposely maintained, nurtured, and grown. In my case, it was my spouse who was there for me. Not everyone is that fortunate; regardless, find your supporter. It will greatly improve your outlook and ultimate resolution of living with TN.

With neurosurgeons—as with most any relationship, especially one where you're interviewing someone to cut a hole in your skull and perform microscopic surgery—you want to feel a connection, as well as confidence rooted in knowledge:

- How did they make you feel?
- Did they take the time to carefully explain your options?
- Were they empathetic to your plight?
- How experienced are they with your condition, and how many similar surgeries have they performed?
- Where were they trained, and who did they train under?
- Is MVD surgery their specialty or subspecialty? …

After asking all of these questions and talking through who we "connected" with, Anne and I chose a neurosurgeon.

On November 16, 2015, he performed my MVD, a surgery that lasted 3 hours, to address both arterial and venous compression of the trigeminal nerve. Having been prepared to anticipate about a 90-minute surgery, Anne became worried. My situation was simply a bit more complicated than expected.

The whole premise of the MVD procedure is to "decompress" the trigeminal nerve and, in my case, to keep the artery and vein from touching or compressing the trigeminal nerve. Most neurosurgeons do this through the placement of a simple piece of Teflon-coated fabric or spacer between the nerve and, in most cases, artery. Although this sounds simple, it is far from it. The neurosurgeon must weave his way through the base of the brain, avoiding other nerves, including the auditory nerve for hearing, to reach the compressed area. Think of that classic childhood board game "Operation," in which you "play" surgeon, removing as many objects as possible from the body without touching the sides of an electrified "cavity." If you touched the side, a buzzer sounded, and the nose of the clown-like figure on the game board lit up to let you know you had lost your turn. Similarly, with MVD surgery, too many touches of nerves are not good, and there are, in fact, probes used to effectively monitor activity to best ensure that the surgeon is steering clear. Yes, it's a delicate surgery.

My surgery went well, with no complications and a speedy recovery, and even with me returning to work within 2 weeks. Pleased, I was completely off my medications within the next 3 years. Relief, at last.

Unfortunately, I was an outlier, and my MVD procedure did not keep the condition from returning as long as most.

In 2018, my pain returned—with a vengeance. This time, I probably waited too long to up my carbamazepine dosage, and as a result, I had a hard time getting the pain back under control. My local neurologist referred me to a neurological specialist in the noninvasive treatment of TN. He was also a renowned researcher, working to find new paths to alleviate the pain associated with TN. He prescribed several new medications, most of which required the use of a "compounding" pharmacy. These new meds helped me get my pain under control, so much so that I could get back on my normal dosage of carbamazepine. The new meds consisted of a compound nasal spray of a small dose of ketamine. This proved extremely helpful in "settling" the nerve, so that the carbamazepine could do its more regimented work. Through this experience, I learned of the correlation between high blood pressure and pain. Pain, unabated, will cause blood pressure to increase, starting what I call a "pain spiral," where one plays off the other, especially in TN. Getting blood pressure under control is an important side aspect of controlling TN pain.

In addition to the neurological specialist, I returned to the neurosurgeon. Even though the MRI scan he ordered showed that the Teflon spacer was still in place, he recommended that we try a nerve ablation procedure known as a gamma knife procedure to partially ablate (destroy) the trigeminal nerve. The key here is to burn and scar the nerve just enough to stop the pain—but not deaden the nerve. For most TN cases, the procedure is expected to offer temporary relief with relatively low levels of risks—say, perhaps, up to 5 years, on average, before any pain recurs. But should it recur, the pain would most likely be less.

For me, this was worth trying, so in 2018, I had the gamma knife procedure. The outpatient procedure itself is rather benign; the only discomfort—despite Novocain injections just under the scalp—came with the mounting of a stabilizing "halo" device into the skull. The halo locks your head in place during surgery. For obvious reasons, you don't want your head wiggling around while a pinpoint laser beam is directed at it! In all, this lasted only 30 minutes and was akin to an MRI scan, although in a much more open setting.

Free of the halo, I drove myself home around midday.

Unfortunately, I cannot say that the gamma knife procedure produced great results for me. In the end, I could not stop my medication, as I had after my prior surgery. But I was able to get the pain under control and avoid all but the carbamazepine. So, there were some positive effects.

I have since sought an additional neurosurgical opinion from a well-respected neurosurgeon. After reviewing my nearly 4-year-old MRI results, he determined that my Teflon spacer was most likely not fully decompressing the trigeminal nerve. Simply put, the nerve and artery were still in contact with one another, just what the initial surgery hoped to correct. To confirm this, I would need new MRI imagery, and if these images proved definitive, the possible "fix" would be a second MVD surgery. By this point, I'm not of the mindset to pursue a second MVD. I tolerate the carbamazepine well, and for the most part, I remain pain-free at a dosage of 900 mg/day.

I've learned many lessons over the past 12 years.

The first was to take the time to do more research. For example, I did not learn of the FPA until well after my second procedure. I'm not sure that having this resource would have changed the course of my condition or the decisions I made to treat it, but the information most likely would have allowed me the option of consulting ultraspecialist neurosurgeons who are nationally—and, in some cases, internationally—known for their surgical treatment of TN.

Perhaps more importantly, however, I would have learned that I am not alone in this condition. Even though it is rare, there are still thousands of people with TN like me, and we all need a support system and educational offerings for treatment options. The FPA provides that. I wish I had found it sooner.

Second, I wish one of my physicians had informed me that any improvement is a win, something I realize and appreciate now. I incorrectly thought that I could have the surgery and that would be it, at least for a long while. Although statistically correct, that's not always the case.

But after all the treatments, my condition has improved and is better than when it started. I'm now relatively pain-free, have few side effects, and enjoy a full life. I have a wonderful family and have enjoyed a great career in aging services.

So, life is good!

For me, TN was just one of those bumps in life's journey. I empathize with those who have experienced complete debilitation from TN. I hope and pray they find treatment options that provide at least some relief. Through the work of the FPA and many others, research is ongoing to assist with this most painful condition.

Finally, I want to thank my neurologist and neurosurgeon who provided me with a better quality of life.

My wish is that you find that, too.

6.5
Persistent Pain, Unshakable Faith
Jan Stubbs

"... a thorn was given to me in the flesh ... to harass me ..."

2 Corinthians 12:7b (ESV)

For the past 60+ years of my life I have lived in pain—most of it quite bearable, but some extremely difficult to deal with. But through all of it, my faith was—and is still—strong, and I knew that, no matter the outcome, I could count on God's grace to get me through it.

My first adult experience with a condition that caused an enormous amount of pain was when I developed rheumatoid arthritis (RA) at the age of 20 years. I can remember not being able to sleep and walking the floor at night in pain, with a facecloth held to my mouth to muffle my sobs so I would not wake up anyone else in the house. As time went on, the initial pain dimmed and morphed into other physical issues that hurt no less, but at least hurt differently. My tendons were subject to tearing, and eventually, many years of RA led to peripheral neuropathy in all four of my extremities.

When I lost a tendon in my left foot, I had a series of surgeries that gave me a stable foot for a while, but then the foot started to turn under, and I was almost walking on its side. A small sore on the side of my foot developed methicillin-resistant *Staphylococcus aureus* (MRSA), which eventually, after many debridements, led to a below-knee amputation.

An amputation can put a lot of strain on a body; the following year, I had to have my right knee replaced and, several years after that, my right hip. I have also developed scoliosis.

But none of them produced the depth and persistence of the pain that I encountered when TN became a part of my life. And, like many of you, I continued in pain completely alone, trying to find out what had happened to me and, more importantly, what could be done about it.

My introduction to TN started one morning when, after breakfast, I got an electric jolt in the right side of my tongue every time I brushed my teeth. I tried feeling my tongue to see if it was cut or had something stuck in it but could find nothing.

I called my dentist, who sent me to an oral surgeon, who took X-rays and said he found nothing. I asked him what he thought it was, and he said it sounded as if it was an atypical case of burning tongue syndrome. Ever the person who is predisposed to take action to fix a problem, I said, "Okay … so what can I do for it?" "Nothing," he replied. "You just have to learn to live with it." And so, I did. At least I tried.

That time in my life is a big blur. I was home from work, recuperating from one of my foot surgeries, and a friend's daughter came in and said to get into the wheelchair, as she had made an appointment with her dentist. The dentist was terrific; she looked up burning tongue syndrome and ordered a solution from a compounding pharmacist for me. Of course, it did not work, but she was also so kind and gentle that she became my dentist until she retired.

All this time, the pain had been getting worse. I sometimes could not even swallow my own saliva, and I was living on clear broth that I dropped down my throat by quarter teaspoonfuls, bypassing my tongue. Many times, I couldn't even talk, and the pain often worked its way into my jaw as well.

Taking the bull by the horns sometime after that, I went to my primary care provider (PCP) to see what he could do for me. He sent me to an ear, nose, and throat specialist, who said it sounded like some kind of neuralgia and he, in turn, was sending me to a neurologist who would not just send me home to "learn to live with it."

Sitting down in the neurologist's office was so affirming. He not only gave a name to my facial pain (trigeminal neuralgia) but also told me that there were a range of drugs that could help me live with the condition. As I was already on gabapentin for my peripheral neuropathy, we would have to try something else in addition, so he prescribed oxcarbazepine, which turned out to be perfect for me. For years, I lived well with this drug—until I did not.

In the neurologist's office, I had found a copy of TN Quarterly (now Quarterly Journal) and learned so much about the condition that I immediately subscribed. It was there that Anne Ciemnecki found my name and introduced me to a support group she was starting and that I attended until cataracts prevented me from driving at night. (Several years later, through her, I joined an online support group that I still attend.)

One day a few years ago, I walked into my PCP's office feeling extremely weak and just not "with it." She ordered blood work for me. I had to wait for the next day to have blood drawn. The following night, she called me and told me to get to the hospital immediately. If I didn't have a ride, I would have to take an ambulance and tell the emergency medical technicians that my sodium count was 123 [in milliequivalents per liter, mEq/L; normal is 135–145 mEq/L]. By the time I reached the hospital, the sodium count was 119 [mEq/L], so low that they had to pump saline into me. My oxcarbazepine was no longer helping but was hurting me.

I did not know where to go from there. My neurologist began trying other drugs, but none seemed to work. I called my son, who is a Bible study teacher in a Christian school, and asked that he and his family pray for me. He assured me that they would and that he would ask his prayer group, meeting that night, to pray as well. When one of the pastors asked what my issue was and my son explained, they realized that one of their congregants had TN and had had surgery, after which he was pain-free. My son connected me with this man. I learned who his surgeon was, and I knew something good could happen from that. I felt that God was leading me in this.

A brain surgeon who had studied under Dr. Janetta performed my MVD, and I have had no TN pain since (5 years). I wish I could say that I have had little pain in the rest of my body as well, but with my TN pain halted—at least for now—and with God's help, I have the strength to deal with my other issues. After all, who at 81 years of age, can expect to be completely free of pain?

6.6
Pregnancy and Motherhood with Trigeminal Neuropathic Pain
Ally Kubik, MEd, MS, BCBA

Although many women dream of having children, nobody dreams of having to navigate pregnancy and motherhood with facial pain. I am here to tell you that it is possible. It may look different, but it is possible. I was diagnosed with facial pain at the age of 13 years. As I began to navigate my life with pain, I feared two things: that I would never be able to get married and that I would never be able to have children of my own. Fast forward 13 years from my diagnosis, and I got married. Eighteen years after my diagnosis, I had my first child.

My experience with pregnancy and facial pain may look different than yours. There is no right answer. My experience with facial pain has taught me that, if one thing does not work, try, and try again. My experience with motherhood is that, once you think you have things figured out, you don't. Although I have had multiple surgeries over the years and my pain is better, I am not pain-free and still require medication daily. My husband has been with me through some of my worst and best times with facial pain. For context, our wedding vows included the challenges of facial pain. We knew that starting a family would be different for us. Before we were ready to have children, I asked my obstetrician (OB) about what this process might be like. He referred me to a consultation with a high-risk OB. The high-risk OB shared that additional ultrasounds and tests would need to be done once I was pregnant. This was a scary, but it was also comforting to know that the team would be monitoring my baby frequently. The doctor continued to explain that one of the three medications I was taking was not safe for conception or pregnancy. Next, I visited my pain management doctor, and we went to the drawing board. I opted to wean off the medication without replacing it with either a higher dose of one of my other medications or another medication altogether. I was able to successfully titrate off the medication that was not safe for pregnancy.

Pregnancy with medication is a difficult pill to swallow. (No pun intended.) When my high-risk OB asked me if coming off all medication was an option for me, I explained that it was not. I did not want to risk my pain flaring uncontrollably during pregnancy. In fact, I have never been off medication completely in the 20+ years I have been living with facial pain. Yet, every woman and pregnancy is different. I have spoken with women with facial pain who were able to stop taking all medications while pregnant. It is difficult for doctors to know what is safest. Often, their only guidance is from animal studies. Hearing this scared me. My high-risk OB found some human case studies, but they were limited to women reporting what medications they took and how their child was developing. There was no scientific study.

When I met with the high-risk OB, I asked what I could do if my pain flared during pregnancy. I have a specific regimen of medications that I take if my pain becomes out of control when I am not pregnant. My high-risk OB and I developed a plan for each trimester because certain medications were safer later in pregnancy. Having a plan beforehand was comforting. I knew that I could carry out the plan if necessary. Some of the questions that are important for a pregnant person to ask at their high- risk OB appointment are as follows:

- Are the medications I am on safe for conception and/or pregnancy?
- What does the research say about this medication during pregnancy?
- What extra will you do to monitor my baby?
- What can I do if my pain flares? Do I need to check with you before I take medication?

Often, people ask what their pain will be like during and after pregnancy? For me, my pain was not much different during pregnancy than at other times. Managing pregnancy side effects was key, especially in the first trimester. With my first pregnancy, I was extremely nauseated for much of the first and third trimesters. Vomiting is a trigger for my facial pain, so keeping that at bay was a priority. Determining what would alleviate the nausea and other normal pregnancy concerns often took trial and error. Making sure I was drinking enough water and getting enough sleep was of supreme importance. Being overly tired is a pain trigger for me. Rest and paying close attention to what my body was telling me was paramount.

What about the actual birthing process? My pain management doctor had suggested that I opt for a C-section so that I was not risking a pain flare while "pushing." I adamantly explained that I had had enough surgery in my life and that I was going to do everything in my power to avoid a voluntary C-section. Prior to my delivery, I created a "cheat sheet" for the labor and delivery staff. It contained a list of my medications, what my pain felt like, my daily pain level, the names and contact information of my pain management doctor and facial pain surgeon, and my pain triggers. (Cold on my face and mouth is a trigger, so don't even offer me ice chips or an ice pack!) I also included the "cocktail" of rescue medications I take if I have a major pain flare. In addition, I added my surgical history, noting that opioid-based medications do not work. Handing the staff this paper when I walked in to deliver was extremely helpful so that everyone was on the same page. When I was ready to push, we requested that my rescue medications be in the delivery room so that there was zero delay if I needed them. During both of my deliveries, I did not feel like my face pain was any worse than normal.

What about my baby? When I was delivering my first, neonatal intensive care unit (NICU) staff were present because my child had been exposed to medication in utero. The NICU staff checked out my baby as soon as he was born. For my second child, the NICU staff was on-call, not present. My labor was much shorter. It was important to my husband and me that delivery was at a hospital with a NICU, just in case something adverse had happened. We did not want to be separated if there was an issue. Thankfully, there was no need for the NICU staff, but I was thankful that they were there.

Breastfeeding was important to me. Not all medications are safe for breastfeeding, and not everyone wants to breastfeed. Your child's pediatrician is the best person to ask. Check prior to delivery. There are also websites that can be checked. One, Infant Risk Center (www.infantrisk.com), is a great resource and even provides opportunities to participate in studies.

Regardless of whether you choose to breastfeed, babies will wake frequently in their early months. This is difficult for someone like me, whose triggers include sleep deprivation and schedule changes. I vividly remember one early morning when I was just gripping the rocker as my son nursed because my face pain was so bad. I thought that it was all going to go downhill from there. I told my husband that I needed to get some sleep that day. We made it happen, and my pain levels retreated. Juggling a new baby is hard; juggling a new baby while experiencing facial pain is even more difficult. I took the new experience with the same attitude: Advocate and rely on your supporters. If someone needs to watch the baby so you can sleep, that needs to happen. If you have to take extra medication, take it. There were a handful of times when I did need to take extra medication, but a quick call to my child's pediatrician (while I was still nursing) confirmed that it was okay or explained how I should feed my child. I try to remember that I cannot take care of others if I am not taking care of myself. I am terrible at following this advice, even though it sounds helpful.

Pregnancy and motherhood are journeys. No two journeys will look the same. No two pregnancies are the same. The important takeaway from my story is that, if your dream is to have children, you can and should.

Chapter 7

Clinical Trials and Cutting-Edge Research

Anne B. Ciemnecki, MA

Chapter 7 of this book focuses on research. We begin with a discussion of clinical trials. Clinical trials are a critical part medical research and the underpinning of all medical advances. They are designed to determine whether a new drug or treatment is safe and effective. Advances in drugs and treatments can improve quality of life for people with chronic diseases.

When a new drug's manufacturer has enough evidence on the drug's safety and effectiveness (from clinical trials), the manufacturer submits a new drug application (NDA) to the U.S. Food and Drug Administration (FDA). This is a long, complicated process. The important takeaway for this discussion is that the drug is approved for a very specific use or disease. Most of the drugs that offer relief from trigeminal neuropathic pain (TNP) are used off-label. This means the drugs were approved for a condition other than TNP. In fact, there has not been a drug approved specifically for TNP since carbamazepine in the 1960s.

The good news is that a clinical trial for a drug developed specifically for classical trigeminal neuralgia, Basimglurant, began in 2022 and is expected to be completed in 2024. In Section 7.1, Anne Ciemnecki presents the nuts and bolts of clinical trials. In Section 7.2, Dr. Raymond Sekula and his colleagues describe the Basimglurant clinical trial. (His office in New York City is one of the clinical trial sites for Basimglurant.) You may be wondering how people can be assured that a clinical trial of a drug does not pose extraordinary risk. In Section 7.3, Dr. Jeffrey Brown answers that question by describing his experience on an "Independent Data Monitoring Committee" (IDMC), also called a "Safety Data Monitoring Committee."

Long before a drug enters a clinical trial, scientists conduct basic research to understand the mechanisms leading to diseases and propose possible targets and therapeutic strategies. Dr. Michael Lim and his colleagues do just that in Section 7.4, as they explain their investigation of the nuclear factor erythroid 2-related factor (NRF2) network.

All of the research described thus far has been prospective, looking toward the future. Another type of research, called retrospective, takes a "look back." Dr. Giulia Di Stefano, a researcher in the Department of Human Neuroscience at Sapienza University in Rome, discusses retrospective research on familial TN. She and I were in a meeting about the Facial Pain Association (FPA) Patient Registry. We connected immediately when I learned that she researched familial TN, and I told her about my family history. I wondered whether she would contribute to this book and am so pleased that she enthusiastically agreed.

7.1
What Is a Clinical Trial, and Should You Participate?
Anne B. Ciemnecki, MA

A clinical trial is a medical research study in which a new or existing drug, device, or treatment is tested to answer a specific health question. If you have trigeminal neuropathic pain (TNP), you might hear about a clinical trial from a doctor who practices at an institution that is taking part in the trial, from a social media site such as https://www.facebook.com/groups/FPAnetwork/, or through the FPA directly as a result of information you provided through the facial pain registry.

A clinical trial is always voluntary. You will never have to pay to be part of a legitimate clinical trial. In fact, you will be reimbursed for some types of expenses you incur as part of the trial. At the very least, you will be paid for some travel expenses, or travel will be arranged for you. You will receive the trial drug or procedure for free. You will also receive free medical examinations and care. The federal CLINICAL TREATMENT Act, which took effect January 1, 2022, stipulated that Medicaid pay for the medical expenses of clinical trials. Medicare also pays some of those costs. The researchers may also provide a small remuneration or stipend to thank you for your time and effort. All of these payments are either reimbursements for expenses or thank you gifts. You will never be paid to provide a specific response to study questions.

Each clinical trial comprises five phases. The phase refers to the stage of the trial, as defined by the U.S. Food and Drug Administration (FDA). You will most likely participate in a phase III clinical trial.

The first phase is called the early phase (formerly called phase 0). The early phase establishes that a small dose of the test medication (or treatment or procedure) is not harmful to humans. This early phase is conducted with no more than 15 trial participants. If the medication is not yet suitable for use with humans, the clinical investigators will do additional research before deciding to continue the trial. Phase I is next. During phase I, investigators spend several months analyzing the effects of the medication on about 20 to 80 people who have no underlying health conditions. During phase I, clinical investigators want to determine the highest dose humans can take without serious side effects. Researchers follow participants very closely to see how their bodies react to the medication during this phase. In addition to evaluating safety and ideal dosage, investigators also assess the best way to administer the drug, such as orally, intravenously, or topically. The FDA reports that 70% of medications tested in phase I move on to phase II.

For the next phases, statisticians calculate how many trial participants are necessary to make statistically significant conclusions about the trial drug. The numbers in the paragraphs below are estimates for drugs that treat common conditions. Because rarer conditions, such as TNP, are found in fewer participants, not as many are needed to reach statistically significant conclusions.

During phase II, several hundred participants who are living with the condition that the new medication is meant to treat are given the same dose as was found to be safe during phase I. Investigators monitor participants for several months or years to determine how effective the medication is and to gather more information about any side effects it might cause. Phase II is not large enough to demonstrate the overall safety of a medication. Therefore, the investigators use the information gathered during phase II to determine methods for conducting phase III. The FDA reports that about one-third of medications tested in phase II move on to phase III.

Phase III of a clinical trial evaluates how the new medication works in comparison to existing medications for the same condition. It usually lasts for several years and involves up to 3000 participants who have the condition that the new medication is meant to treat. Because of the larger number of participants and longer duration of phase III, rare and long-term side effects are more likely to show up. If the investigators demonstrate that the medication is at least as safe and effective as others already on the market, the FDA will usually approve the medication. About 25% to 30% of medications move on to phase IV.

Phase IV clinical trials occur after the FDA has approved a medication. This phase includes the most participants, often thousands, and lasts the longest, often years. During phase IV, investigators learn about the medication's long-term safety and effectiveness.

Many drugs used to treat TNP are used "off-label." This means that the drug has been tested for another condition, usually epilepsy, depression, anxiety, or pain caused by neuropathic conditions such as diabetes, but not trigeminal neuralgia (TN). Because the drug has had both a phase I and a phase II trial, the drug has been proven safe for human use. When a drug is used off-label, it is unknown whether this drug is better than other drugs for TN.

To protect research participants, also called human subjects, a clinical trial requires approval from an Institutional Review Board (IRB). The FDA sets the requirements for the creation and on-going work of all IRBs.

The IRB will initially review proposed research protocols, such as consent forms and materials used in recruiting research participants. Based on individual IRB members' reviews and a group discussion, the IRB will approve the proposed project, require modifications, or not grant approval because the rights and well-being of research participants are at risk. Once approved, the IRB will review the project periodically, usually once a year, to assure that research participants continue to be protected.

If you would like to participate in a clinical trial, the IRB will require that you learn about the study and your role in it, including any risks and benefits you may incur. This is the informed-consent process and is one of the most important components of an IRB review. Note that informed consent is a process, not merely a signature on a piece of paper. If you are considering participation in a clinical trial, you must speak with the study staff, usually a clinical trial coordinator in a physician's office, to learn about the study and its purpose. That person will give you, both orally and in writing, all of the information you need to consent to participate or not. This written document is called the informed-consent document. It should be written in clear language that you understand. Although the FDA does not require specific language for the consent form, it does require that the consent contains the following elements:

- *Information about the study.* This includes the number of participants enrolled, all of the procedures, exactly what you will be required to do, and your length of participation.
- *The meaning of "trial."* The consent form must include a clear statement that you may get the drug being studied or you may not. Further, even if you do receive the study drug, it may not be a drug that helps you.
- *Risks and benefits of participation.* As a prospective study participant, you must be notified of predictable risks and discomforts, benefits to you, and a clear statement that there may be no benefits to you personally, although your participation may provide benefits for others in the future.
- *Voluntary participation.* You have the right to refuse participation or stop participating at any time without losing benefits to which you are entitled.
- *Security and confidentiality of data.* The researchers must provide an assurance of confidentiality and an explanation of how records that could identify you will be kept.
- *Contact information for questions that arise later.* Telephone numbers and email addresses for the study investigators and for a person on the IRB. You would call the IRB if you thought the study was causing harm to participants.

Most importantly, you should be able to ask questions and have them answered clearly. You will need to sign the informed-consent document, but you do not need to sign it on the spot. You may take it home to discuss with family and/or friends. The decision to participate is yours. No one—neither study staff nor your friends or family—should pressure you to participate.

The next step in a clinical trial is to determine if you are eligible for the trial. Clinical trials are designed to test a drug or procedure for a particular group of people. You must be one of those people to take part in the study. The study staff will ask you screening questions to determine if you are eligible to participate. They screen for either, or both, inclusion and exclusion for the study. Women who are pregnant or planning to become pregnant during the study period may be excluded. This exclusion is to prevent unnecessary harm to an unborn baby. People with intermittent TNP may be included in a particular study, whereas people with constant pain may be excluded. This is to test the drug on people for whom it is intended to help. Because of diversity and inclusion initiatives by the government and private companies, studies are expanding to include people who have typically been excluded in the past. Drugs are no longer tested only on men. Companies actively recruit participants of all races, ethnicities, and socio-economic socioeconomic statuses for clinical studies. Even though the research team will ask personal questions to determine your eligibility for a study, the eligibility decision is not a personal one. It is determined in advance of your screening. Even if you are eligible to participate in a study, your participation is voluntary, and you can change your mind at any time during the study.

Perhaps you have heard the term "randomized controlled trial" or RCT study. RCT studies are the gold standard in medical research. RTCs are the most rigorous methods for determining whether a cause–effect relationship exists between an intervention and an outcome. In the simplest form of RCT study, once your eligibility has been determined, you will be randomly assigned to a treatment or control group. The treatment group will receive the drug that is being tested. The control group will not. The control group stays on currently available medication. Sometimes, studies have more than one treatment group, for example, a high-dose group and a low-dose group. You will not know which group you are in. Your doctor may not know either. The drugs distributed to participants in each group are designed to look the same. Randomization prevents bias in clinical trials.

Using random methods, usually a computer program, to assign participants to a study group ensures that all groups are the same at the start of a study. Differences between the groups are due to random factors, not research biases such as sampling bias or selection bias. With all environmental and other factors remaining the same, the outcomes for the treatment and control groups will be compared at the end of the study. Researchers can determine which treatment, the new one or the existing one, is more effective and has fewer side effects. You may hear some of the following terms in relation to RCT studies:

- A *single-blind* study is a type of clinical trial in which one party, either the researcher or the participant, does not know whether the new drug or the existing drug is administered to the participant.
- In a *double-blind* study, neither the researcher nor the participant know who gets which drug.
- In a *triple-blind* study, even the analysts do not know who gets which drug.
- *Parallel studies* compare two or more treatments. Participants are randomly assigned to just one group or the other, treatments are administered, and then the results are compared.
- By contrast, in a *crossover* clinical trial, study participants receive each treatment in a random order. Essentially, every patient serves as their own control group. Crossover studies are used when researchers are unable to recruit enough study participants for statistical validity. In Section 7.2, Dr. Raymond Sekula describes the details of a crossover clinical trial of Basimglurant for TNP. The crossover study is an appropriate design because of TNP's low prevalence.

Clinical trials have preset guidelines on the number of visits, treatments, or procedures that each participant must have. The trial is intended to end when the last patient has completed all of their activities. Sometimes, clinical trials end early. Early terminations focus on the trial drug's safety and effectiveness. Large trials have a committee, called the Independent Data Monitoring Committee (IDMC), that conducts interim analysis as the trial progresses to determine the trial drug's efficacy and safety. After each analysis, the committee decides whether the trial should continue, be modified, or terminate early. Following are some of the reasons a trial may end early:

- Interest in the trial has fallen. Perhaps, the market for the drug is not sufficient or new drugs have been approved for the same condition.
- The researchers were unable to recruit enough participants.
- The benefit of the trial drug is proven early in the trial period. In this case, it is unethical to withhold the trial drug from the control group.
- The drug's lack of effectiveness is proven early.
- Most importantly, the interim analysis demonstrates that the drug is harmful and the risk to participants is too high to continue. In Section 7.3, Dr. Jeffrey Brown describes his participation on an IDMC.

A trial can end for you any time you decide to drop out.

In conclusion, clinical trials are regulated, voluntary, and safe. Such trials represent the only way new drugs or treatments can be tested on human participants. Participation is rewarding and worthwhile.

For more information on current clinical trials, visit clinicaltrials.gov, a worldwide, interactive database of clinical trials.

7.2
Basimglurant: A Drug Trial for Trigeminal Neuralgia
Celine Shon and Raymond F. Sekula, Jr., MD

Overview of Trigeminal Neuralgia. The term trigeminal neuralgia (TN) encompasses a number of facial pain entities of varying severity. When all forms of facial pain are considered together, these conditions affect nearly 10% of the world's population. According to the International Headache Society, the International Association for the Study of Pain, and the European Academy of Neurology, TN is "classical" if the pain consists of "recurrent unilateral brief electric-shock-like pains, abrupt in onset and termination, limited to the distribution of one or more divisions of the trigeminal nerve and triggered by innocuous stimuli" (Headache Classification Committee of the International Headache Society 2013). Magnetic resonance imaging of the brain or intraoperative inspection should show contact or deformation of the trigeminal nerve root adjacent to the brain stem. Idiopathic TN presents in a manner similar to classical TN but without evidence of morphometric or structural changes to the trigeminal nerve. The U.S. National Institutes of Health (NIH) considers classical and idiopathic TN to be "rare" disorders. Most often, oral anticonvulsant medications are the first treatments prescribed. Carbamazepine (Tegretol) is the only drug approved by the FDA for TN treatment in the United States. Other off-label drug treatments include lamotrigine, topiramate, pregabalin, gabapentin, phenytoin, fosphenytoin, and baclofen, which are second-in-line treatments or add-on therapies to carbamazepine or oxcarbazepine. Unfortunately, many of these alternatives do not provide adequate pain relief or may cause bothersome or debilitating side effects.

What Is Basimglurant? Basimglurant is a drug on a trial sponsored by the FDA that may be helpful for people with various types of TN and orofacial pain. Basimglurant has the potential to be an effective treatment because it could decrease neuronal excitability, thereby reducing the pain and abnormal firing of the nerve. Visually, Basimglurant is a white to yellowish powder. It is also soluble in acidic aqueous solutions.

Editor's Note: Some of this section is quite technical. The following paragraph is an example. Whereas the technical information may be of interest, it is not necessary for the understanding of Basimglurant or its clinical trial.

On a molecular level, Basimglurant is a strong and selective negative allosteric modulator of the metabotropic glutamate receptor 5 (mGluR5 receptor). This means that the drug's molecules bind to the mGluR5 receptor site, thus inhibiting mGluR5's function. This inhibition occurs either by altering the drug's receptor structure (thus affecting its ability to act) or by reducing its attraction to other substances that enhance its function.

During phase I of a clinical trial, investigators examine the effects of the medication on people with no underlying health conditions to determine the highest dose that can be taken without serious side effects. When the phase I trials of Basimglurant began, the drug was formulated as an immediate-release (IR) hard gelatin capsule developed to provide a rapid onset of action. However, its tolerability was improved by changing the formulation to a moderate-release (MR) pill, which provides a steady and controlled drug release. Basimglurant has been demonstrated to be the most effective mGluR5 negative allosteric modulator, as it has promoted analgesic activity in three independent preclinical models, namely, in animals with neuropathic pain. Its pain-relieving effect is similar to that of standard morphine and duloxetine (Cymbalta). Because the activation of mGluR5 increases neuronal excitability, overactivation of mGluR5 has been indicated to cause multiple central nervous system diseases.

Prior Clinical Studies. To date, 20 clinical studies have been completed to determine this drug's safety. One study considered adults with major depressive disorders. Most of the study participants reported that the undesirable effects of the drug were mild, with three of the side effects reported to be moderate in intensity. Some of the common adverse events were dizziness, insomnia, somnolence, disturbance in attention, headaches, and psychiatric and gastrointestinal disorders. Two severe adverse events were acute psychotic reaction and mania with suicidal ideation. However, 413 healthy volunteers were treated with single or multiple doses of Basimglurant IR or the placebo to show that the drug was generally well-tolerated and safe.

Phases of the Study. The current study with Basimglurant is a phase II/III multicenter study, with a 4-week screening period followed by an 8-week run-in period; a 12-week parallel-group, double-blind, randomized withdrawal, placebo-controlled study; and a 52-week open-label extension. The purpose of the study is to evaluate the efficacy and safety of a daily dose of 1.5–3.5 mg of Basimglurant in participants who have TN with a suboptimal response to their current anti-pain therapy. The consent period, including screening assessments, will be counted as period 0. Figure 7-1 presents the screening criteria for exclusion and inclusion in the clinical trial. Individuals who are not eligible for the trial, which has strict inclusion criteria, will be able to take Basimglurant if it goes to market and their doctor prescribes it. Note that the most important criterion for inclusion in the study is a willingness to discontinue the use of current pain-relieving drugs, especially gabapentin (Neurontin) or pregabalin (Lyrica). Participation in a clinical study is voluntary, and participants who are in unbearable pain can drop out at any time with no consequences. Those who can "hold out" until the open-label phase of the study will receive Basimglurant at no cost for 1 year.

The run-in phase, or period 1, is between the screening and randomization periods. During the run-in phase, which lasts 8 weeks, all participants receive the Basimglurant treatment. Only those who benefit from the Basimglurant at the end of period 1 can move on to the double-blind period.

During the double-blind period, or period 2, which lasts 12 weeks, participants are randomly assigned to a treatment group, which receives Basimglurant, or a control group, which receives a placebo (i.e., a sugar pill). Neither the researchers nor the participants know who is taking Basimglurant and who is taking the placebo. The double-blind period is randomized through an interactive voice/web response. The participants will take the same daily dose of Basimglurant or the placebo as they were taking at the end of period 1. The participants will take the Basimglurant at home, and their compliance with the study treatment will be assessed at each visit. The medication intake should occur at the same time every day within a margin of 2 hours. Up to 200 people will participate in the study; however, it is estimated that about 70 eligible participants will be randomized and enrolled to obtain enough participants with pain recurrence during the double-blind period. During periods 0 through 2, the investigator will meet the participants weekly, with a follow-up visit 28 days after the participant finishes the study.

Finally, the open-label extension will end the study and last for 52 weeks. During the open-label extension period, all remaining participants will receive Basimglurant.

Exclusion Criteria. Individuals meeting any of the following criteria are excluded from participating in this study.

1. Expressing suicidal ideation; having a recent history of suicidal behavior; or in the opinion of the investigator, being at risk of harming themselves
2. Current or prior history of diagnosis of schizophrenia or chronic psychotic disorders
3. History of substance dependence or substance abuse in the past 6 months, except for nicotine
4. Being unwilling to discontinue current analgesics
   a. Gabapentin or pregabalin should be discontinued during the first 2 weeks of period 1 at the latest
5. Use of opioids, except for pain control on a need basis as long as it does not exceed 2 days per week
6. Known allergic reaction to Basimglurant or one of its components
7. Previous treatment with Basimglurant
8. Treatment with antipsychotics within 6 months prior to screening
   a. Treatment of depressive symptoms with selective serotonin reuptake inhibitors is permitted if treatment started more than 6 weeks before screening
9. Use of any investigational drug within 90 days before initiation of Basimglurant
10. Evidence of clinically significant, uncontrolled, unstable medical conditions or recently diagnosed cardiovascular disease
11. History of gastric or small intestinal surgery or presence of a disease that causes malabsorption
12. Body mass index greater than 33 kg/m^2 (for example, a 5'7" person weighing more than 211 pounds would fall into this category)
13. Severe impaired hepatic function
14. Severe renal impairment

Inclusion Criteria. Individuals meeting all of the following requirements are eligible to participate in this study:

1. Ability and willingness to provide written informed consent and comply with study procedures
2. Fluency in the language of the investigator, study staff, and informed consent
3. Age between 18 and 75 years
4. Diagnosis of primary TN confirmed by a study neurologist
   a. Classical TN, purely sudden attacks
   b. Classical TN with accompanying continuous pain
   c. Idiopathic TN, purely sudden attacks
   d. Idiopathic TN with accompanying continuous pain
5. Experience pain defined as at least three sudden attacks per day, each rated at an intensity of 4 or more on the self-reported pain rating scale on at least 4 days per week
   a. The pain should be present at least 2 months prior to study entry and can be associated with or without continuous pain
6. Females with childbearing potential are eligible to participate if not currently pregnant or breastfeeding and one of the following conditions applies:
   a. Use of acceptable contraceptives during the study intervention period (The investigator should also evaluate the potential for contraceptive method failure in relationship to the first dose of the study intervention)
   b. Negative result of a highly sensitive pregnancy test within 28 days before the first dose of the study intervention

Figure 7-1.   Exclusion and inclusion criteria in the Basimglurant clinical trial.

Throughout the study, all participants will keep a daily diary of the number of pain attacks, the severity of the worst attack, the duration of the pain, the average pain over the preceding 24 hours, and functioning. Participants will also answer the Penn Facial Pain Scale–Revised, a self-report measure of pain intensity, and the Patient

Global Impression of Change questionnaire, which reflects the participant's belief about the efficacy of treatment.

Restrictions. Although there are no dietary or activity restrictions, the consumption of alcohol during treatment is advised not to exceed an average of 2 units per day, where 1 unit is about the equivalent of 330 mL of beer, 125 mL of wine, or 25 mL of spirits. Participants are also instructed not to consume alcohol for at least 1 hour before and 1 hour after intake of the medication. In terms of other drugs or substances that can be used, because Basimglurant is a substrate, the substance that an enzyme acts upon, consuming substances that are strong inducers of the CYP1A2 and CYP3A4 drug-metabolizing enzymes is prohibited. Carbamazepine (Tegretol) and phenytoin (Dilantin) are examples of strong CYP3A4 inducers. Moderate or strong inducers of these enzymes can significantly reduce Basimglurant exposure and compromise the efficacy of the Basimglurant treatment, or they can increase Basimglurant exposure and increase the risk of side effects. Heavy cigarette smoking is not recommended during the study period as smoking also induces CYP1A2 activity. Participants will record any other medications or vaccines, such as over-the-counter medicines, prescriptions, recreational drugs, vitamins, or herbal supplements, taken during their study enrollment. They will also record the reason for use; administration dates, including start and end dates; dosage information; and administration frequency.

Scientific Rationale for Study Design. This study's design has been successfully used in several neuropathic pain studies, including those involving individuals with TN. Without the presence of a pain rescue medication, a substantial portion of the placebo-treated participants with TN during the second period would be expected to discontinue the treatment early, as the pain will likely recur. Hence, rescue medication will be provided to participants with a severe exacerbation of their pain, but only until the pain is resolved or for a maximum of 7 days. Because clinical trials are voluntary, if the participant requests to discontinue the study drug, has any occurrence of any medical condition that causes them to be unable to comply with the requirements, or has a severe adverse event, they are free to discontinue the treatment. The starting dose of 1.5 mg was selected on the basis of prior studies completed on adults with major depressive disorders, as the drug was safe, well-tolerated, and effective. The dose increment of 0.5 mg daily every 7 days was chosen to establish an optimal daily dose with respect to tolerability and response for individuals. The maximum dose of 3.5 mg met the target goal of the study, and a slow titration to this dose was expected to be safe.

Risk Assessments. The highest identified risk in past studies was dizziness, so even though no lifestyle restrictions exist, participants will be warned about carrying out hazardous activities such as driving and operating machinery. Some other potential risks of Basimglurant are hallucinations, delusions, mania, euphoria, mood elevation, a burning or prickling sensation (paresthesia), numbness (hypoesthesia), loss of consciousness (syncope), inability to move normally (catatonia), effects on the liver, cardiac disorders, gastrointestinal disorders, endocrine disorders, reproductive system disorders, breast disorders, and potential for abuse or dependence. All of these potential risks have not yet been confirmed, and participants will be monitored continuously for possible abnormalities.

Conclusion. The study trial for the drug Basimglurant began at the start of 2022 and is expected to run until August 2024, as participants are still being entered into the trial. If the U.S. FDA approves its use in treating subtypes of TN, such as classical TN and idiopathic TN, this will be the second drug for TN to be approved by the FDA since the 1960s.

7.3
Clinical Trials: A Safety Story
Jeffrey A. Brown, MD, FACS, FAANS

How are research protocols monitored? — or — "Is it safe[1]?"
In the late 1990s, because of my recent publications on the treatment of high-velocity missile and shrapnel injuries to the brain, I was appointed to an Independent Data Monitoring Committee (IDMC)

---

[1] Famous line from the movie *Marathon Man*, in which an unprepossessing avid jogger finds himself in the hands of an evil dentist whose human experiments were unspeakable.

for an international study of an innovative medical treatment for severe head injury. A year later, I became the chair of that committee. The study was unique. The patients to be treated could not give consent. They were in coma. Consent to enter the research trial had to be obtained as an emergency from their legally authorized representative, an unusual situation that would require careful control to protect the patient who lacked the ability to consent.

Institutional review boards (IRBs) must approve any investigation that is defined as "research." If a physician wishes to publish a review of a single patient who is treated in a unique manner that the physician believes deserves calling to the attention of his colleagues, this is not considered research. Neither is a review of two or three patients with similar conditions. More than that becomes the study of a series of patients and reaches the definition of research.

Research studies can be prospective or retrospective. In a retrospective study, the physician takes a look back at patients' medical records that already exist and may have been recorded for reasons not relating to the current project. These studies do not follow patients into the future. They do not need to have patients' written consent. However, they do need to have the permission of the IRB. This is because the data being reviewed need to be protected so that patients' identities are not mistakenly revealed by the study publication or during its ongoing evaluation period. Data must be stored in a secure site in a secure manner with limited access granted only to authorized individuals. Consent from the patients is not required in this case because it is presumed that they were treated by accepted standards of care without experimentation or thought of future publication.

Prospective studies look forward and do require patient consent. Prospective studies review a form of treatment that is yet to be accepted as a standard of care and that has not yet been shown to provide a clear advantage. Often, the study will include different arms. One arm may be a placebo that is not expected to provide benefit and is to be given "blindly." This means that neither the patient nor the treating physician knows that the placebo treatment is not going to be effective and is designed so that the effect of the treatment being studied can be compared to that of the placebo. This can be a problem for consenting patients, and a complex study design is required to deal with this issue. Often, there is an option for "crossover," such that patients who received the placebo will also receive the experimental treatment at some point.

Clinical research studies have different levels. They start with smaller reviews once some laboratory work suggests a benefit from the treatment; then a study commences to determine the safety of the treatment in humans with some attention to efficacy, followed by larger studies intended to define the extent of efficacy.

In the case of the study in which I was involved, there was what is called "equipoise." That is, the drug worked in laboratory studies, but in real life, no one knew whether the treatment being offered would help, so that denying it did not put the patient at risk. Only if the treatment is given is there risk in this case, and those risks must be made known to the consenting party.

So, what is the role of an IDMC?

My job was to recruit experts in the field of head injury to join me in reviewing the results of the ongoing research project. The doctors who are the principal investigators in the study and are performing the work of caring for the patients with the head injuries will not have access to the data as the trial progresses. They will not know, for example, whether the medication that they have given to a patient is the placebo or the study drug. They will, however, be required to treat each patient the same.

I recruited to my committee a renowned senior laboratory research expert and a neurosurgeon in the field of head trauma, a neurologist also known for her expertise in caring for patients with head injuries, and a statistician. The statistician would be the only "unblinded" individual involved in the study. His job was to keep constant track of any deaths in this population and determine whether those individuals had been given the drug or not. He would also become aware if it was statistically clear that the drug being studied was saving lives and, therefore, that it was ethically unreasonable to deny it to patients by continuing the study.

On a midweek afternoon, I was in my office when I received an urgent phone call from the statistician. His words still reverberate with me. This is what he said:

"The lines have crossed."

And he waited for me to catch my breath.

What were these lines?

There is a form of statistical analysis that makes use of aptly named Kaplan–Meier Survival Curves. I had studied with Dr. Meier in medical school at The University of Chicago, where he was a professor. A survival curve keeps track of, in this case, the number of patients still alive day-by-day after a certain treatment has been given. In this case, it was either the placebo or the investigational drug. One graphical line was a day-by-day look at those patients who received the drug; the other line was for those who had not.

The lines crossed when the number of deaths among patients who had received the drug exceeded the number of deaths among those who had not.

Could it be that something about the drug was killing people? It was the job of the monitoring committee to find out if that was true and to do it fast.

I convened an emergency meeting of the committee at the headquarters of the drug company conducting the study for the pharmaceutical firm that manufactured the trial drug. The pharmaceutical firm had hired this second company to design and run the study. It was a well-known and well-respected firm. Hiring an outside firm to conduct a clinical trial removes bias or the optics of bias.

We all flew or drove in and arrived early on the following Saturday morning to be faced with a large stack of charts in a room without windows—but with plenty of coffee. We went through every chart of every patient who had died. We took all day to do it.

This is what we discovered:

The drug being infused was known to inhibit the formation of highly reactive species called free radicals. Free radicals are leaked by brain cells with weakened membranes and can cause a cascade of further brain injury to other cell membranes after they are released into the region between cells, called the extracellular space. Another effect of the drug, however, was that it could lower blood pressure, but this was to be controlled by infusing the drug slowly over a defined period. If blood pressure is lowered in a patient with brain injury and swelling, then the only partially injured brain cells would not be receiving adequate oxygenation and could be at risk of further cell death and further brain swelling. This is a cascade of contrary consequences.

What we learned was that, in some hospitals, the drug was being infused more rapidly than in other hospitals. When the infusion was faster, blood pressure dropped. Regardless, despite efforts to control the infusion rates by study design, in the real world, this parameter was not being adequately controlled. In many patients, blood pressure was dropping to levels causing irreparable brain injury.

And patients were dying because of it.

We could not allow this to continue, so, we called a halt to the study worldwide.

The concept of the study of this drug was sound. The drug had been studied well before starting the clinical experiment, but the therapeutic window was too tight to control with safety when doctors were providing emergency treatment to patients with such serious injuries that they were already in coma.

What works in the laboratory may not translate into the real world of health care.

Yet, in the real world of research there is a built-in safety net designed to protect each person with the courage to enter a research project that may help them, along with thousands of others like them.

Coda: The drug being studied in the trial I described is still being used today but for a very different reason and in a very different manner than in that case. Indeed, it has made its mark to the benefit of many other patients in a safe and efficacious translation of its usefulness.

I am glad for it and for what my committee was forced to do.

7.4
The NRF2 Network: A Potential Therapeutic Target for Trigeminal Neuralgia

Risheng Xu, MD, PhD; Collin B. Kilgore, MD; and Michael Lim, MD

Editor's Note: In 1756, Nicolaus Andre, a French physician, in his text, maladies de l'urethre et sur plusies fait, convulsitts, coined the term "tic douloureux" when commenting on other convulsive movements he

observed in the body. His proposed treatment for this "Maladie cruelle and obscure" was to gradually drip mercury water and apply cauterizing stones over the face at the site of pain. It was an innovative form of nerve ablation. The cauterizing stones were added to ensure that no blood clots formed that might put pressure on the offending nerve, a hypothesized cause of nerve injury. It was not until 1962, 2 centuries later, that an oral anticonvulsant medication, carbamazepine (Tegretol), was discovered to be an effective therapy for trigeminal pain. The FDA approved the drug. Since then, no further drugs have been approved because so little effort has been made to investigate any. The study summarized so well by Xu, Kilgore, and Lim is remarkable because it represents the first modern laboratory investigative leap into the medical treatment of trigeminal neuropathic pain. Bravo to the authors for this work, and cross our fingers that it will lead to an effective alternative to the seizure medications that currently compose our mainstay medical therapy.

Typical trigeminal neuralgia (TN) is thought to result from pulsatile vascular compression of the trigeminal nerve, the principal sensory nerve of the face. This compression can injure the nerve, leaving it prone to sending painful signals to the brain. The only drug approved by the U.S. Food and Drug Administration (FDA) for managing TN is carbamazepine, an anticonvulsant, which reduces signaling throughout the nervous system. Patients who do not find relief from medication may undergo surgery, in which microsurgical dissection frees the nerve from the offending blood vessel. Microvascular decompression (MVD) is 90% effective, with a recurrence rate averaging 15% after 15 years.

We still have an incomplete understanding of the molecular mechanisms behind TN. Not all patients with TN have an identifiable vascular etiology causing the short circuits felt as stabbing pain. People with multiple sclerosis, for example, most often do not have one because the disease can cause sclerotic plaques in the trigeminal white matter that jumble normal neural transmission. A common consequence of nerve injury and inflammation is the generation of reactive oxygen species (ROS). ROS are unstable molecules that, when uncontrolled, can damage signaling proteins through a process of oxidative stress. Several studies have found that ROS may contribute to neuropathic pain signaling. In animal models of sciatica, it has been found that pain relief can occur by blocking ROS with antioxidants. However, the sciatic and trigeminal nerves are very different, and it was necessary to do more work to investigate what these results could mean for TN.

We first collected cerebrospinal fluid (CSF) from patients with TN when they were undergoing an MVD procedure. We discovered that most of these patients had elevated CSF markers of oxidative stress. To validate these findings, we worked with an animal model for TN and found the same elevated markers for oxidative stress as we saw in humans.

After we had established that oxidative stress occurs in TN, we wanted to know which pain pathway is activated. We hypothesized that TRPA1, a well-known pain-producing channel located in both pain- and itch-encoding sensory neurons, was activated in TN. To confirm our hypothesis that the channel was activated by ROS, we first created a line of cells containing TRPA1. We then introduced patient CSF samples from our TN patients to the TRPA1 cell line. To our surprise, we found that TRPA1 was activated by our patients' CSF. Furthering this hypothesis, we treated our TN mice with compounds blocking TRPA1 and found that we could reduce their pain.

Now that we knew that blocking TRPA1 had pain-reducing effects, we believed that this could be a promising therapeutic strategy in managing TN. However, current approaches to block TRPA1 in diabetic neuropathy and postoperative pain have been disappointing. This pushed us to try a new approach, namely, to go back to the cause of the pain, namely, the oxidative stress, and to reduce it. For this, we turned to NRF2, a known transcription factor that the body uses to create natural antioxidants. As TRPA1 seems central to pain in the mouse model of TN, we hypothesized that activating the NRF2 antioxidant network may lessen pain by reducing the level of ROS.

We now had a goal. If we could somehow find a drug that could turn on the NRF2 antioxidant network, perhaps we could have a new treatment for TN. Using complex state-of-the-art drug screening tools (which are also being used for cancer, diabetes, and inflammatory bowel disease, for example), we focused our efforts on two compounds with a high likelihood of activating the NRF2 antioxidant network: exemestane and JQ-1. When we applied the two drugs to

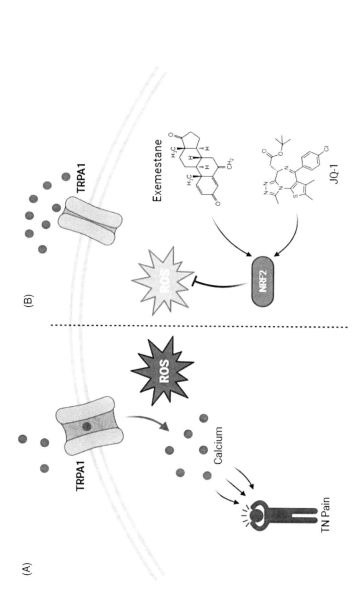

Figure 7-2. Schematics depicting (A) the involvement of TRPA1 and ROS in the generation of TN pain and (B) proposed mechanism by which the candidate drugs exemestane and JQ-1 could reduce TN pain by blocking TRPA1 and activating the NRF2 antioxidant network to reduce the level of ROS. Abbreviations: NRF2, nuclear factor erythroid 2-related factor 2 (used by the body to create natural antioxidants); TN, trigeminal neuralgia; TRPA1, transient receptor potential ankyrin 1 (channel located in pain-encoding sensory neurons); ROS, reactive oxygen species.

our TN cells, we observed that exemestane elevated NRF2 activity better than JQ-1, but both still reduced oxidative stress. When we applied either exemestane or JQ-1 to our TN mice, we were excited to see that the mice experienced much less pain, suggesting that these drugs have promising potential. We even found that applying exemestane directly to branches of the trigeminal nerve lessened pain—a technique that could potentially be harnessed by surgeons as a more targeted form of therapy. Figure 7-2 presents schematics illustrating the roles of TRPA1 and ROS in generating TN pain, as well as the potential effects of the candidate drugs exemestane and JQ-1 in blocking TRPA1 and reducing the level of ROS.

By leveraging a combined clinical, molecular, and computational approach, our study identified the NRF2 antioxidant network as a potential therapeutic target for TN pain. Using a transcriptome-guided drug discovery approach, we identified exemestane and JQ-1 as two candidate NRF2 network modulators for treating TN pain. In contrast to current pharmacologic agents, which mask pain by blunting nerve firing, increasing the NRF2 transcriptional network may provide a therapeutic approach that improves pain through oxidative control. These drugs are still in the very early stages of investigation, but we hope that they represent a promising new direction for TN therapy. Should they succeed in future clinical trials, the compounds we found could represent a new line of medications that patients and providers could use in TN management.

7.5
Familial Trigeminal Neuralgia
Giulia Di Stefano, MD, PhD

Trigeminal neuralgia (TN) is a neuropathic facial pain condition that causes unilateral paroxysmal pain, in the region of one or more divisions of the trigeminal nerve, usually described as an electric-shock-like sensation or stabbing pain. This paroxysmal pain is typically triggered by innocuous stimuli on the face or intraoral trigeminal territory. The incidence of this condition increases with age and is higher in women than in men. Unlike migraine and other pain conditions that are influenced by hereditary factors, TN is considered to be a sporadic condition, despite the description of rare familial cases. Recent publications have opened new perspectives. Case series and cross-sectional studies have reported a familial occurrence, thus supporting the presence of genetic factors. In a recent cross-sectional study of a large cohort of people with TN, the authors identified 12 occurrences of TN with positive family history out of 88 enrollees. (Di Stefano et al, 2020). These study participants reported at least one first- or second-degree relative affected by what was described as TN. Individuals with familial occurrence had either classical TN, from a neurovascular conflict, or idiopathic TN, without a clear etiology. Some of them reported an onset of TN at an early age, an extremely rare condition in classical and idiopathic TN. Clinical characteristics in the patients examined, including affected divisions, trigger factors, the development of concomitant continuous pain, and refractory periods, did not differ between those with sporadic and familial TN, making the two forms of TN clinically indistinguishable. In people with a familial history of TN, the authors observed a higher frequency of refractoriness to pharmacological treatment in comparison with previous data collected on a large sample of people with TN. This finding suggests that the possible pathophysiological mechanisms underlying familial TN might reduce the effectiveness of first-line drugs (carbamazepine and oxcarbazepine). A better comprehension of genetic factors would be helpful for the development of the most appropriate treatment. Because paroxysmal pain in TN is related to an abnormal hyperexcitability of trigeminal ganglion neurons, the authors of one study performed a genetic analysis of the neuronal electrogenisome in these patients and identified rare variants of genes encoding voltage-gated channels and transient receptor potential (TRP) channels (Di Stefano et al., 2021).

In one patient with familial history, the authors identified a known mutation in the sodium channel gene SCN10A (Nav1.8, p.Ala1304Thr), which was previously reported in a patient with neuropathic pain related to peripheral neuropathy (Faber et al., 2012).

Another study reported abnormal expression of voltage-gated sodium channels Nav1.7, Nav1.3, and Nav1.8 in patients with TN, thus supporting the hypothesis that a channelopathy might concur to the pathophysiology of this facial pain condition (Siqueira et al, 2009).

The identification of rare variants of gene-encoding TRP channels opened the way to in vitro functional studies to assess their possible pathogenetic role. Gualdani and colleagues assessed two of the previously identified TRPM7 and TRPM8 mutations through patch-clamp analysis (Gualdani et al, 2021). The authors found that the TRPM7 mutation (A931T) produces a destabilization of the transmembrane domains of the channel, leading to an abnormal sodium ion influx. The authors also found that the expression of TRPM7-mutant channels increases the hyperexcitability of trigeminal ganglion neurons, possibly contributing to the development of TN in patients carrying this mutation. The same authors found that the mutation in TRPM8 (R30Q) modifies the channel properties, enhancing the activation, increasing the basal current amplitude and intracellular calcium ion concentration in cells carrying the mutant channel, and enhancing the channel response to menthol.

A familial occurrence of TN supports the hypothesis of a multihit model in which genetic factors contribute to the pathophysiology. Genetic factors may increase the vulnerability of trigeminal axons and predispose an individual to the development of TN in response to vascular compression.

Genetic factors may affect a person's response to pharmacological treatment, especially in those without severe neurovascular conflict. Further studies will be needed to clarify this hypothesis.

Editor's Note: Whereas the signature patient in whom a genetic variant was found was evaluated for TN, the two relatives who also had the variant and were said to have TN were not evaluated clinically to confirm the diagnosis of TN. Their facial pain may have been from another cause. One should wait, as is stated in the conclusion of this discussion, for clarification of the issue of genetic factors in trigeminal neuropathic pain.

Chapter 8
A Letter to My Sons

Anne B. Ciemnecki, MA

We conclude this volume with a heartfelt letter that I have written to my sons about familial trigeminal neuralgia (TN). Familial TN is rare. I do not want this to cause undue concern. Take the good advice from the letter along with the message that I love my sons mightily.

In 1979, when I sat in neurosurgeon Dr. Alan Gardner's office, I was worried. My grandmother had TN, and so, now, did my mother. Would I? Dr. Gardner assured me that three direct descendants with TN would be the most gargantuan coincidence ever. He might even write a journal article about us! Nearly half a century later, I am doing the writing. Here is what we know about familial TN.

There are about 30 articles in the medical literature about familial TN. Most have been published within the past 3 years. In 2020, Dr. Jaydev Panchwagh wrote, "Familial TN is unusual by all means. It is likely to be less than 2% or 3% of all TN patients. It is possible that patients inherit their certain anatomical variations in either the brain and skull, or in the 'make-up' of blood vessel contours, laxity, or lengths that predispose them to both have TN. We don't know" (Panchwagh, 2020). He did notice that, generally, the familial type of TN is on the same side in all affected family members.

In another 2020 study, the first of its kind, Giulia Di Stefano and colleagues considered a large cohort of patients with TN to ascertain the occurrence of familial cases and to provide a systematic description of clinical features of the familial form of the disease (Di Steffano 2020). She found 12 occurrences of TN in her sample of 88 study participants, for a rate of 11%. Her group concluded that familial TN is more common than once thought and hypothesized that ion channel variants might contribute to the pathology in at least some cases of TN.

In a systematic review that ended with publications available in January 2021, Mari Aaroe Mannerak , Aslan Lashkarivand , and Per Kristian Eide looked at 71 studies (Mannerak 2021). Only a few studies provided information about the prevalence of familial TN. Those studies indicated that about 1% to 2% of people with TN have the familial form. The available human studies suggest that 15 genes are possible contributors to the development of TN. The list reads like alphabet soup: CACNA1A, CACNA1H, CACNA1F, KCNK1, TRAK1, SCN9A, SCN8A, SCN3A, SCN10A, SCN5A, NTRK1, GABRG1, MPZ gene, MAOA gene and SLC6A4. Their roles in familial TN still need to be addressed.

Although experimental animal studies suggest an emerging role of genetics in trigeminal pain, the animal models may be more relevant for trigeminal neuropathic pain than for TN. In summary, this systematic review suggests a more significant role of genetic factors in TN pathogenesis than previously assumed.

Per Kristian Eide did a deeper dive later in 2021 (Eide 2022). He looked at 268 patients with either classical or type 2 TN. I have not seen a description of the sample of patients. The familial form of TN was present in 41 of the 268 or 15.3% of the patients. Of those, 15.2% had classical TN, and 16.7% had type 2 TN. Of the 41 families, 38 families had two affected members, five have three affected members, and one had four affected members. Rare indeed, and not necessarily direct descendants! In comparison to those without familial connections, the 41 people with familial TN showed significantly earlier onset of TN and a significantly higher occurrence of right-sided pain. In the familial cases, there was no difference in gender distribution, hypertension, or the branch of the nerve involved. Eide concluded that "The occurrence of the familial form of the disease is more frequent than traditionally assumed" (Eide 2022).

A few additional articles on familial TN have been published. A 2022 study in PAIN by Gambeta et al. claims that CaV3.2 calcium channels contribute to TN (Gambeta 2022). Another 2022 study by our own Medical Advisory Board member, Wolfgang Liedtke, does not support that finding. (Liedtke 2022) The one thing that many believe in now, thanks to research by Giulia Di Stefano is that it is not the gene itself that correlates with TN, but a mutation in the gene. You can find Dr. Di Stefano's work in Chapter 7.5 of this book.

In summary, we have a lot to learn about familial TN. We hope that science will enlighten us on the form of TN that exhibits itself amongst relations and that we will all be the better for knowing it.

Dear Brian Charles and David Andrew,

This is your mother speaking, your Jewish mother. You know what comes with the territory: worry—fear—fretting—concern—apprehension—nervousness—and most of all, caring and loving you.

So, Brian, I worried when you moved to Oklahoma City at just 22 years old to begin your career as a meteorologist. You knew no one. I was not sure you could cook or do laundry. Most of all, I worried that you would miss us as much as we missed you. Within 6 months, you met people who would become your friends. Of course, your friends influenced you to take part in activities that caused me to worry. Were you drinking or doing drugs? No, you were chasing tornadoes! How did you think I would feel when you sent me a selfie that looked like you were holding a tornado in your hand? I will tell you what I thought: I thought you would find yourself in the land of Oz talking to Glinda, the Good Witch of the North. She would explain that you were in Munchkinland. You might think of donuts—I was thinking of flying monkeys.

And David, was it necessary to kayak around the Statue of Liberty—twice—in an inflatable kayak? Is that water clean? Didn't you worry about the ferries? What if you had a close encounter with a sharp rock? You even watched from your office window, in 2009, when US Airways Flight 1549 crash-landed on the Hudson River shortly after taking off from LaGuardia. Was Captain Chesley ("Sully") Sullenberger III in that kayak with you? No, it was your friend Anthony, whose mother worries as much as I do. What were you thinking? You were thinking that it was a great adventure. I was thinking that there might not be second "Miracle on the Hudson."

Guys, I have worried about you since before you were born. Would you have 10 fingers and 10 toes? Would you hit all your first-year milestones? Would you smile, sit up, babble, walk, and talk on time? Would you like preschool? Could you color within the lines when necessary? Would you learn to read, write, and do arithmetic? Would you survive middle school without too much bullying? Would you be able to work the locker combination in high school and climb the ropes in gym class? Would you have a nice group of friends? Would you be accepted at the college of your choice? (David, I worried a lot when you applied to only one school because you were so sure you would be accepted. You were!) Would you meet a life partner? Would you have respect for others, and would others respect you? Would you be a mensch (a person of integrity and honor)?

I worried for nothing. You both grew up to be respectable, responsible young (well, now middle-aged) men. You have beautiful, kindhearted wives and sons whom I love with all my being.

Yet, one worry stays in my heart. As you know, both my maternal grandmother, Nana Linder, and my mother, your Grandmommy, had classic trigeminal neuralgia. Nana Linder managed her pain with glycerol injections, Dilantin, and later Tegretol, as well as her after-dinner joint. She grew the marijuana plants in her garden. She suffered. I was not aware of it until my mother's pain began. Nana Linder lived to the age of 79 and had complications from cirrhosis of the liver. Her doctors thought that she abused alcohol. The truth was that her body could not process the required pain medications.

My mother suffered miserably. Her pain was intense, and she took high doses of Dilantin and Tegretol. The drugs barely helped. She could not bite, chew, or brush her teeth easily. Eventually, she had a right-sided rhizotomy that relieved the pain but left her numb. Soon after, she experienced left-sided pain and had another rhizotomy. After that, the pain returned to a different branch of the nerve on the right side. She was not well enough for another rhizotomy and treated the new pain with high doses of medication. Along with difficulty eating, she had Crohn's disease, which caused problems digesting food and absorbing nutrients. She died at the age of 70, weighing just 85 pounds. She probably starved to death.

Our family history of facial pain leaves much to be desired. You could say that effects of trigeminal neuralgia killed both my mother and grandmother. I have been more fortunate. Medical procedures have progressed. The two microvascular decompressions that helped me were not available to either of them. Neither was gamma knife radiosurgery. Today's medications are somewhat safer. The internet makes us smarter. Rare diseases are recognized and supported by organizations like the Facial Pain Association (FPA). There is even more progress. Clearer, three-dimensional MRIs and virtual reality mean more exact surgical procedures. Basimglurant, a new drug in phase II/III clinical testing, was developed specifically for trigeminal neuralgia. Doctors are exploring the NRF2 network. More will come over the next decades.

I pray that you do not inherit this horrific scourge of a disease. You may not. It affects females in our family. But our family's course of trigeminal pain is unusual. If you are affected, it might be long after I am gone. So, as you have surmised, I have nuggets of wisdom for you. You should heed the first, fourth, and seventh ones RIGHT NOW!

1. If trigeminal neuralgia strikes (no pun intended), you will feel like you have a tooth problem and seek the advice of a dentist. Check in with your dentist now. Be sure they are aware of trigeminal neuralgia and your family history. Guide them to the website of the Facial Pain Association (FPA), https://www.facepain.org/exactlyzero/. If they have not taken continuing education courses in neuropathic facial pain, encourage them to do so. The FPA sponsors such courses periodically, often at no cost. If they are not interested, or if they say they know everything there is to know about neuropathic facial pain, find a new dentist! Oh yeah—and do not have any root canals, extractions, or other dental (or sinus) surgeries until you rule out trigeminal neuralgia.

2. How do you rule out trigeminal neuralgia? Visit an orofacial pain specialist. Orofacial pain is the specialty of dentistry that encompasses the diagnosis, management, and treatment of pain disorders of the jaw, mouth, face, head, and neck. An orofacial pain doctor is trained in the evidence-based

understanding of the underlying pathophysiology, etiology, and prevention of this pain, along with its treatment. They are in the best position to differentiate between a dental problem and a trigeminal nerve problem. To find an orofacial pain dentist, search under the "Find a Member" tab of the American Academy of Orofacial Pain's website, https://aaop.org. Select someone who is a Fellow of the Academy. These specialists bill under your medical rather than dental insurance. If you are not sure, ask the office to file the claim with your medical plan. Usually, dental benefits are more limited than medical benefits.

3. Even if facial pain strikes, keep up your general dental work. Ask the dentist to use both short- and long-lasting injectable anesthesia even for a prophylactic exam. The last thing you need is extensive dental work because you are not taking care of your teeth. There are dentists, usually associated with dental schools, who specialize in working with patients with facial pain. Call a faculty practice associated with a dental school to find one.

4. Develop a relationship with a primary care physician who will work with and "play well" with your facial pain specialist. You are likely to need blood tests and medical examinations before taking drugs or having certain procedures. You will want all results documented in your general medical record and in the records of specialists who are treating your trigeminal neuropathic pain. Seeing one primary care specialist with whom you have a great relationship facilitates this. Using patient portals helps you and your doctors share information. (Try to select a physician who is younger than you. You do not want the doctor to retire before you die! Same goes for the orofacial pain specialist.)

5. Once you begin to take medication, use one, and only one, pharmacy unless you need drugs that are only available outside that pharmacy. Compounded drugs are an example. If possible, work with the same one or two pharmacists. Many drugs are used off-label and will seem odd to the pharmacist. A pharmacist may not even fill your prescriptions without an

explanation. Keeping to the same pharmacy will ensure that all your drugs are documented in one place and that the pharmacist can check for hazardous drug interactions.

6. Avoid opiates except in extremely acute situations and for brief time periods. Opiates do not protect against neuropathic pain, and you are likely to become addicted. If you must, ask your doctor for a plan to titrate off the opiates. Or ask your new best friend, the pharmacist. Many doctors are incredibly good at prescribing drugs to ease your pain, but not particularly good at getting you off the drugs. Drug withdrawal is ugly and painful. Have a plan. Do not try to do much else while weaning off.

7. Keep working. No matter how much pain you are in, keep working. You cannot get through this disease without health insurance benefits. Do not do anything that will compromise your health benefits. Level up to the best, most flexible health insurance coverage you can afford now. Treatments and drugs for neuropathic facial pain are expensive. It may be too late to get better coverage if your pain is considered a preexisting condition. If you need to, ask for accommodations under the Americans with Disabilities Act (https://www.ada.gov).

8. Do not be afraid of treatments. Brain surgery sounds scary, but it might be easier than years and years of drugs—and it could mean more relief. Just be sure that any procedure you select is evidence-based. Select a trusted, experienced doctor. Start with the list of FPA Medical Advisory Board members. Travel to reach the right specialist if you need to. Remember, there is no magic bullet. You may need to take medication after surgery or have acupuncture along with medication. Use whatever evidence-based combinations of treatments and drugs are necessary to relieve the pain and allow you to live your life. As a researcher and a person with facial pain, I will come back and haunt you if you do not select evidence-based drugs and treatments. Although there is some disagreement about when to have surgical procedures, I recommend getting them as soon as possible. Trigeminal neuralgia progresses. The longer you wait, the more damage the vascular

compression does. The risk with waiting is that you will be in more pain and surgical outcomes will be less effective.

9. Know your triggers. Then, avoid them. You know that my triggers are cold drinks and cold air, especially cold blowing air, on my face. If you pay attention, triggers will be obvious. If brushing your teeth triggers pain, you may need to switch to a smaller, softer toothbrush. If indoor cold air is a trigger, choose a seat that is out of the breeze. If outdoor chilly air is a trigger, invest in a collection of scarves. Avoiding triggers is not always easy, but if you are creative, you can make yourself much more comfortable.

10. Tell people. Let me tell you how I learned to be honest about my pain. One day, I was having a conversation with a valued colleague. I was not at my best and told him what was wrong. He said, "Okay then, all this time I thought you were just a bitch." Being honest about your pain has many advantages. First, the pain shows on your face. People will assume something is wrong and not know what it is. They may think you are angry but do not know why. If you fess up about your pain, people will support you. That does not mean they will pity you. It means they will help you out in small, but important, ways. We were not supposed to block the air ducts in our offices. When the facilities staff learned why I taped a piece of cardboard over the air vent, they looked the other way. Be sure to tell your children also. They know, and even when they are small, they can be accommodating. When Kyle was a baby, before kissing me, he would ask, "Which side is your boo-boo face, Didi?"

11. Seek support. You cannot get through this disease by yourself. Find a support group that meets at least once a month. Support group members will share their feelings, experiences, coping strategies, and firsthand treatment information. They tell you about helpful resources. Your relationship with a doctor or other medical professional may not provide adequate emotional support, and your family and friends may not understand the impact of trigeminal neuropathic pain. Your support group will fill the emotional support gap. Participating

in a group provides you with an opportunity to be with people who have a common purpose and understand one another. The best support group conversations are ones that are not related to facial pain, but instead, are pleasant discussions with like-minded people. You can find support groups on the FPA website. Some are location-based and meet in-person. Others are virtual. Some are for people with a particular kind of facial pain, for example, people with facial pain and multiple sclerosis or people whose pain is/was due to a brain tumor. Some are for young people. Find a group that works for you. If you cannot find one, start one!

Most of all, show that you are grateful for the support that you get from your family and friends. No one signs up to have a partner, friend, or parent in chronic pain. People who stick with you for a lifetime of trigeminal neuralgia are gems.

12. Do not let trigeminal neuralgia take over your life. The disease will be as devastating as you allow it to be. Try not to stop going places, seeing people, and doing things you love. Distraction is a great pain reliever. Will I take a vacation if I am in pain? Heck, yes! I would be in pain if I stayed home, so why not relax on a beach, or look at mountains? If I could bottle up the joy I get from my grandchildren, I would. I am never in pain when I am with them. Pets also relieve pain, as do hobbies. Try to keep your medication levels low enough to be in the land of the living. I have had times when my medication levels were too high to allow driving. This was when I was taking methadone, an opiate for pain relief. Other medications do not take the same toll on your body or mind. Tell your doctor what you value most so they can prescribe drugs or treatments that allow you to engage in those valued activities.

13. Be kind to yourself. Do, but do not overdo. Fighting pain is hard and consumes your energy. Rest when you need to. Try not to overschedule yourself. Get enough sleep. Eat nutritious meals even if you need to eat soft foods.

14. Nothing will give you as much of a sense of empowerment, control, or hope as giving to others. You both make financial contributions to the FPA, and I am so proud of and grateful for

those contributions. Give of yourself also. Become a peer mentor, a support group leader, or a holiday Phone a Pain Pal buddy. Think about how much you can support others who see their parents or friends in pain. If you want to volunteer for an organization other than the FPA, that is okay. Just give of yourself.

I will end this letter with one last thought. You are the strongest people I know. Living in a household with a primary caregiver in constant pain is very, very unsettling. All you want to do is take the pain away, and of course, you cannot. I have been on both sides of this pain. It is much harder to watch someone in pain than to be someone in pain. Emotionally, you have been through the worst of trigeminal neuralgia. I pray that you never experience this pain yourself. Would I have wanted children if I knew they might inherit the pain? First, understand that researchers did not consider trigeminal neuralgia hereditary in the 1970s and 1980s. Daddy and I did not make a conscious decision to start a family despite the pain. I am glad I did not know. I cannot imagine life without either one of you.

All my love, forever,
Mom

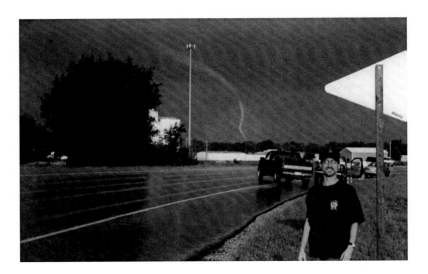

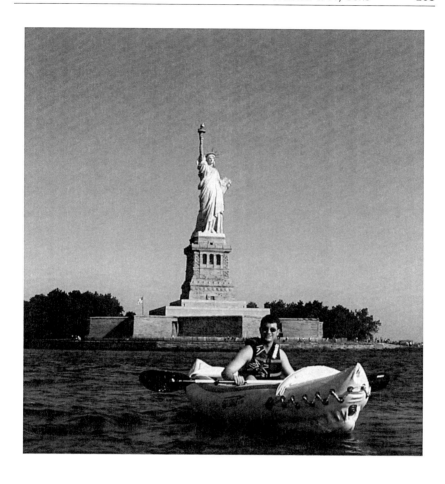

Glossary

Ablation	Surgical injury to a nerve.
Acceptance and Commitment Therapy (ACT)	An action-oriented approach to psychotherapy that uses acceptance and mindfulness strategies along with commitment and behavior-change strategies for acknowledging and accepting pain and moving on with other aspects of life.
Acetylcholine	The neurotransmitter produced by neurons referred to as cholinergic neurons. In the peripheral nervous system, acetylcholine plays a role in skeletal muscle movement, as well as in the regulation of smooth muscle and cardiac muscle. In the central nervous system, acetylcholine is believed to be involved in learning, memory, and mood.
Acute	Having a sudden onset, sharp rise, and short course. Often contrasted with chronic.
Affective aspects of pain	Pain has two components: sensory and affective. The affective component of pain is cognitive in nature and involves the brain experiencing the sensation of pain as something unpleasant.
Afferent (nerves)	Conducting or conducted inward or toward something (for nerves, toward the central nervous system).
Allodynia	Pain from a stimulus that does not normally provoke pain.
α-2 adrenoceptor agonists	Drugs used to treat high blood pressure. Also called α-2 agonists.
Analgesic	Medication that acts to relieve pain. Unlike medications used for anesthesia during surgery, analgesics do not turn off nerves, change the ability to sense your surroundings, or alter consciousness.
Anesthesia dolorosa	Pain associated with significant numbness.
Anesthetic	Medication that acts to prevent the sensation of pain during medical procedures or surgery.
Angiotensin-converting enzyme (ACE) inhibitors	A group of medicines used to treat and manage high blood pressure and heart failure and to reduce complications of a heart attack.
Anterior inferior cerebellar artery (AICA)	One of the three main arteries that supplies blood to the cerebellum.
Anti–calcitonin gene-related peptide (anti-CGRP) antibodies	Antibodies that detect or target CGRP, a neuropeptide that acts as a vasodilator and may play a role in migraine. There are two types of CGRP antibodies: monoclonal antibodies that prevent migraines and CGRP receptor antagonists, which are used for acute migraine treatment.

Anti-convulsive drugs	Medications used to prevent seizures that are also prescribed for trigeminal neuropathic pain.
Antihypertensive drugs	Medications that lower blood pressure.
Anti-inflammatory drugs	Medications that help to reduce inflammation, which often helps to relieve pain. Also called nonsteroidal anti-inflammatory drugs (NSAIDs).
Antinociceptive	The action or process of blocking the detection of a painful or injurious stimulus by sensory neurons.
Appendage slings	During microvascular decompression surgery, the blood vessel compressing or pulsating on the nerve can be moved away from the nerve and tethered with an appendage sling. This is an alternative to using a Teflon-like substance to separate the vessel and the nerve.
Apprehensive cognitions anxiety	An intense or extreme sense of fear or dread about everyday situations or tasks based on worry about potential but improbable threats.
Atherectomy	A minimally invasive procedure for removing plaque from blood vessels, opening up the arteries so blood can flow normally. Also called an atherectomy.
Arterial contact	Compression of the trigeminal nerve by an artery, the most common being the superior cerebellar artery and anterior inferior cerebellar artery. This is the primary cause of trigeminal neuralgia (TN).
Asymmetrical	Having two sides or halves that are not the same.
Atypical tetracyclic antidepressants	A class of medications that differ from other classes of antidepressants, in that they ease depression by affecting chemical messengers (neurotransmitters) used to communicate between brain cells. Like most antidepressants, atypical antidepressants work by ultimately effecting changes in brain chemistry and communication in brain nerve cell circuitry known to regulate mood, thereby helping to relieve depression.
Atypical trigeminal neuralgia	A constant burning or aching sensation (rather than overwhelming jolts of pain) that lasts for prolonged periods and the pain encompasses a wider area of the face. Trigeminal neuralgia is classified as atypical when atypical pain is present more than half the time or when just atypical pain is present. Also called persistant idiopathic facial pain.
Auricular acupuncture	The stimulation of the auricle of the external ear for the diagnosis and treatment of health conditions in other parts of the body. Also known as ear acupuncture when the stimulation is achieved by the insertion of acupuncture needles, whereas the term auriculotherapy often refers to electrical stimulation on the surface of the ear.

Autoimmune diseases	Conditions in which the immune system mistakenly attacks healthy body cells.
Autoimmune trigeminal neuropathic pain	Trigeminal neuralgia (TN) is not generally considered an autoimmune disease. However, TN can be a symptom of the autoimmune condition multiple sclerosis.
Autonomic effect	Effects of the autonomic nervous system (ANS), which controls involuntary actions. It has the following effects on your body's systems: controls the tear system around your eyes; controls how your nose runs and when your mouth waters; controls your body's ability to sweat; accelerates heart and lung action; inhibits stomach and upper-intestinal action to the point where digestion slows down or stops; constricts blood vessels in many parts of the body.
Autosomal dominant inheritance	One way in which genetic traits pass from one parent to their child. When a trait is autosomal dominant, only one parent needs to have an altered gene to pass it on.
Axon	The long threadlike part of a nerve cell along which impulses are conducted from the cell body to other cells.
Behavioral pain medicine	A specialty area of medicine that focuses on how thoughts and behaviors impact health and disease. It is designed to help patients talk through their pain experience, identify negative thoughts and behaviors that might be contributing to their condition, and develop skills or coping mechanisms to help provide pain relief. Behavioral pain medicine can help patients learn self-management techniques to better regulate sensory experience. The goal is to help patients build a pain coping "toolkit," which can include pain science education, relaxation and mindfulness, time-based activity pacing, and developing more balanced thoughts.
Benzodiazepines	A class of agents that work in the central nervous system and are used for a variety of medical conditions, such as anxiety disorders, insomnia, and seizures. They act on specific receptors in the brain, called γ-aminobutyric acid A (GABA-A) receptors. Benzodiazepines attach to these receptors and make the nerves in the brain less sensitive to stimulation, which has a calming effect.
Bidirectional	Capable of reacting or functioning in two, usually opposite, directions.
Bilateral	Occurring on both sides of the body.
Binocular vision	A type of vision in which two eyes face in the same direction to perceive a single three-dimensional image of the surroundings.
Biofeedback	A type of therapy that uses sensors attached to your body to measure key body functions. Biofeedback is intended to help you learn more about how your body works. This information may help you to develop better control over certain body functions and address health concerns.

Biomedical science	The intersection of biology and medicine. This field involves the application of biological and physiological principles to advance knowledge in health care and medicine. It typically relates to research, theories, techniques, and technology used in areas such as diagnostic medical testing, treatment of diseases and health conditions, genetics, and biomedical engineering.
Biopsychosocial model	An approach to understanding mental and physical health through a multisystem lens, understanding the influence of biology, psychology, and social environment.
Blepharospasm	A neurologic disorder affecting the muscles controlling the eyelids. It starts off as twitching and can progress to an inability to open the eyes.
Blood pressure	The pressure of circulating blood against the walls of blood vessels. Blood pressure is usually expressed in terms of the systolic pressure over diastolic pressure in the cardiac cycle. It is measured in millimeters of mercury above the surrounding atmospheric pressure or in kilopascals.
Board certification	A process by which a physician or other professional demonstrates a mastery of advanced knowledge and skills through written, oral, practical, and/or simulator-based testing. The American Board of Medical Specialties (ABMS) is one of the most well-known organizations that provides board certification to physicians and practitioners in various specialties. ABMS board certification serves two primary roles: as an independent evaluation of a physician's or specialist's knowledge and skills to practice safely and effectively in a specialty and as a trusted credential patients can rely on when selecting a provider for their needs.
Bolus	A discrete amount of medication, drug, or other compound that is administered within a specific time, generally 1–30 minutes, to raise its concentration in the blood to an effective level.
Botulinum toxin, botulinum neurotoxin, Botox (BoTN)	A medication used for therapeutic and cosmetic purposes. Medicinal uses include chronic migraine, spastic disorders, cervical dystonia, and detrusor hyperactivity. Botulinum toxin is in the neurotoxin class of medications.
Brain stem	The stalk-like part of the brain that connects the brain to the spinal cord. It sits toward the bottom of the brain and is part of the central nervous system.
Brain-stem auditory evoked potential (BAEP) monitoring	Tests that monitor the function of the auditory nerve and auditory pathways in the brain stem during neurosurgery to prevent injury. Also known as brain stem auditory evoked response (BAER).
Burning mouth syndrome (BMS)	A painful, complex condition often described as a burning, scalding, or tingling feeling in the mouth that may occur every day for months or longer. Dry mouth or an altered taste in the mouth may accompany the pain.

Burning tongue	A condition that causes a chronic or recurrent burning sensation in the tongue, gums, lips, inside cheeks, and mouth. The symptoms include a burning sensation in the mouth, dry mouth, increased thirst, loss of taste, bitter or metallic taste, and sore throat. The causes can be classified as primary or secondary. Primary causes are related to problems with taste or sensory nerves, whereas secondary causes include various medications that cause dry mouth, fungal infections of the mouth, a lack of nutrients, dentures that are ill-fitting or that contain materials that irritate mouth tissues, allergies or reactions to foods and additives, reflux of acid from the stomach, endocrine disorders such as diabetes, overbrushing of the tongue, use of an abrasive toothpaste, overuse of mouthwashes, and more.
Calcium channel blockers	A group of medications that limit how your body uses calcium. By slowing down how your cells use calcium, these medications can lower your blood pressure, prevent heart rhythm problems, and more.
Calcium phosphate cement (CPCs)	A type of bone substitute used in a variety of applications, including craniofacial and dental defect repair, neurosurgical burr hole repair, bone defect repair, and bone tissue engineering.
Cannabinoid	The cannabis plant produces more than 480 compounds, dozens of which are known as cannabinoids. These compounds are the active ingredients that are responsible for the way marijuana affects people, whether they are enjoying it recreationally or using it to treat an illness.
Central nervous system	The brain and spinal cord.
Central pain	Central pain, also known as centralized pain syndrome, is a disorder of the central nervous system (CNS). It occurs due to changes in how the brain and spinal cord interpret pain signals, resulting in heightened sensitivity. The primary symptom of centralized pain is pain with no known cause that lasts for 3 months or more. The pain is usually constant, but it can also be intermittent. People with centralized pain may experience pain in response to light forms of touch, such as from wind, sheets, or clothing. Other symptoms include itchiness, numbness, difficulty sleeping, and mood changes. Centralized pain can occur after damage to the spinal cord, brain stem, or other parts of the CNS. It can also result from dysfunction in how the CNS sends and receives pain messages. Causes include stroke, brain tumors, spinal cord injury, multiple sclerosis, and other risk factors. Treatment for centralized pain may involve medications and stress reduction. Managing chronic pain is essential for improving quality of life.

Cerebellar hemorrhage or hematoma	A type of intracranial hemorrhage in which the bleeding is located in the posterior fossa or cerebellum.
Cerebellum	Located in the lower back part of the brain, the cerebellum plays a vital role in most physical movements, including eye movements. Problems with the cerebellum can lead to coordination difficulties, fatigue, and other challenges. The cerebellum accounts for about 10% of total brain weight but contains as many as 80% of all neurons in the brain.
Cerebrospinal fluid (CSF)	A type of clear liquid that surrounds, protects, and cushions the brain and spinal cord. The fluid is held in place by spider-like membrane called arachnoid and a second layer called dura mater, a dense tissue that sits directly under the skull and makes up the outermost layer of the brain. A CSF leak can occur if there is a tear or hole in the dura mater.
Cervical spondylosis	A general term for wear and tear that affects your cervical spine. If you have cervical spondylosis, your neck may ache, hurt, or feel stiff. Also called arthritis of the neck.
Cervicogenic headaches	A type of headache that results from problems with the neck or spine, such as osteoarthritis or injury. Symptoms of a cervicogenic headache may include pain on one side of the head or face, a stiff neck, pain around the eyes, and pain while coughing or sneezing. Cervicogenic headaches can mimic migraines. The primary difference is that a migraine headache is rooted in the brain, whereas a cervicogenic headache is rooted in the neck or base of the skull.
Chiari malformation	A rare congenital condition in which the brain tissue extends into the spinal canal, which causes severe headache and neck pain.
Chronic	Persisting for a long time or constantly recurring. Often contrasted with acute.
Cicatricial	Associated with scarring.
Classical trigeminal neuralgia (cTN)	A type of chronic pain disorder that involves sudden, severe facial pain. It affects the trigeminal nerve, or fifth cranial nerve, which provides feeling and nerve signaling to many parts of the head and face. Trigeminal neuralgia (TN) is a type of neuropathic pain that is typically caused by a nerve injury or nerve lesion. The classical form of the disorder causes extreme, intermittent, sudden burning or shocklike facial pain. The pain lasts anywhere from a few seconds to 2 minutes per episode. These attacks can occur very close together, in stretches that can last for long periods.

Clinical trial phase I	Usually, the first part of a clinical trial that involves people. Phase I studies are undertaken to determine the highest dose of a new treatment that can be given safely without causing severe side effects. Although the treatment has been tested in laboratory and animal studies, the side effects in people are not yet known for sure.
Clinical trial phase II	Second part of a clinical trial that involves several hundred participants who are living with the condition that a new medication is meant to treat. The participants are usually given the same dose as was found to be safe in the previous phase. Investigators monitor participants for several months or years to determine how effective the medication is and to gather more information about any side effects it might cause. Although a phase II trial involves more participants than earlier phases, it is still not large enough to demonstrate the overall safety of a medication. However, the data collected during this phase help investigators design methods for conducting phase III.
Clinical trial phase III	Third part of a clinical trial that usually involves up to 3000 participants who have the condition that a new medication is meant to treat. Trials in this phase can last for several years. The purpose of phase III is to evaluate how the new medication works in comparison to existing medications for the same condition. To move forward with the trial, investigators need to demonstrate that the medication is at least as safe and effective as existing treatment options. To do this, investigators use a process called randomization. This involves randomly choosing some participants to receive the new medication and others to receive an existing medication. Phase III trials are usually double-blind, which means that neither the participant nor the investigator knows which medication the participant is taking. This helps to eliminate bias in the interpretation of the trial results.
Clinical trial phase IV	Final part of a clinical trial that occurs after the Food and Drug Administration (FDA) has approved a medication. This phase involves thousands of participants and can last for many years. Investigators use this phase to collect more information about the medication's long-term safety, effectiveness, and any other benefits.
Cluster headache	A type of headache that occurs in periods of frequent attacks known as clusters. Cluster headaches cause intense pain in or around one eye on one side of the head and can be severe enough to wake people from sleep. Cluster periods can last from weeks to months. Then, the headaches usually stop for a period of time, which may last for months or years.

Cognition	The mental process of gaining knowledge and comprehension. Involves thinking, knowing, remembering, judging, and problem-solving.
Cognitive aspects of pain	Pain is a subjective perceptive phenomenon involving cognitive processing, rather than a purely sensory phenomenon. Cognition is composed of critical elements such as attention, perception, memory, motor skills, executive functioning, and verbal and language skills. Cognition is a vital component of the subjective perception of pain requiring cognitive evaluation, learning, recall of past experiences, and active decision making.
Cognitive behavioral therapy (CBT)	A form of psychological treatment. CBT considers psychological problems to be based on faulty or unhelpful ways of thinking and learned patterns of unhelpful behavior. CBT treatment usually involves efforts to change thinking patterns, including recognizing one's distortions and then reevaluating them in light of reality, gaining a better understanding of the behavior and motivations of others, using problem-solving skills to cope with difficult situations, and learning to develop a greater sense of confidence in one's own abilities. CBT treatment also involves learning to calm one's mind and relax one's body.
Comorbid insomnia and sleep apnea (COMISA)	A highly prevalent and debilitating disorder that results in additive impairments to patients' sleep, daytime functioning, and quality of life.
Comorbidity	The existence of more than one disease or condition within an individual at the same time.
Compounded medications	A drug that is specifically mixed and prepared for an individual patient, based on a prescription from their doctor.
Compression	A squeezing together; the exertion of pressure on an object to increase its density; a decrease in the dimensions of an object under the action of two external forces directed toward one another in the same straight line.
Computed tomography (CT)	A diagnostic imaging procedure that uses a combination of X-rays and computer technology to produce images of the inside of the body. CT scans can show detailed images of any part of the body, including the bones, muscles, fat, organs and blood vessels. In CT, the X-ray beam moves in a circle around the body. This allows many different views of the same organ or structure and provides much greater detail. The X-ray information is sent to a computer, which interprets the X-ray data and displays it in two-dimensional form on a monitor.
Concomitant continuous pain	Trigeminal neuralgia (TN) is a neuropathic facial pain condition, characterized by unilateral paroxysmal pain in the distribution territory of one or more divisions of the trigeminal nerve, triggered by innocuous stimuli. A subgroup of patients with TN also suffer from concomitant continuous pain, that is, a background pain between the paroxysmal attacks.

Constructive interference in steady state (CISS)	An advanced imaging technique used for magnetic resonance imaging (MRI) that consists of a fully refocused fast-gradient echo sequence. Considered to be superior to conventional MRI. CISS is used in the assessment of the anatomical variations and various pathologies involving the cranial nerves and central nervous system. Any high-strength MRI machine with magnetic strength of at least 1.3 T can produce CISS images. CISS has different names according to different brands and manufacturers, including "fast imaging employing steady-state acquisition" (FIESTA) by General Electric and "volumetric interpolated brain examination" (VIBE) by Siemens.
Continuous	Characterized by continued occurrence or recurrence. Often implies a close prolonged succession or recurrence. Usually implies an uninterrupted flow or spatial extension.
Copay/Copayment	A fixed amount for a covered service, paid by a patient to the provider of the service before receiving the service. The percentage of a copayment is the ratio indicating the relative share of the amount paid by the patient, with the insurer covering the remainder of the reasonable and customary costs for covered services in a particular geographical area.
Corticosteroids	A class of drugs that can reduce inflammation and treat various medical conditions.
COX-2 inhibitor (coxibs)	A type of nonsteroidal anti-inflammatory drug (NSAID) that directly targets cyclooxygenase-2 (COX-2), an enzyme that is responsible for inflammation and pain. Targeting selectivity for COX-2 reduces the risk of peptic ulceration and is the main feature of this drug class.
Cranial nerves	Twelve pairs of nerves (CN I through CN XII) that serve various areas and functions of the head. The trigeminal nerve is the fifth cranial nerve (CN V). The names and functions of the cranial nerves are as follows:

Cranial nerve 1	Olfactory nerve – sensory
Cranial nerve 2	Optic nerve (CN II) – sensory
Cranial nerve 3	Oculomotor nerve (CN III) – motor
Cranial nerve 4	Trochlear nerve (CN IV) – motor
Cranial nerve 5	Trigeminal nerve (CN V) – mixed
Cranial nerve 6	Abducens nerve (CN VI) – motor
Cranial nerve 7	Facial nerve (CN VII) – mixed
Cranial nerve 8	Vestibulocochlear nerve (CN VIII) – sensory
Cranial nerve 9	Glossopharyngeal nerve (CN IX) – mixed
Cranial nerve 10	Vagus nerve (CN X) – mixed
Cranial nerve 11	(Spinal) Accessory nerve (CN XI) – motor
Cranial nerve 12	Hypoglossal nerve (CN XII) – motor.

Craniocervical dystonia (also called spasmodic torticollis)	A condition that causes the muscles in the neck to contract, resulting in involuntary movements of the head and neck, such as bending and turning. These movements can be painful and may prevent participation in preferred activities. Treatment can help manage symptoms.
Crossover study/ crossover trial	A longitudinal study in which subjects receive a sequence of different treatments (or exposures). In a randomized clinical trial, the subjects are randomly assigned to different arms of the study, which receive different treatments. A crossover trial has a repeated measures design in which each patient is assigned to a sequence of two or more treatments, one of which may be a standard treatment or a placebo.
Decompression	Release from pressure, or a surgical procedure that relieves pressure such as the pressure of a blood vessel on a nerve.
Deep brain stimulation	A procedure in which surgeons insert a thin electrode through a small opening in the skull into the thalamus, a part of the brain where pain sensation occurs. A stimulation device attached to the electrode delivers low-grade electrical signals to override pain signals.
Demyelination	The process involving the loss or destruction of myelin, the protective sheath around nerve fibers.
Denervation	Any loss of nerve supply, regardless of the cause.
Dermatome	An area on the body that relies on a specific spinal or cranial nerve.
Diagnosis of exclusion	A diagnosis of a medical condition reached by a process of elimination. It is used when the presence of a medical condition cannot be established with complete confidence from history, examination, or testing. A diagnosis of exclusion is an expression that applies to the diagnosis that is left over after all other possible differential diagnoses have been excluded. Medical conditions that are classified as diagnoses of exclusion are those for which there is no definitive test.
Diastolic	Relating to the phase of the heartbeat when the heart muscle relaxes and allows the chambers to fill with blood. Diastolic blood pressure is the bottom number of the blood pressure reading. It is important for the supply of oxygen to the heart muscle. A normal diastolic blood pressure for most healthy adults is usually less than 80 mmHg.
Differential diagnosis	A method used to determine the root cause of a patient's symptoms or medical condition. It entails assessing a variety of probable diagnoses and removing or confirming them methodically based on the patient's clinical history, physical examination, and diagnostic testing. To narrow the probable diagnoses, health care practitioners compare the patient's symptoms and test findings to a list of possible illnesses. Health care experts arrive at an accurate diagnosis and establish an appropriate treatment strategy by analyzing and ruling out illnesses.

Diplopia	Double vision, or the simultaneous perception of two images of a single object that may be displaced horizontally or vertically in relation to each other.
Disorder	An abnormal physical or mental condition.
Dissociative	Mental health condition involving the loss of a connection between thoughts, memories, feelings, surroundings, and identity.
Distal	Situated away from the center of the body or from the point of attachment. The opposite of proximal.
Dopamine reuptake inhibitor (DRI)	Drug that functions by preventing the reuptake of the neurotransmitter dopamine. The fact that such a drug prevents dopamine reuptake leads to increased concentrations of dopamine between synapses. This increases stimulation of the central nervous system and tends to improve cognitive function, alertness, and performance.
Doppler ultrasound	An ultrasound that monitors blood flow.
Double-blind study	A research method commonly used in clinical trials where both the participants and the experimenters are unaware of who is receiving a particular treatment. This is done to prevent biased results, especially due to cues that convey an experimental hypothesis to the subject.
Dura mater	The strong, thick outer layer of tissue that covers and protects the brain and spinal cord and is closest to the skull and spinal vertebra.
Duration	The length of time that something exists or lasts.
Duration of action	The length of time that a particular drug is effective.
Dysesthesia	A numbness or abnormal sensation severe enough that a patient considers it disturbing.
Efferent	Conducting outward from a part or organ; conveying nerve impulses to an effector.
Efficacy	How well a particular treatment or drug works under carefully controlled scientific testing conditions.
Electromyography (EMG)	A technique used to measure muscle response or electrical activity in response to a nerve's stimulation of the muscle. The test is used to help detect neuromuscular abnormalities. One or more small (electrodes) are inserted through the skin into the muscle. The electrical activity detected by the electrodes is displayed on an oscilloscope.
Emotional awareness and expression therapy (EAET)	A form of psychological therapy that targets the trauma, stress, and relationship problems that are found in many people with chronic pain, especially "centralized" pain. EAET emphasizes the importance of the central nervous system and emotional processing in the etiology and treatment of chronic pain. EAET targets unresolved trauma or emotional conflicts to reduce or resolve pain symptoms.

Empowered Relief®	A 2-hour intervention that provides individuals with essential pain relief skills, delivered by certified clinicians.
Encephalopathy	A disease that affects brain structure or function, causing an altered mental state and confusion.
Entity	An entity can be anything that is relevant to health care. It usually represents a disease or a pathogen, but it can also be an isolated symptom or an anomaly of the body.
Epidemiology	The study and analysis of the distribution (who, when, and where), patterns and determinants of health and disease conditions in a defined population.
Episodic	Happening only sometimes and not regularly.
Equipoise	A situation in which things are perfectly balanced. Clinical equipoise is important because it ensures that medical research is conducted in an ethical and unbiased manner and that the results of the trial are valid and reliable.
Etiology	The cause, set of causes, or manner of causation of a disease or condition.
Evoked potentials	Electrical signals that are generated by the nervous system in response to a stimulus. Evoked potentials can be used to record the brain's response to different types of stimulation and test the function of the nervous system.
Extended-release (ER)	Medications that last longer in the body. An extended-release medication is usually labeled with "ER" or "XR" at the end of its name. This allows the medication to be taken less often compared to the immediate-release (IR) version.
Extended retrosigmoid approach	Craniotomy approach designed to gain maximal access to the cerebellopontine angle and petroclival region of the brain.
Familial trigeminal neuralgia	Trigeminal neuralgia (TN) that runs in families. Even though most cases of TN are sporadic, it is known that some are familial. The occurrence of familial forms of TN is an indicator of genetic involvement in the condition.
Fascicles	Small or slender bundles (such as nerve fibers).
Fasciectomy	A surgical procedure to remove fascia, or the thin connective tissue that surrounds and supports every organ, muscle, bone, nerve fiber, and blood vessel in the body.
Fast imaging employing steady-state acquisition (FIESTA)	An advanced high-resolution imaging technique used for magnetic resonance imaging (MRI) machines manufactured by General Electric. A FIESTA sequence can reveal whether trigeminal neuralgia is caused by nerve compression. Generally, it is one of the imaging modalities of choice for the assessment of anatomical variations and pathologies involving the cranial nerves and central nervous system. Others are constructive interference in steady state (CISS) and volumetric interpolated brain examination (VIBE) by Siemens. All of these techniques are superior to conventional MRI.

Fibrin glue	A surgical formulation used to create a fibrin clot for hemostasis (clotting), cartilage repair surgeries, or wound healing. It contains separately packaged human fibrinogen and human thrombin. Also used for repairing dura mater.
Fifth vital sign	Pain. Traditionally, four vital signs have been recognized: body temperature, heart rate or pulse, respiratory rate, and blood pressure. A rating of how much pain one is experiencing is the fifth vital sign. Pain is subjective, reported by the patient, and is measured on a 0–10 pain scale.
Flocculus	A small lobe of the cerebellum at the posterior border of the middle cerebellar peduncle anterior to the biventer lobule. Like other parts of the cerebellum, the flocculus is involved in motor control.
Foramen ovale	The opening in the skull through which the mandibular branch of the trigeminal nerve passes on its way into the face.
GABA-B receptor agonist	A drug that is an agonist for one or more of the GABA receptors, producing typically sedative effects, and may also cause other effects such as anxiolytic, anticonvulsant, and muscle relaxant effects
Gabapentinoids	A class of drugs that include gabapentin, pregabalin, and mirogabalin, as well as a gabapentin prodrug, gabapentin enacarbil. Gabapentin is an anti-epileptic drug that is also used to treat partial seizures in adults and children who are at least 3 years old. Pregabalin and gabapentin have traditionally been used to treat epilepsy and neuropathic pain. Gabapentinoids are increasingly being prescribed for pain as alternatives to opioids.
Gadolinium dyes	Intravenous drugs used in diagnostic imaging procedures to enhance the quality of magnetic resonance imaging (MRI) or magnetic resonance angiography (MRA).
Ganglia	Clusters of nerve cell bodies.
Ganglionectomy	The surgical removal of a ganglion cyst.
Gastroesophageal reflux disease (GERD)	A condition in which stomach acid repeatedly flows from the stomach back into the esophagus, creating a burning sensation and potentially irritating the esophageal lining.
Generic drug	A pharmaceutical drug that contains the same chemical substance as a drug that was originally protected by chemical patents. Generic drugs are allowed for sale after the patents on the original drugs expire.
Genetics	The science of genes, heredity, and the variation of organisms.
Geniculate ganglion	A sensory ganglion of the facial nerve (CN VII) containing the cell bodies of the fibers responsible for conducting taste sensation from the anterior two-thirds of the tongue. Also, neurons located at the ganglion contribute to the sensory innervation of other sites, such as the palate, the pinna of the ear, and the ear canal.

Geniculate neuralgia	A rare nerve pain disorder that results in severe ear pain. It is caused by a small nerve (the nervus intermedius) being compressed by a blood vessel. The pain is usually sharp, often described as an "ice pick in the ear," but may also be dull and burning. Ear pain can also be accompanied by facial pain.
Gepants (calcitonin gene-related peptide [CGRP] receptor blockers)	Drugs that block CGRP from binding to CGRP receptors, which is a key contributor to the trigeminal nerve pain and inflammation of migraines. They can be used to treat episodic migraine attacks or as a preventive treatment to reduce migraine frequency and number of headache days. CGRP inhibitors come in two forms: small molecules called gepants and larger molecules called monoclonal antibodies. Some are FDA-approved for preventing migraines, others are FDA-approved for treating acute migraines, and one is approved for both acute and preventive therapy.
Glossalgia	Pain localized in the tongue, especially neuralgic pain in the tongue.
Glossodynia/ glossopyrosis	A painful, complex condition often described as a burning, scalding, or tingling feeling in the mouth that may occur every day for months or longer. Dry mouth or an altered taste in the mouth may accompany the pain.
Glossopharyngeal nerve	The ninth cranial nerve (CN IX), which exits the brain stem from the sides of the upper medulla. As a mixed nerve (sensorimotor), it carries afferent sensory and efferent motor information.
Glossopharyngeal neuralgia (GPN)	A rare condition that can cause sharp, stabbing, or shooting pain in the throat area near the tonsils, the back of the tongue, or the middle ear. The pain occurs along the pathway of the glossopharyngeal nerve, which is located deep in the neck. It serves the back of the tongue, the throat, the parotid gland (one of the salivary glands), the middle ear, and the eustachian tube.
Half-life	A measure of how long it takes for the concentration or amount of a drug in the body to be reduced by half. It is useful for determining the dosing frequency and the time required for a drug to be eliminated from the body. A drug's half-life depends on factors such as the volume of distribution and the clearance of the drug. Different drugs have different half-lives, ranging from minutes to days.
Harm avoidance (HA)	A personality trait characterized by excessive worrying; pessimism; shyness; and being fearful, doubtful, and easily fatigued.

Hematoma	A bruise or area of blood that collects outside the larger blood vessels. Hematomas can be due to injuries or trauma in the area. A hematoma is similar to a hemorrhage, but a hemorrhage refers to ongoing bleeding whereas the blood in a hematoma has typically already clotted.
Hemicrania continua and paroxysmal hemicrania	Two types of headaches not caused by another medical condition. They are characterized by one-sided pain and autonomic symptoms. Hemicrania continua can be remitting or non remitting. Paroxysmal hemicrania has severe bursts of pain.
Hemifacial spasm	A nervous system condition in which the muscles on one side of the face twitch. The cause of hemifacial spasm is most often a blood vessel touching or pulsing against a facial nerve; although it can also be caused by a facial nerve injury or a tumor.
Herpes zoster	Also known as shingles, this is a viral infection caused by the same virus that causes chickenpox. When it strikes the face, it can cause burning pain.
High cervical spinal cord stimulation	A therapeutic intervention to manage various chronic pain conditions. It involves applying electrical current to the posterior aspect of the spinal cord in an attempt to decrease the pain signals traveling to and from the brain.
Hindbrain	Lower back part of the brain that includes most of the brain stem (containing the medulla and pons) and the cerebellum. It is located at the back of the head and looks like an extension of the spinal cord. Also known as the rhombencephalon it is one of the most crucial parts of the central nervous system (CNS), as it connects the brain to the spinal cord so that messages can be sent from the brain, down the spinal cord, to the rest of the body.
Hyperalgesia	An increased response to a stimulus that is normally painful.
Hypersomnolence	A condition marked by excessive chronic daytime and nighttime sleepiness. People who live with hypersomnolence do not enjoy restorative nighttime sleep, even though some sleep up to 7 hours a night, so they tend to nap throughout the day. The condition is akin to the term "hypersomnia," although hypersomnia technically refers to excessive daytime fatigue only. Those with hypersomnolence do not get restorative rest or relief from naps. Hypersomnolence is often experienced among people with depression and is a diagnostic marker of that condition.
Idiopathic facial pain	A pain in the face or mouth that does not have a clear cause.
Incidence	The number of new cases of a disease or condition that develop in a population within a specified period of time.

Independent data monitoring committee (IDMC)	A group of independent experts who conduct periodic reviews of accumulated interim data during a clinical trial. The IDMC is responsible for ensuring the safety of study participants and the validity and integrity of the data. IDMCs are also called Data and Safety Monitoring Boards (DSMBs) and Data and Safety Monitoring Committees (DSMCs).
Induration	When the soft tissue of different parts of the body, especially the skin, becomes thicker and harder due to an inflammatory process caused by various triggering factors.
Inflammation	A natural response of the body's immune system to injury, infection, or irritation. It is a complex process that involves various cells and molecules in the body. Inflammation can be acute or chronic. Acute inflammation is a short-term response to injury or infection, whereas chronic inflammation is a long-term response that can lead to tissue damage and various diseases. Some common symptoms of inflammation include pain, swelling, redness, and heat.
Innervation	The supply or distribution of nerve fibers to any part of the body. The provision of nerve stimuli to a muscle, gland, or other nerve.
Innocuous stimuli	Stimuli that are not harmful or damaging to the body. They are usually benign and do not elicit any pain or discomfort. Examples of innocuous stimuli include light touch, heat produced by the body, and clothing rubbing against the skin.
Insomnia	Also known as sleeplessness. A sleep disorder in which people have trouble falling asleep or staying asleep for as long as desired. Insomnia is typically followed by daytime sleepiness, low energy, irritability, and a depressed mood.
Intermediate-release (IR)	A type of modified-release dosage that is designed to release the medication in a controlled manner over a period of time, usually between 4 and 12 hours. This is in contrast to immediate-release medications, which dissolve quickly and release the medication into the bloodstream immediately.
Intermittent	Coming and going at intervals, not continuous, occasional, stopping or ceasing for a time and then starting again.
International Classification of Diseases-11 (ICD-11)	Eleventh revision of the *International Classification of Diseases* (ICD). It replaces the 10th edition (ICD-10) as the global standard for recording health information and causes of death. The ICD-11 is a large taxonomy consisting of about 85,000 entities, also called classes or nodes. An entity can be anything that is relevant to health care. It usually represents a disease or a pathogen, but it can also be an isolated symptom or (developmental) anomaly of the body. There are also classes for reasons someone may contact health services, social circumstances of the patient, and external causes of injury or death.

Interposition	The surgical placement of one body structure between two others.
Interventional	A branch of medicine that uses minimally invasive techniques to diagnose and treat various conditions, such as pain, cancer, vascular diseases, and more. Interventional medicine can offer benefits such as less risk of infection, less pain, faster recovery, and lower cost compared to traditional surgery.
Intracranial	Within the skull.
Intractable	Not easy to fix, cure, or relieve. For example, intractable pain is pain that does not get better with medication or other treatments.
Intraoperative electromyography (EMG)	A technique that measures the electrical activity of muscles and nerves during surgery. It can help diagnose and prevent nerve or muscle damage, as well as monitor the function of the nervous system.
Intraoperative neurophysiological monitoring (IONM)	Procedures used during surgery to monitor neural pathways during high-risk neurosurgical, orthopedic, peripheral nerve, and vascular surgeries. These procedures assist surgeons in preventing damage to and preserving functionality of the nervous system.
Intravenous	Existing or taking place within, or administered into, a vein.
Institutional Review Board (IRB)	A committee at an institution that applies research ethics by reviewing the methods proposed for research involving human subjects, to ensure that the projects are ethical. The main goal of IRB reviews is to ensure that study participants are not harmed or that harms are minimal and outweighed by research benefits. Such boards are formally designated to approve (or reject), monitor, and review biomedical and behavioral research involving humans, and they are legally required in some countries under certain specified circumstances. Also known as an independent ethics committee (IEC), ethics review board (ERB), or research ethics board (REB).
Jugular foremen	One of the two (left and right) large openings in the base of the skull, located behind the carotid canal. It is formed by the temporal bone and the occipital bone and allows many structures to pass, including the inferior petrosal sinus, three cranial nerves, the sigmoid sinus, and meningeal arteries.
Kaplan–Meier survival curve	The Kaplan–Meier curve is commonly used to analyze time-to-event data, such as the time until death or the time until a specific event occurs. For medical applications, the Kaplan–Meier curve graphically represents the survival rate or survival function. Time is plotted on the x axis, and survival rate is plotted on the y axis.

Lacrimation

The process or act of producing and secreting tears.

Lancinating

A type of pain that is sharp, stabbing, or piercing. It is often associated with nerve damage or irritation, such as in trigeminal neuralgia. Lancinating pain is very intense and debilitating and may require medical treatment to relieve the underlying cause.

Loop

Refers to a condition in which a blood vessel compresses the trigeminal nerve as it exits the brain stem, causing intense electric-shock-like pain or debilitating spasms.

Lower cranial nerves

A group of four cranial nerves (IX X, XI, and XII) responsible for various functions such as swallowing, speech, taste, respiration, and sensation in the head and neck regions.

Lupus/systemic lupus erythematosus (SLE)

An autoimmune disease in which the body's immune system mistakenly attacks healthy tissue in many parts of the body.

Magnetic resonance imaging (MRI)

A noninvasive imaging technology that produces detailed three-dimensional images of the interior of the body. Instead of using radiation as in X-ray imaging, MRI uses a large magnet, radio waves, and a computer to take a rapid series of pictures while the patient is inside a magnetized chamber. An MRI brain scan is painless and is useful in detecting vessels compressing the trigeminal nerve, multiple sclerosis, and brain tumors.

Meckel's cave

A pouch of dura mater that contains cerebrospinal fluid and serves as a conduit for the trigeminal nerve. Also known as the trigeminal cave or cavum trigeminale.

Meige's syndrome

A rare neurological movement disorder characterized by involuntary and often forceful contractions of the muscles of the jaw and tongue (oromandibular dystonia) and involuntary muscle spasms and contractions of the muscles around the eyes (blepharospasm).

Microvascular decompression (MVD)

A type of brain surgery used to treat trigeminal neuralgia in which a compressing blood vessel is lifted off the trigeminal nerve. A small cushion is or glue is used to prevent the blood vessel from returning to its original position.

Microvascular transposition (MVT)

A type of brain surgery that involves transposing the offending blood vessel onto the dura with fibrin, rather than performing microvascular decompression with Teflon.

Migraine headache

A type of headache characterized by recurrent attacks of moderate to severe throbbing and pulsating pain on one side of the head. The pain is caused by the activation of nerve fibers within the walls of brain blood vessels traveling inside the meninges (the three layers of membranes protecting the brain and spinal cord).

Mindfulness	The practice of maintaining a moment-by-moment awareness of thoughts, feelings, bodily sensations, and the surrounding environment, through a gentle, nurturing lens. Mindfulness also involves acceptance, meaning that we pay attention to our thoughts and feelings without judging them—without believing, for instance, that there is a "right" or "wrong" way to think or feel in a given moment. When we practice mindfulness, our thoughts tune into what we're sensing in the present moment rather than rehashing the past or imagining the future.
Mindfulness meditation	A type of meditation that involves focusing on the present moment and being aware of thoughts, feelings, and sensations without judgment. Such meditation helps reduce stress, anxiety, and depression and improve overall well-being. There are many ways to practice mindfulness meditation, including breathing methods, guided imagery, and other practices that help to relax the body and mind.
Mindfulness-based intervention (MBI)	A form of treatment that uses a mindfulness approach, focusing on concepts such as self-awareness, nonjudgment, and acceptance.
Mindfulness-based stress reduction (MBSR)	An effective, scientifically researched method for reducing physical and psychological suffering while building resilience, balance, and peace of mind through the practice of mindfulness.
Modified-release (MR)	A mechanism used in tablets and capsules to dissolve a drug over time so that it is released more slowly and steadily into the bloodstream, while having the advantage of being taken at less frequent intervals than immediate-release (IR) formulations of the same drug.
Motor cortex stimulation	A surgical procedure in which small contact plates are attached to an electrical stimulation device and placed on the surface of the brain covering over the cortex region. Stimulating this region with low-grade electrical current reduces activity in the thalamus, where pain is felt.
Motor fibers	Axons of motor neurons that carry information from the central nervous system to peripheral organs, muscles, and glands.
Motor function	The abilities and mechanisms through which muscle movements are controlled and coordinated. It involves various brain regions, including the motor cortex, basal ganglia, and cerebellum.
Multiple sclerosis (MS)	A chronic autoimmune disorder that affects the central nervous system. The immune system attacks the myelin, which is the protective layer around nerve fibers, causing inflammation and lesions. This makes it difficult for the brain to send signals to the rest of the body.

Musculoskeletal pain	Pain that affects the muscles, bones, ligaments, tendons, or nerves.
Myectomy	Surgical excision of part of a muscle.
Myelin	A white fatty material, composed chiefly of lipids and lipoproteins, that encloses certain axons and nerve fibers. Like insulation around an electric wire. It allows electrical nerve impulses to travel quickly and efficiently throughout the body.
Name-brand drug	A drug sold by a drug company under a specific name or trademark that is protected by a patent. Brand-name drugs may be available by prescription or over the counter.
Narcolepsy	A chronic neurological disorder that involves a decreased ability to regulate sleep–wake cycles. Symptoms often include periods of excessive daytime sleepiness and brief involuntary sleep episodes.
Neoplastic	Of, relating to, or constituting a tumor or neoplasia. A neoplasm is an abnormal growth of cells, also known as a tumor. Neoplastic diseases be benign (noncancerous) or malignant (cancerous) tumor growth.
Nerve block	Use of a drug, chemical, or surgery to stop a nerve signal from getting through to the brain. In the case of trigeminal neuralgia, these can be used for temporary pain relief or to diagnose the exact nature and location of a pain.
Nerve conduction studies	Medical diagnostic tests that evaluate the function and electrical conduction of the peripheral nerves. The test involves stimulating the nerve with electrodes attached to the skin and measuring the speed and strength of the nerve signal.
Nerve root	The initial segment of a nerve leaving the central nervous system.
Nerve root level injury	A condition that occurs when nerves in the spine are damaged or compressed. This can cause pain, increased sensitivity, numbness, and muscle weakness
Nervus intermedius	A branch of the geniculate nerve. When compressed by a blood vessel, it can cause pain deep in the ear.
Nervus intermedius neuralgia	A rare condition characterized by brief paroxysms of pain felt deeply in the auditory canal. Other terms previously used for this condition include geniculate neuralgia and Hunt neuralgia.
Neurectomy	A nerve resection. A neurosurgical procedure in which a peripheral nerve is cut or removed to alleviate neuropathic pain or permanently disable some function of a nerve. The nerve is not intended to grow back. For chronic pain it may be an alternative to a failed nerve decompression when the target nerve has no motor function and numbness is acceptable.

Neurodestruction	The damage or death of neurons. In ablative procedures to treat neuropathic facial pain, nerves are destroyed on purpose with the goal of relieving pain and resulting in as little numbness as possible.
Neuroendocrine system	A network of glands and nerve cells that make hormones and release them into the bloodstream. The neuroendocrine system consists of two main components: the hypothalamus and the pituitary gland. The hypothalamus is a part of the brain that receives signals from various parts of the body and translates them into hormonal messages. The pituitary gland is a small organ at the base of the brain that secretes different hormones in response to the hypothalamic signals.
Neurologist	A medical doctor who specializes in treating diseases of the nervous system, including the brain and spinal cord and is distinct from a neurosurgeon who also performs invasive procedures.
Neuroma	A tangle of poorly developed nerve endings that resprout following a nerve injury.
Neuromodulation	Electrical stimulation of a peripheral nerve, the spinal cord, or the brain for relief of pain.
Neuromyotonia (NMT)	A form of peripheral nerve hyperexcitability that causes spontaneous muscular activity resulting from repetitive motor unit action potentials of peripheral origin.
Neuropathic facial pain	Facial pain resulting from injury to the trigeminal nerve.
Neuropathic pain	Pain that originates in the nerve, due to injury or disease.
Neuropathy	Disturbance of function or pathologic change in a nerve, causing numbness when it occurs in a sensory nerve.
Neurotomy	The application of heat (as in radio frequency nerve lesioning) or freezing to sensory nerve fibers to cause their temporary degeneration, usually to relieve pain. Neurotomy and neurolysis (where the degeneration is caused by the application of chemical agents) are forms of neurolytic block. "Neurotomy" is sometimes used as a synonym for neurectomy, the cutting or removal of nervous tissue.
NMDA-receptor blockers	A class of drugs that work to antagonize, or inhibit the action of, the N-methyl-d-aspartate (NMDA) receptor. They are commonly used as anesthetics for humans and nonhuman animals; the state of anesthesia they induce is referred to as dissociative anesthesia.
Nociception	Perception of pain caused by a physical injury that is detected by the body's nerve endings. Normal perception of pain.

Nociceptive pain	Pain caused by potentially harmful stimuli being detected by nociceptors around the body. Nociceptive pain is one of the two main types of physical pain. The other is called neuropathic pain.
Noninflammatory diet	A diet based on whole, nutrient-dense foods that contain antioxidants. These diets work by reducing levels of free radicals, which are reactive molecules that may cause inflammation when they are not held in check.
Non-rapid eye movement (NREM) sleep	An essential part of the sleep cycle. It involves three stages, denoted N1, N2, and N3, with N3 being the deepest. NREM sleep stages are vital for physical and mental restoration. Sleep deprivation and fragmented sleep can limit the amount of time spent in NREM sleep and lead to health problems.
Non-REM sleep stage 1 (stage N1)	The first sleep stage a person enters when nodding off. This sleep stage is when one's heartbeat, eye movements, brain waves, and breathing activity begin to taper down. Motor movements also diminish, although one may experience muscle twitches called hypnic jerks. The first episode of stage N1 sleep usually lasts for only a few minutes.
Non-REM sleep stage 2 (stage N2)	Sleep stage in which a continued slowing of one's heartbeat, breathing, muscle activity, and eye movements occurs. During this stage, a reduction in body temperature also occurs. Throughout the course of the night, a person spends about half the time in stage N2 sleep.
Non-REM sleep stage 3 (stage N3)	Sleep stage during which one's heartbeat, breathing, muscle activity, and brain waves are at their slowest. This sleep stage is otherwise known as deep sleep, because experts believe it to be the most critical stage for regenerating the body and brain.
Nonsteroidal anti-inflammatory drugs (NSAIDs)	Drugs that help reduce inflammation, which often helps to relieve pain.
Norepinephrine and dopamine reuptake inhibitors (NDRIs)	Drugs that function by inhibiting the reuptake of the neurotransmitters norepinephrine and dopamine. This leads to increased neural concentrations of these activating neurotransmitters, resulting in increased stimulation of the central nervous system. Certain NDRIs inhibit the reuptake of norepinephrine to a greater extent than dopamine (and vice versa).
Novelty seeking	A personality trait associated with exploratory activity in response to novel stimulation, impulsive decision making, extravagance in approach to reward cues, quick loss of temper, and avoidance of frustration.

Nuclear factor erythroid 2-related factor 2 (NRF2)	A transcription factor that regulates the cellular defense against toxic and oxidative insults through the expression of genes involved in oxidative stress response and drug detoxification. NRF2 activation renders cells resistant to chemical carcinogens and inflammatory challenges.
Nucleus solitarius (or solitary nucleus)	A series of purely sensory nuclei forming a vertical column of gray matter embedded within the medulla oblongata and is involved in autonomic functions. Through the center of the solitary nucleus runs the solitary tract, a white bundle of nerve fibers, including fibers from cranial nerves VII, IX, and X.
Numerical rating scale (NRS)	Pain screening tool that requires the patient to rate their pain on a defined scale, for example, from 0 to 10, where 0 is no pain and 10 is the worst pain imaginable.
Obstructive sleep apnea (OSA)	The most common sleep-related breathing disorder; characterized by recurrent episodes of complete or partial obstruction of the upper airway, leading to reduced or absent breathing during sleep.
Occipital nerve stimulation (ONS)	A procedure that implants a device with electrodes near the occipital lobe that can stimulate nerves to help manage head pain. It is used as a treatment option for headaches and facial pain.
Occipital nerves	A group of nerves that originate in the cervical spine and innervate the area along the back of the neck and the sides and back of the head. Their primary function is to deliver sensory information to the skin on the back and side of the scalp and the skin of the external ear.
Occipital neuralgia	A condition associated with the occipital nerves. Symptoms include shooting or stabbing pain along the greater occipital nerve. The pain can travel along the back of the head, neck, and scalp and be triggered by turning the head or pushing on the area. The pain is typically on one side, and the site can be so sensitive that it is difficult to lie down or wash your hair.
Occiput	The back of the head or skull.
Ocular migraine headache	A type of migraine aura that affects only one of the eyes. It causes temporary changes in vision that may or may not be accompanied by a headache. The visual symptoms during an ocular migraine usually do not last as long as symptoms of a migraine with aura. The headache pain tends to be right behind the affected eye. These episodes can be scary, but they are mostly harmless and short-lived.
Oculocardiac reflex (OCR)	A decrease in heart rate by greater than 20% caused by pressure or traction on the eye or its muscles. It is a response to irritation of the trigeminal nerve.

Off-label	Use of an FDA-approved medication in a way that has not been approved by the FDA. This can include using a drug for an unapproved indication, age group, dosage, or route of administration. Although legal, when a medication is used off-label, the drug's efficacy and safety has not been reviewed by the FDA.
Oligodendroglia cell	A type of glial cell found in the central nervous system of vertebrates and invertebrates that produces myelin. Also known as an oligodendrocyte.
Open-label extension (OLE) of a clinical trial	A type of clinical trial that typically comes after an initial double-blind, randomized controlled trial (RCT). In an OLE study, participants are offered access to an investigational drug or product that was shown to be effective in the preceding controlled trial. An open-label extension study is one that will lie between a double-blind, randomized controlled drug trial and the request for FDA approval.
Opioid	One of the pain-killing agents that originate from the poppy flower and its product opium. Morphine and codeine were two of the earliest opioids. Opioids are sometimes used to treat persistent facial pains that have not responded to other therapies. Opioids are most effective for nociceptive pain.
Opioid NMDA-receptor modulator	NMDA-receptor antagonists have been studied for their role in pain management. They are believed to be effective in reducing pain by blocking the N-methyl-d-aspartate (NMDA) receptor, which is involved in the development of chronic pain. Some of the NMDA-receptor antagonists that have been studied include ketamine, memantine, dextromethorphan, and magnesium.
Oral dysesthesia	A painful, burning feeling in the mouth.
Orbicularis oculi muscle	A muscle in the face that closes the eyelids.
Orofacial pain dentistry	A specialty of dentistry that encompasses the diagnosis, management, and treatment of pain disorders of the jaw, mouth, face, and associated regions.
Osteotomy	A surgical procedure that involves cutting bone (and sometimes adding bone tissue) to reshape or realign bones.
Oxidative stress	Excess levels of free radicals in the body, leading to the inability of antioxidants to get rid of the unstable and excess free radicals.
Oxytocin	A hormone that is a natural pain reliever. It acts by activating the endorphin receptors and by blocking nerve impulses between the brain and spinal cord. Oxytocin is released into the blood by a small population of neurons that also stimulate cells in the spinal cord. It surges in a woman's body at the time of delivery to provide pain relief. People with chronic pain have lower levels of oxytocin in their blood.

Pain psychology	A specialty area of psychology that studies and treats the psychological and behavioral aspects of chronic pain. Pain psychology can help individuals cope with the challenges and consequences of living with chronic pain, such as emotional distress, reduced functioning, and impaired quality of life. Pain psychology is also a branch of medical psychology, as chronic pain can affect various medical conditions and outcomes.
Pain self-management	A person's ability to manage their pain symptoms and treatment, as well as the physical, emotional, and social consequences and lifestyle changes caused by chronic pain. It means coping with the day-to-day tasks needed to get a person dealing with chronic pain back to life.
Painful posttraumatic trigeminal neuropathic pain (PPTTNP)	A painful condition that may result from injury to the sensory division of the trigeminal nerve. Treatment of this condition is challenging, and consensus on treatment to resolve neuropathic pain has yet to be standardized. Equally challenging is the identification of surgical outcome variables to guide surgical treatment of PPTTNP. This is partly due to the variability in pain characteristics, severity of nerve injury, location, and duration from injury to surgery.
Palate	The roof of the mouth separating the mouth from the nasal cavity.
Pan-COX inhibitor	A type of nonsteroidal anti-inflammatory drug (NSAID) that inhibits the activity of both cyclooxygenase-1 (COX-1) and cyclooxygenase-2 (COX-2) enzymes. The COX-1 and COX-2 enzymes are responsible for producing prostaglandins, which cause inflammation, pain, and fever. COX-2 inhibitors, which selectively inhibit COX-2 enzymes, are more commonly used than pan-COX inhibitors because COX-2 inhibitors cause fewer stomach and intestinal problems.
Parallel studies	A type of clinical trial in which participants are randomly assigned to a single treatment. The treatment can include placebo, a specific dose of the drug being investigated, or a standard-of-care treatment. A parallel design compares two or more treatments and evaluates their effects. It is the "gold standard" for phase III clinical trials.
Parasympathetic nervous system (PNS)	One of the two functionally distinct and continuously active divisions of the autonomic nervous system (ANS). It is in opposition to the other division, the sympathetic nervous system (SNS). The PNS predominates under quiet "rest and digest" conditions, whereas the SNS drives the "fight or flight" response in stressful situations. The main purpose of the PNS is to regulate bodily functions and to conserve energy to be used later.

Parotid gland	One of the bilateral pair of salivary glands located on each side of the face, just in front of and below each ear.
Paroxysm	Sudden recurrence or intensification of symptoms, such as a spasm or seizure.
Partial (or focal) motor seizure	A type of seizure that begins in only one part of the brain and causes unconscious or involuntary movements. They often affect the face, hands, and toes on one side of the body. They can involve twitching or jerking muscle movements, uncontrolled tightening of muscles, or repetitive or automatic movements (e.g., smacking the lips, blinking or tapping a hand or finger).
Pathophysiology	The study of abnormal changes in body functions that are the causes, consequences, or concomitants of disease processes.
Peak effect	The effect of a drug when its level in a patient's blood is the highest.
Penetrance	The extent to which a particular gene or set of genes is expressed in the phenotypes of individuals carrying it, measured by the proportion of carriers showing the characteristic phenotype.
Percutaneous	Passed, performed, or effected through the skin.
Periodic limb movement disorder (PLMD)	Repetitive cramping or jerking of the legs during sleep. The only movement disorder that occurs only during sleep. Also called "periodic limb (or leg) movements of sleep" (PLMS).
Peripheral level injury	An injury resulting from a systemic disease (e.g., diabetes, autoimmune disease) or localized damage (e.g., trauma, compression, tumor) that manifests with neurological deficits distal to the level of the lesion.
Peripheral nerve stimulation (PNS)	A method used to treat chronic pain. It involves surgery that places a small electrical device (a wirelike electrode) next to one of the peripheral nerves. (These are the nerves that are located beyond the brain or spinal cord). The electrode delivers rapid electrical pulses that are felt as mild tingles (called paresthesias). During the testing period (trial), the electrode is connected to an external device, and if the trial is successful, a small generator is implanted into the patient's body. The patient is able to control stimulation by turning the device on and off and adjusting the stimulation parameters as needed.
Peripheral nerves	Nerves outside the brain and spinal cord. In the case of trigeminal neuralgia (TN), these include the many branches of the trigeminal nerve that serve the teeth, gums, and other parts of the face.

Persistence	The act of continuing drug treatment for the prescribed duration. It can be defined as "the duration of time from initiation to discontinuation of therapy."
Personality structure	The organization of the various features of personality as based on theory or empirical findings.
Petrous temporal bone	From the Latin word "petrosus," meaning "stonelike," the petrous temporal bone is one of the densest bones in the body. It is pyramid-shaped and is wedged in at the base of the skull between the sphenoid and occipital bones. It has a base, an apex, three surfaces, and three angles, and it houses the components of the inner ear.
Pharyngeal	Relating to or located in the region of the pharynx.
Pharynx	The muscular tube that connects the mouth and the throat.
Photobiomodulation	A form of light therapy that uses light sources including lasers, light-emitting diodes, and broadband light for the relief of pain and inflammation.
Physical therapy	A health care modality that addresses the illnesses or injuries that limit a person's abilities to move and perform functional activities in their daily lives. Physical therapists promote, maintain, and restore health through physical examination, diagnosis, management, prognosis, patient education, physical intervention, rehabilitation, disease prevention, and health promotion.
Polysomnography	A sleep study or test used to diagnose sleep disorders. During the test, brain waves, blood oxygen levels, heart rate, and respiration are recorded during sleep. Eye and leg movements are also measured. The test is usually conducted at a sleep disorders unit within a hospital or at a sleep center but may be conducted at home. A sleep study can help diagnose sleep apnea, periodic limb movement disorder (PLMD), restless legs syndrome, narcolepsy, rapid eye movement (REM) sleep behavior disorder, unusual behaviors during sleep, and unexplained long-lasting insomnia.
Polytetrafluoroethylene (PTFE) felt	A non-bioabsorbable perforated patch made of polytetrafluoroethylene (PTFE), a synthetic fluoropolymer of tetrafluoroethylene that has numerous medical applications. The commonly known brand is Teflon.
Pons	The part of the brain stem that lies inferior to the midbrain, superior to the medulla oblongata, and anterior to the cerebellum. This region of the brain stem includes neural pathways and tracts that conduct signals from the brain down to the cerebellum and medulla, as well as tracts that carry the sensory signals up into the thalamus.

Postherpetic neuralgia	A condition that causes burning pain in the nerves and skin. It is the most common complication of shingles, and it occurs when nerve fibers become damaged during an outbreak of shingles. The pain lasts long after the rash and blisters of shingles go away. The risk of postherpetic neuralgia rises with age, and the condition mainly affects people older than 60 years of age.
Posttraumatic stress (PTS)	A mental health condition that develops following a traumatic event and is characterized by intrusive thoughts about the incident, recurrent distress or anxiety, flashbacks, and avoidance of similar situations. Note that one can experience posttraumatic stress without having posttraumatic stress disorder (PTSD).
Posterior fossa	The part of the cranial cavity located between the foramen magnum and the tentorium cerebelli. It is formed by the sphenoid bones, temporal bones, and occipital bone. It houses the cerebellum and parts of the brain stem.
Posterior inferior cerebellar artery (PICA)	The largest branch of the vertebral artery. It is one of the three main arteries that supply blood to the cerebellum. Blockage of the posterior inferior cerebellar artery can result in a type of stroke called lateral medullary syndrome.
Prevalence	The number of existing cases of a disease or condition during a given period of time regardless of when the disease or condition started.
Primary (or idiopathic) burning mouth syndrome	A condition related to problems with taste or sensory nerves but with no known cause, whereas causes of secondary BMS include various medications, fungal infection, lack of nutrients, dentures, allergies or reactions to foods and additives, reflux of acid from the stomach, endocrine disorders, overbrushing of the tongue, use of an abrasive toothpaste, overuse of mouthwash, and more.
Prior authorization	A health plan cost-control process that requires physicians and other health care professionals to obtain advance approval from a health plan before a specific service is delivered to the patient to qualify for payment coverage.
Prospective study	A type of experimental design that looks forward in time and observes events as they arise. Participants begin the study without having a condition of interest, and researchers gather data and take measurements at regular intervals to identify the occurrence of specific outcomes, along with other data that might relate to them.
Proximal	Near the center of the body or the point of attachment of a bone or muscle. The opposite of distal.
Psychophysiology	The study of the relationship between physiological and psychological phenomena, or the way in which the mind and body interact:

Ptosis	An abnormal but painless eye condition in which the upper eyelid droops, potentially obstructing vision. Also known as blepharoptosis.
Pulsatile	Pulsating; relating to pulsation.
Quality of life (QOL)	Defined by the World Health Organization as "an individual's perception of their position in life in the context of the culture and value systems in which they live and in relation to their goals, expectations, standards, and concerns."
Radio-frequency ablation (RFA)	The use of radio waves to create a current that heats a small area of nerve tissue, so that the heat destroys that area of the nerve, stopping it from sending pain signals to the brain. RFA can provide lasting relief for people with chronic pain Also called radio-frequency neurotomy.
Ramsay Hunt syndrome	An acute peripheral facial neuropathy that occurs as a complication of shingles. It causes hearing loss and facial paralysis.
Randomized controlled trial (RCT)	A form of scientific experiment used to control factors that are not under direct experimental control. Examples include clinical trials that compare the effects of drugs, surgical techniques, medical devices, diagnostic procedures, or other medical treatments. By randomly allocating participants among compared treatments, an RCT enables statistical control over these influences. RCTs are the "gold standard" for clinical research.
Rapid eye movement (REM) sleep	A unique phase of sleep characterized by random rapid movement of the eyes, accompanied by low muscle tone throughout the body and the propensity of the sleeper to dream vividly.
Rapid eye movement (REM) sleep deprivation	Lack of REM sleep leads to fatigue, irritability, changes in mood and memory, and issues with cognition and problem-solving. It can also affect cardiovascular health; increase the risk of type 2 diabetes; and contribute to cancer, stroke, and neurodegenerative diseases such as Alzheimer's.
Raynaud's phenomenon	A condition in which the body's normal response to cold or emotional stress is exaggerated, resulting in abnormal spasms (vasospasms) in small blood vessels called arterioles. The disorder mainly affects the fingers but can also involve the ears, nose, nipples, knees, and toes. The vasospasms reduce blood circulation, leading to discomfort and changes in skin color.
Reactive oxygen species (ROS)	Byproducts of the normal metabolism of oxygen. ROS have roles in cell signaling and homeostasis. During times of environmental stress, ROS levels in the body can increase dramatically, resulting in significant damage to cell structures. This is known as oxidative stress.

Referred pain	Pain perceived at a location other than the site of the painful stimulus. It is the result of a network of interconnecting sensory nerves that supplies many different tissues.
Refractory	Not responding to treatment.
Remission	Reduction or disappearance of the signs and symptoms of a disease. Also refers to the period during which this reduction occurs.
Research-based	Refers to practices that were developed in accordance with the best research available. Users can feel confident that the strategies and activities included in the program or practice have a strong scientific basis for their use.
Restless leg syndrome (RLS)	A condition that causes an uncomfortable feeling in the legs and a strong urge to move them. It typically occurs in the evening or at night when sitting or lying down, and moving the legs can ease the discomfort for a short time.
Retrolabyrinthine presigmoid approach	A surgical technique used to remove medium to large vestibular schwannomas (acoustic neuromas), which are noncancerous tumors on the main nerve leading from the inner ear to the brain. This is a minimally invasive surgical option that provides direct access to the cerebellopontine angle and preserves hearing function.
Retromastoid craniectomy	A surgical technique that uses a small window behind the ear as the main approach for microvascular decompression of the cranial nerves (for trigeminal neuralgia or hemifacial spasm).This operation is augmented by the introduction of an endoscope, allowing for visualization around corners, limiting the need for extensive tissue removal or brain retraction.
Retrospective study	An experimental design that looks back in time and assesses events that have already occurred.
Reward dependence	A personality trait or temperament that responds markedly to signals of reward, particularly to verbal signals of social approval, social support, and sentiment. When reward dependence levels deviate from normal, several personality and addictive disorders appear.
Rhizotomy	A surgery to cut or damage a nerve root so as to interfere with the transmission of pain signals to the brain.
Risk–benefit considerations	An important aspect of decision-making that involves the assessment of risks and benefits. In the context of health-related research, risk–benefit analysis is a critical part of the process of evaluating the ethical acceptability of proposed research.
Root canal	A procedure that involves removal of the pulp to repair a decaying or infected tooth.

Root entry zone (REZ)	The section of the trigeminal nerve near the brain stem where the myelin covering is thinnest.
Safety monitoring committee	A group of experts who review data from a particular study to ensure the safety of participants and the validity and integrity of the data.
Scalded mouth syndrome	Another name for burning mouth syndrome (BMS).
Schwann cells	A type of large neurological cell responsible for forming the thicker myelin sheath around the neurons of the peripheral nervous system and supplying nutrients to individual axons. Also called neurilemma cells.
Scleroderma	A group of autoimmune diseases causing hardening and tightening of the skin and connective tissues. It occurs as a result of the overproduction of the protein collagen in skin tissues.
Sclerotic plaques	A symptom of atherosclerosis, which is the buildup of fats, cholesterol, and other substances in and on artery walls. Plaques can cause arteries to narrow, blocking blood flow, and can also burst, leading to a blood clot. Sclerotic lesions, on the other hand, are an unusual hardening or thickening of the bones, which can be either benign or malignant.
Sectioning of the nervus intermedius (NI)	An ablative procedure for treating geniculate neuralgia.
Sensory aspects of pain	The physical sensation of pain, including the location, intensity, and quality of the pain. Pain also has an affective dimension, or emotional experience.
Sensory fibers	Nerve fibers that carry information from different receptors of sensory neurons in the peripheral nervous system to the central nervous system. Also called afferent nerve fibers.
Sensory function	The sensory system is responsible for detecting and processing sensory information from the environment and converting it into electrical signals that can be interpreted by the brain.
Seroma	A buildup of bodily fluids in a tissue or organ after surgery, usually at the site of the surgery. The skin appears as a swollen lump.
Shingles	A viral infection that causes a painful rash or blisters on the skin, usually in one area of your body. Caused by the same virus that causes chickenpox.
Sialometry	A diagnostic tool used to measure saliva flow. It can be used in two ways: for the collection of whole saliva (that is, combined secretions of all salivary glands) and for the collection of glandular saliva (that is, gland-specific saliva).

Sigmoid sinus	A dural venous sinus that lies deep within the human head and connects with the jugular foramen and the petrosal sinus, so named because of its "S" curve.
Single blind study	A type of experiment or clinical trial in which the participants of the study are not aware of which treatment they are receiving but the researchers are.
Sjögren's syndrome	A long-term autoimmune disease that affects the body's moisture-producing glands and often seriously affects other organ systems, such as the lungs, kidneys, and nervous system. It can lead to facial pain.
Sleep apnea	A potentially serious sleep disorder in which breathing repeatedly stops and starts.
Sleep bruxism	Grinding or clenching teeth during sleep.
Sleep efficiency (SE)	Ratio of the total amount of time spent asleep in a night compared to the total amount of time spent in bed.
Sleep fragmentation	The interruption of nocturnal sleep.
Sleep quality (SQ)	One's subjective perception of how well they slept, which is often based on how rested they feel in the morning.
Serotonin and norepinephrine reuptake inhibitors (SNRIs)	A class of medications that are effective in treating depression. SNRIs are also used to treat anxiety disorders and long-term (chronic) pain, especially nerve pain. SNRIs may be helpful for individuals who have chronic pain in addition to depression.
Social Security Disability Income (SSDI)	A government-sponsored benefits program that provides financial assistance to people with qualifying disabilities. Payment depends on work and earnings history.
Sodium channel blocker	Drug that impairs the conduction of sodium ions through sodium channels. Used in the treatment of cardiac arrhythmias. Also used as a local anesthetic and anticonvulsant.
Somatosensory system	The network of neural structures in the brain and body that produces the perception of touch, temperature, body position, and pain.
Sore tongue	Pain or tenderness in the tongue, making it difficult to eat or drink.
Spasm	A sudden involuntary contraction of a muscle; a group of muscles; or a hollow organ, such as the bladder.
Spinal cord stimulation	A treatment for neuropathic pain that uses a mild electric current to block nerve impulses in the spine.
Spinal fluid	A clear, colorless body fluid found within the tissue that surrounds the brain and spinal cord.

Spinal tap	A medical procedure in which a needle is inserted into the spinal canal to collect cerebrospinal fluid for medical testing. Also called a lumbar puncture.
Stages of sleep	There are four stages of sleep, which are categorized into two main types: rapid eye movement (REM) sleep and non-REM (NREM) sleep. Non-REM sleep is further divided into three stages as follows:

- NREM stage 1 (N1) corresponds to the transition from wakefulness to sleep and is a very light sleep stage. It usually lasts for a few minutes. During stage N1, muscle activity decreases, and eye movements are slow.
- NREM Stage 2 (N2) is a slightly deeper sleep stage. It is characterized by a reduction in heart rate and a decrease in body temperature as the body prepares for deeper sleep. Stage N2 makes up a significant portion of a full night's sleep.
- NREM Stage 3 (N3) or deep sleep is important for physical restoration and growth, immune function, and building up energy for the next day.

The fourth stage is REM sleep, which is associated with dreaming and is characterized by rapid eye movements, increased brain activity, and a temporary paralysis of voluntary muscles to prevent the acting out of dreams.

Step therapy	A requirement implemented by prescription drug insurance providers of using the most cost-effective drugs for a given condition as a first try before stepping up to a more expensive or risky therapy. Also known as step protocol or a "fail-first" requirement.
Stevens–Johnson syndrome	A rare, acute, and serious disorder of the skin and mucous membranes. It usually occurs as an adverse reaction to medication that starts with flu-like symptoms, followed within a few days by a painful rash that spreads, blisters, and peels. Stevens–Johnson syndrome is a medical emergency that usually requires hospitalization.
Stomatodynia/ stomatopyrosis	A painful, complex condition often described as a burning, scalding, or tingling feeling in the mouth that may occur every day for months or longer. Dry mouth or an altered taste in the mouth may accompany the pain.
Stroke	A medical condition in which poor blood flow to the brain causes cell death. There are two main types of strokes: ischemic, due to lack of blood flow, and hemorrhagic, due to bleeding. Also known as a cerebrovascular accident (CVA) or brain attack.
Subcutaneous	Situated or applied under the skin.

SUNCT	An acronym for "short-lasting, unilateral, neuralgiform headaches with conjunctival injection and tearing." SUNCT leads to a sharp intermittent pain centering around the eye along with a red eye, tearing, and a runny nose.
Superior cerebellar artery (SCA)	An artery of the head that arises near the end of the basilar artery and supplies parts of the cerebellum, midbrain, and other nearby structures. Compression or pulsing of the SCA near the trigeminal nerve is the cause of trigeminal neuralgia in some people.
Supplemental Security Income (SSI)	A government program that provides monthly payments to people with disabilities and older adults who have little or no income or resources. The monthly SSI payment depends on income, living situation, resources.
Support group	A group of people with common experiences or concerns who provide each other with encouragement, comfort, and advice.
Supraorbital foramen	Part of the frontal bone of the skull. A bony elongated opening located above the eye socket and below the forehead that lies directly under the eyebrow. The nerve providing sensation to the forehead runs through it.
Surgical neurectomy	A neurosurgical procedure in which a peripheral nerve is cut or removed to alleviate neuropathic pain or permanently disable some function of a nerve. The nerve is not intended to grow back. For chronic pain, this procedure may be an alternative to a failed nerve decompression when the target nerve has no motor function and numbness is acceptable Also called a neurectomy.
Symmetrical	Having, involving, or exhibiting symmetry; correspondence in size, shape, and relative position of parts on opposite sides of a dividing line or plane.
Sympathetic nervous system (SNS)	A branch of the autonomic nervous system (ANS) that prepares the body for "fight or flight" responses during stressful situations. A network of nerves that increases the body's activity and mobilizes its resources when in danger, under stress, or engaged in physical activity. Its effects include increasing the heart rate, breathing ability, and eyesight and inhibiting digestion, among other functions.
Synapse	A structure that allows a neuron to pass an electrical or chemical signal to another neuron or to the target effector cell. Synapses are essential to the transmission of nervous impulses from one neuron to another, playing a key role in enabling rapid and direct communication by creating circuits. In addition, a synapse serves as a junction where both the transmission and processing of information occur, making it a vital component of communication between neurons.

Synaptic neuromuscular junction	A chemical synapse between a motor neuron and a muscle fiber that allows the motor neuron to transmit a signal to the muscle fiber, causing muscle contraction.
Syndrome	A set of medical signs and symptoms that are correlated with each other and are often associated with a particular disease or disorder. When a syndrome is paired with a definite cause, this becomes a disease.
Synkinesis	A neurological symptom in which a voluntary muscle movement causes the simultaneous involuntary contraction of other muscles.
Systemic approach	In psychotherapy, a systemic approach is a form of psychotherapy that focuses on how an individual's personal relationships, behavior patterns, and life choices are interconnected with the issues they face in their life.
Systolic	Relating to the phase of the heartbeat when the heart contracts, forcing blood onward through the body. Systolic blood pressure is the top number of the blood pressure reading, which measures the force the heart exerts on the walls of the arteries each time it beats. A normal systolic blood pressure for most healthy adults is usually less than 120 mmHg.
Tai chi	An ancient Chinese martial art that combines slow and graceful movements, breathing, and meditation.
Temperament traits	Consistent individual differences in behavior that are biologically based and are relatively independent of learning, system of values, and attitudes.
Temporomandibular disorders (TMDs)	A group of more than 30 conditions that affect the jaw joint and surrounding muscles and ligaments. Can cause several issues, including jaw pain, headaches, and difficulty opening and closing the mouth. "TMJ" refers to the actual temporomandibular joint (jaw) joint, whereas "TMDs" refer to disorders or dysfunctions of the joint.
Temporomandibular joint (TMJ) pain	Pain in the temporomandibular jaw joint; sometimes confused with trigeminal neuralgia (TN).
Tension headache	A headache that causes mild to moderate pain 'that is often described as feeling like a tight band around the head.
Tesla (T)	Unit of magnetic field strength. Important for magnetic resonance imaging (MRI), as MRI machines with stronger magnets (higher T) can provide clearer images with more intricate details.
Therapeutic window	Dose range of a drug that provides safe and effective therapy with minimal adverse effects; determined as the range between the minimum effective therapeutic concentration and the minimum toxic concentration.

Tinnitus	A condition in which a constant ringing sound is sensed in the ear in the absence of an external source.
Topical medication/ topical therapy	A medication applied to a particular place on or in the body. Most often, use of a topical medication involves application to body surfaces such as the skin or mucous membranes (creams, foams, gels, lotions, and ointments.) May also be inhaled or applied to the surface of tissues other than the skin, such as eye or ear drops or medications applied to the surface of a tooth.
Transcranial magnetic stimulation	A noninvasive procedure that uses magnetic fields to stimulate nerve cells in the brain to improve symptoms of depression.
Transcutaneous electrical nerve stimulation (TENS)	A method of pain relief and muscle relaxation involving the use of a mild electrical current applied to the skin.
Transdermal	A route of administration in which active ingredients in a medication are delivered across the skin for systemic distribution, as in a transdermal patch, for example.
Transected/transection	A cross section or cutting across something.
Transient receptor potential (TRP) channels	Sensors for a variety of cellular and environmental signals. These channels are responsible for various sensory responses including heat, cold, pain, stress, vision, and taste and can be activated by a number of stimuli.
Transient receptor potential ankyrin 1 (TRPA1)	The sole member of the TRPA gene subfamily.
Transpose/ transposition	A change in order or relative position of something, often through an exchange of position.
Trigeminal Autonomic Cephalgias (TACs)	Primary headaches involving the trigeminal vascular system. In addition to single sided pain have autonomic effects. Cluster headches, paroxysmal nemicranias and SUNCT/ SUNA are TACs. Hemicrania continua, while related, is not.
Trigeminal nerve nucleus	The largest of the cranial nerve nuclei, which extend through the whole of the midbrain, pons, and medulla and into the high cervical spinal cord.
Trigeminal neuralgia (TN)/trigeminal neuropathic pain (TNP)	A long-term pain disorder that affects the trigeminal nerve, the nerve responsible for sensation in the face and motor functions such as biting and chewing. It is a form of neuropathic pain. There are two main types. One results in episodes of severe, sudden, shocklike pain on one side of the face that last for seconds to a few minutes. Groups of these episodes can occur over a few hours. The other form results in a constant burning pain that is less severe. Both forms can occur in the same person. TN is regarded as one of the most painful disorders known to medicine.

Trigeminocervical complex (TCC)	An area in the brain stem and upper cervical spinal cord where neurons from different sources converge. The TCC is involved in the transmission of pain signals from the neck, jaw, face, and head. The TCC can be associated with various conditions that affect these regions, such as headache, migraine, and TMJ disorders.
Trigger	To cause something to start.
Trigger points/trigger sites	Hyperirritable spots in the skeletal muscle associated with palpable nodules in taut bands of fibers. The trigger point model states that unexplained pain frequently radiates from these points of local tenderness to broader areas, sometimes distant from the trigger point itself. Also called myofascial trigger points.
Triple-blind study	A study in which knowledge of the treatment assignment(s) is concealed from subjects and investigators, as well as from the researchers who organize and analyze the study's data.
Tumor	A solid mass of tissue that forms when abnormal cells group together. Tumors can affect bones, skin, tissue, organs, and glands.
Typical trigeminal neuralgia (TN)	A painful facial condition caused by an impingement of the trigeminal nerve by a blood vessel. Characterized by sudden, severe, electric-shock-like pain that can occur without warning. These episodes can last for just seconds or for prolonged periods. Symptoms can be triggered by talking, brushing teeth, chewing, or even just touching a "trigger point" on the face while shaving or applying makeup.
Unilateral	One-sided.
Vagoglossopharyngeal neuralgia	An uncommon presentation of glossopharyngeal neuralgia in which the typical symptoms of pain are associated with cardiac symptoms including arrhythmias, asystole, and syncope. This condition is believed to be due to complex interconnections between the nervus intermedius, the vagus nerve, and the glossopharyngeal nerve.
Vagus nerve/vagal nerve	The 10th cranial nerve. This is the longest of the cranial nerves, serving as the main nerve of the parasympathetic nervous system (PNS). This system controls specific involuntary body functions such as digestion, heart rate, and immune system.
Varicella zoster virus (VZV)	Causes chickenpox (varicella), commonly affecting children and young adults, and shingles (herpes zoster) in adults but rarely in children. Also known as human herpesvirus 3.
Vascular	Relating to blood vessels.

Vascular compression	A common cause of trigeminal neuralgia. The condition is caused by a blood vessel pressing against the trigeminal nerve, which can wear away the insulation of the nerve over time, leaving it exposed and highly sensitive. Also known as neurovascular compression.
Vascular malformations	Irregularities in arteries or veins, throughout the body.
Vasculature	The blood vessels or arrangement of blood vessels in an organ or body part.
Virtual reality	A simulated experience that employs pose tracking and three-dimensional near-eye displays to give the user an immersive feel of a virtual world.
Visual analog scale (VAS)	A scale used to determine the pain intensity experienced by individuals. It consists of a line, approximately 10–15 cm in length, with the left side signifying no pain with a smiling face image and the right side signifying the worst pain ever with a frowning face image.
Voltage-gated channels	Any of the gated ion channels that open in response to a change in the membrane potential of a cell membrane. These channels give muscle fibers and neurons their ability to generate and propagate impulses. Also called voltage-regulated channels.
Volumetric Interpolated Brain Examination (VIBE)	An advanced imaging technique used for magnetic resonance imaging (MRI) machines manufactured by Siemens that consists of a fast-gradient echo sequence and is considered to be superior to conventional MRI. VIBE is used in the assessment of anatomical variations and various pathologies involving the cranial nerves and central nervous system. Any high-strength MRI machine with magnetic strength of at least 1.3 T can produce VIBE images. VIBE has different names according to different brands and manufacturers, including "fast imaging employing steady-state acquisition" (FIESTA) by GE and "constructive interference in steady state" (CISS).
Yoga	A physical, mental, and spiritual practice that originated in ancient India and involves a combination of physical postures, breathing techniques, and meditation. Yoga can help build strength and flexibility, manage pain, and reduce stress. There are various styles of yoga, each with its own unique set of postures and breathing techniques.

Author Biographies

Hossein Ansari, MD, FAAN, FAHS, is a board-certified neurologist and fellowship-trained certified headache specialist with board certification by the United Council of Neurological Subspecialties (UCNS). After finishing his fellowship, Dr. Ansari created a multidisciplinary headache and facial pain clinic at Neurology & Neuroscience Associates, Inc. (NNA) in Akron, OH, where he also served as the medical director of NNA's headache clinic. He was also an assistant professor of medicine at Northeastern Ohio Medical University and a consulting neurologist at Summa Health System in Akron. In June 2015, Dr. Ansari moved to San Diego, CA, to start a headache and facial pain clinic for the University of California, San Diego (UCSD), where he served as director of the headache clinic. In July 2020, Dr. Ansari joined Kaizen Brain Center, also in San Diego, CA, to develop a multidisciplinary Headache Clinic and Facial Pain Clinic, where he currently conducts clinical trials for migraine and trigeminal neuralgia. He has also continued both his clinical and teaching career at UCSD.

Dennis R. Bailey, DDS, D-ABOP, FAAOP, D-ABDSM, is an orofacial pain specialist who also manages sleep-related breathing disorders (snoring and sleep apnea) through the use of oral appliances. He is a visiting lecturer in the Orofacial Pain and Sleep Medicine Program at UCLA School of Dentistry and is an Associate Professor at the LECOM School of Dental Medicine in Bradenton, FL. He was the lead author of the textbook ***Dental Management of Sleep Disorders***, 2nd edition, and he is an Associate Editor for the ***Journal of Oral & Facial Pain and Headache***.

Molly Becker is a doctoral student in Suffolk University's Clinical Psychology PhD program. She has extensive experience in mindfulness through participation in research and clinical training. Her research interests lie at the intersection between health and social justice with a focus on the reproductive health of marginalized women.

Jeffrey A. Brown, MD, FACS, FAANS, is the immediate past chair of the Medical Advisory Board of the FPA and is coeditor of this book and its first volume, *Facial Pain: A 21st Century Guide* (Lulu, 2020). He has edited a previous book on facial pain; is coeditor of the textbook *Functional Neurosurgery: The Essentials* (Thieme, 2020); has published more than 60 peer-reviewed articles in the neurosurgical literature, including more than 25 articles on trigeminal neuropathic pain, 45 abstracts, and 40 book chapters; and has delivered more than 220 invited lectures and practical course directorships on the subject. He has served on the Board of Directors of the American Association of Neurological Surgeons (AANS) and has been Chair of the Joint Section on Pain of the AANS and the Congress of Neurological Surgeons (CNS), the two major societies representing organized American neurosurgery. He represented neurosurgery as a member of the Advisory Board to the American College of Surgeons. Dr. Brown currently maintains a teaching position as Assistant Clinical Professor at NYU Langone Long Island School of Medicine. In 2023, he retired from the active clinical practice of neurosurgery. He now serves as an editor and reviewer for several neurosurgical publications and is most proud of his 17 years of service as an honorary surgeon for the NYPD. Perhaps related to that position, on the side, he writes crime fiction.

Kenneth F. Casey, MD, is an associate professor at Michigan State University and Associate Professor of Physical Medicine and Rehabilitation at Wayne State University. Dr. Casey, certified by the American Board of Neurological Surgery, was trained as a neurosurgical generalist at the University of Pittsburgh under Dr. Peter Jannetta. He completed his undergraduate and surgical training at Georgetown University; The University of Medicine and Dentistry of New Jersey; and Queensquare Hospital in London, England. He is a past Chairman of the FPA Medical Advisory Board. Dr. Casey generously shares his time and knowledge with the facial pain community.

Rachel Chance is a high school student in New York City. Previously, she has done work experimenting on the neurological effects of nicotine in the form of vaping compared to that in the form of oral pouches. Most recently, Rachel spent her summer at Columbia Presbyterian interning for neurosurgeon Dr. Raymond F. Sekula.

Hemamalini Chandrashekhar, BDS, MDS (OMFS), PgD (Adv Clin Rsch), is a trained oral and maxillofacial surgeon with more than 15 years of expertise spanning clinical dentistry, oral and maxillofacial surgery, academics, and clinical research. She served as an Assistant Professor in the Department of Oral & Maxillofacial Surgery at Government Dental College, Mumbai, India, and was Medical Advisor in Immuno-Oncology for Roche India. Soon to graduate with her second Master's degree in Orofacial Pain from Rutgers University, she received extensive training from Nair Hospital Dental College in India and UCLA, Boston University, and Rutgers in the United States. Driven by a passion for academia and research, she has actively participated in numerous research projects and contributed to publications in international journals.

QiLiang "Q" Chen, MD, PhD, is a pain management anesthesiologist and system neuroscientist at Stanford University and VA Palo Alto Healthcare System (VAPAHCS). His research focuses on delineating the neural mechanism of chronic pain and characterizing the physiological changes in the descending pain-modulating circuits after head injury and other forms of trauma, a topic especially relevant to Veterans and other individuals with chronic posttraumatic pain. Clinically, his interests include integrating advanced image guidance into pain procedures and exploring novel pharmacological and minimally invasive interventions for chronic posttraumatic pain, complex headaches, and craniofacial pain conditions.

John Choi, MD, is currently a fourth-year neurosurgery resident at Stanford. His research focuses on the intersection of immunology and neurosurgical disease. Prior to residency in California, he graduated from the Johns Hopkins School of Medicine. He is committed to offering a high level of care and education for all of his patients.

Anne Brazer Ciemnecki, MA, is a retired senior fellow from Mathematica, where she specialized in health and economic policy. Her mother and grandmother had trigeminal neuralgia. Anne has seen treatment evolve from the ineffective alcohol injections her grandmother used to the high-tech magnetic resonance imaging, microvascular decompression (MVD), and gamma knife ablation that alleviated her pain. She serves on the New Jersey Commission on National and Community Service and the Womanspace Advisory Counsel. She is a member of the Mercer County Medical Reserve Corps, an advocate for domestic violence victims, and a therapy dog handler. Anne is Secretary of the FPA Board of Directors and has been a peer mentor and support group leader for the FPA. She has been instrumental in designing the FPA Patient Registry. Anne is the coeditor of this book and its first volume, *Facial Pain: A 21st Century Guide* (Lulu, 2020).

Michele Cohen, LCSW, FIPA, is a psychotherapist/psychoanalyst in private practice, based in New York City, with an interest in group work as well as individual adult treatment. She is a graduate of the Psychoanalytic Training Institute of the Contemporary Freudian Society (CFS) in New York City and a Fellow of the International Psychoanalytic Association. Michele is a Training and Supervising Analyst at the Contemporary Freudian Society. She has taught in both CFS's Psychoanalytic Training Institute and its 2-year Psychoanalytic Psychotherapy Program. She has also supervised and taught at the Metropolitan Institute for Training in Psychoanalytic Psychotherapy (MITPP). Michele also has an ongoing interest in understanding the mind–body duality as it interfaces with patients suffering from physical pain conditions, an area of practice that is often misunderstood by physicians as well as by mental health professionals. She has presented her work in this area at NEFESH International (2018) and at the FPA's National Conference (2019). She currently facilitates online support groups for individuals with neuropathic facial pain.

GianCarlo Colloca, MEd, MS, holds a Master's degree in Software Engineering with a specialization in artificial intelligence and a Master's degree in Music Education, with a focus on classical guitar. His commitment to education led him to embrace interdisciplinary educational projects, which parallel the coordination of various activities within cultural associations. GianCarlo's blend of technical expertise and artistic proficiency enables him to bridge the gap between technology and creativity. In particular, with his extensive background in the arts and spatial sound and digital image processing, he contributes to the development of technical tools with a strong artistic vision and aesthetics in digital-media-based projects.

Luana Colloca, MD, PhD, MS, holds an MD, a Master's degree in Ethics, and a PhD in Neuroscience. As a physician-scientist and an MPower Distinguished Professor at University of Maryland, Baltimore, she leads an NIH-funded research portfolio focused on the phenotypes of temporomandibular joint disorders and the development of nonpharmacological interventions for chronic pain. In particular, her research incorporates virtual reality technology for symptoms management, which holds promise for personalized medicine to decrease suffering and disability.

Beth Darnall, PhD, is Professor at Stanford University School of Medicine in the Department of Anesthesiology, Perioperative, and Pain Medicine where she directs the Stanford Pain Relief Innovations Lab. She is creator of Empowered Relief® and serves on the Medical Advisory Board of the FPA. She has delivered keynote addresses in Australia, New Zealand, The Netherlands, the United States, and the United Kingdom and has briefed the U.S. Congress three times on patient-centered pain care. Her work has been featured in media outlets such as *Scientific American, The Guardian* (Australia), National Public Radio (NPR), BBC Radio, *The Wall Street Journal, The New York Times,* and *Nature.* In 2018, she spoke on the psychology of pain relief at the World Economic Forum in Davos, Switzerland.

Jordan Dattero is an undergraduate pursuing a Bachelor of Science degree in Biological Engineering with a minor in Brain and Cognitive Sciences at the Massachusetts Institute of Technology (MIT). She has 2 years of experience in the laboratory of Guoping Feng at MIT's McGovern Institute for Brain Research investigating gene therapy as a treatment for Rett syndrome. Currently, Jordan is working under the mentorship of Dr. Raymond Sekula, a neurosurgeon at Columbia Presbyterian.

Giulia Di Stefano, MD, PhD, is a researcher in the Department of Human Neuroscience at Sapienza University of Rome. In the past 10 years, her research projects have focused on the development of new neurophysiological techniques to test the nociceptive afferents upon the application of neurophysiological and morphometric techniques in the study of pathophysiological mechanisms of pain and on the investigation of possible biomarkers to predict drug response in patients with neuropathic pain. In 2013, within the framework of a fellowship at the Department of Neuroscience, Physiology and Pharmacology, University College of London, she focused on the function of the trigeminal nerve and on the brain stem circuitry of defensive responses in humans. One of her main research themes is the study of the pathophysiological mechanisms of facial pain, with a specific focus on trigeminal neuralgia.

Megan Tudor Donnelly, DO, is a United Council for Neurologic Subspecialities (UCNS) board-certified headache specialist. She is Director of Novant Health's Comprehensive Headache Center, as well as the founder and director of their interdisciplinary facial pain clinic. She is a graduate of the Lake Erie College of Osteopathic Medicine (Erie, PA). She completed her residency in neurology at the Cleveland Clinic Foundation, as well as a Fellowship in Headache Medicine at the Cleveland Clinic Foundation. She is a nationally known speaker and has published extensively on various topics related to head and face pain. She resides in Charlotte, NC, with her husband and two boys.

Trish Elliott, BS, grew up in Key Largo, FL, before receiving her Bachelor's degree in chemistry, with minors in neuroscience and business administration, from Southern Methodist University as a Hunt Leadership Scholar. She is currently obtaining her Master's degree in Ethics and Organizational Behavior at Palm Beach Atlantic University (West Palm Beach, FL), as she assists in neuroscience research at Florida Atlantic University, with aspirations to attend medical school and pursue a career in neurology.

Stephen P. Fleming, MBA, is President and CEO of The Well Spring Group, a nonprofit aging services provider based in Greensboro, NC. Steve is the past Chair of the Board of LeadingAge, the nation's largest aging services provider association, and has held positions on numerous governmental, professional, civic, and faith-based boards including the FPA. Steve developed TN in 2009 and had MVD surgery in 2015. Steve currently manages his recurrent TN with medication. Steve had a 15-year stint as a college football official, and today, he enjoys golf, hiking, and time in the garden. Steve and his wife, Anne, a retired public-school teacher, have two adult daughters, and a beautiful new granddaughter.

Saige Fong is a medical student at the University of Hawai'i John A. Burns School of Medicine. She received her BA degree in Psychology and an MS degree in Medical Sciences from Boston University. Her research and practice interests include primary care with a focus on immigrant and refugee mental health services.

Maria Merlano Gomez was raised in Venezuela and migrated to the United States to pursue her Bachelor's degree in medical biology at Florida Atlantic University. She cofounded Friends of MSF, a chapter affiliated with Médecins Sans Frontières (Doctors Without Borders), as she proceeded with neuroscience research during her undergraduate studies. Her goal is to go to medical school.

Jonathan Greenberg, PhD, is an Assistant Professor of Psychology at Harvard Medical School and a Research Staff Psychologist at Massachusetts General Hospital. His work primarily focuses on developing and testing mindfulness-based and mind–body interventions for individuals with chronic pain and other populations. He frequently shares his knowledge with the facial pain community via webinars and articles in the *Quarterly Journal*. He has been personally involved in mindfulness practice since 2003 and has since integrated his interest in mindfulness into his clinical and academic work.

Gary M. Heir, DMD, is an internationally recognized expert in orofacial pain and temporomandibular disorders. He is the director of the Center for Temporomandibular Disorders and Orofacial Pain in the Department of Diagnostic Sciences at Rutgers School of Dental Medicine, where he holds the Robert and Susan Carmel Chair in Algesiology. Dr. Heir played a significant role in getting orofacial pain recognized as the 12th specialty in dentistry by the American Dental

Association. In addition to his work at Rutgers, Dr. Heir is a highly sought-after lecturer, having delivered nearly 300 presentations on orofacial pain and related subjects throughout the world. He has served as the president of the American Academy of Orofacial Pain and the American Board of Orofacial Pain and as a member of the Commission on Dental Accreditation (CODA) and the Council on Dental Education and Licensure. Dr. Heir has published more than 100 peer-reviewed articles, chapters, and abstracts on orofacial pain and temporomandibular joint disorders. He also serves as the section editor for Orofacial Pain Neuroscience of *The Journal of the American Dental Association*. He is contributing to the FPA's dental education initiative.

Vince Holtmann, MA, MS, is a retired engineer and college mathematics instructor. Diagnosed with a meningioma and trigeminal neuralgia in 2006, he first underwent CyberKnife treatment and ultimately had surgery in 2008 to remove the tumor. Since the surgery, which included an MVD, he has remained pain-free. He is an FPA peer mentor and has been coleader of the St. Louis support group since 2011. He also serves as leader of the recently formed tumors and facial pain support group.

Lilah Keating is an ambitious high school student and aspiring neuroscientist with a passion for learning. For the past few years, she has worked at New York University researching Alzheimer's disease. Currently, Lilah is working under the mentorship of Dr. Raymond Sekula, a neurosurgeon at Columbia Presbyterian. She plans to pursue further scientific research and academic opportunities in the future.

Collin Kilgore, MD, is currently pursuing his PhD at Johns Hopkins University in the laboratory of Dr. Xinzhong Dong, whose group studies the biology of itch and pain and the immune system. He hopes to become a physician-scientist specializing in the treatment of neuroinflammatory diseases.

Lily H. Kim, MD, studied Human Biology and graduated with distinction from Stanford University. She then pursued her MD degree at Stanford School of Medicine, where she developed a passion for surgically treating neurological conditions. She is a current fourth-year resident in the Stanford Department of Neurosurgery.

Gary D. Klasser, DMD, is a Professor in the Division of Diagnostic Sciences at Louisiana State University School of Dentistry. In 2004, he graduated from the University of Kentucky with a Certificate in Orofacial Pain. In 2005, he completed a fellowship in Oral Medicine and Oral Oncology at the University of Illinois at Chicago (UIC). From 2005 to 2011, he was an Assistant Professor and Director of the Oral Medicine and Facial Pain Clinic at the UIC College of Dentistry. Dr. Klasser has published in many peer-reviewed journals and contributed chapters to various textbooks while also serving as an editorial reviewer for a number of journals. He is also coeditor for the 7th edition of the American Academy of Orofacial Pain (AAOP) book *Orofacial Pain: Guidelines for Assessment, Diagnosis, and Management* (Quintessence, 2023).

Ally Kubik, MEd, MS, BCBA, is a boy mom, Special Education teacher, and Board-Certified Behavior Analyst. She has had facial pain since the age of 13 years. Ally has been involved with the FPA for almost 20 years. She was one of the original members of the Young Patients Committee (YPC). She currently serves on the FPA's Board of Directors and is a peer mentor for the FPA.

Laura Launderville is a trigeminal neuralgia and occipital neuralgia warrior. She volunteers with the FPA and serves as a board member for the YPC. As a rare facial pain patient herself, she finds volunteering, advocating, and bringing awareness to other young patients' needs incredibly rewarding. Laura also volunteers with a nonprofit called The Vashti Initiative that supports those who have experienced spiritual and religious trauma. Laura blogs, authors articles, and tries to bring awareness to rare diseases and chronic illnesses by sharing her story. She finds joy from nature, listening to music, watching period dramas, and spending time with her partner and their two kitties, named Luna and Charlotte, at her home in Hampton Roads, VA.

Wolfgang Liedtke, MD, PhD, is a German-American neurologist. He is a corporate executive at Regeneron Pharmaceuticals, Tarrytown,

NY, where he is the Neurology Chair within Regeneron's Global Development – Genetic Medicines research area. Dr. Liedtke also holds positions as an Elected Member of the New York University (NYU) Pain Research Center, an Adjunct Professor at NYU College of Dentistry, and an Adjunct Professor of Neurology at Duke University in Durham, NC. Dr. Liedtke, as a basic research scientist, first described the TRPV4 ion channel in 2000 while at Rockefeller University. Then, after moving to Duke University (where he was an academic professor from 2004 to 2021), his research group made foundational discoveries related to the genetic mechanisms that govern nerve cells' ionic balance and excitability. He has now published more than 150 peer-reviewed articles that have been referenced more than 20,000 times. As a clinician, he founded two clinics within Duke Health to provide care for patients with trigeminal pain, other forms of nerve pain, and refractory pain in the context of comorbidities across the medical and dental spectrum. He has gained patients' enduring trust as a doctor who provides empathetic, yet science-based medical care. A long-term supporter of the FPA and grantee of the Facial Pain Research Foundation (FPRF), in 2021, he was selected to join the Medical Advisory Board of the FPA. His webinars on medications for the treatment of trigeminal neuropathic pain are popular and have been watched over and over again by members of the facial pain community.

Mark E. Linskey, MD, is a Professor of Neurological Surgery at University of California, Irvine (UCI). He is also the Western Regional Director of the Medical Advisory Board of the FPA and an Editor for the British Medical Association's *British Medical Journal* "Clinical Evidence" manual module on trigeminal neuralgia. He was previously the training module editor for the Trigeminal Neuralgia module of the American College of Physicians' "Smart Medicine" physician point-of-care decision support tool before it was discontinued. He currently runs the cranial nerve clinic for the Department of Neurological Surgery at UCI, and he serves as the faculty advisor for the Orange County FPA support group, which is the oldest FPA support group in continuous existence in the United States (dating back to the days when the FPA was known as the Trigeminal Neuralgia Association).

He was trained in MVD for 7 years with Peter Jannetta and in gamma knife stereotactic radiosurgery with L. Dade Lunsford at the University of Pittsburgh.

Michael Lim, MD, is the Chair of the Department of Neurosurgery at Stanford School of Medicine and a board-certified neurosurgeon specializing in trigeminal neuralgia and brain tumors. Before his appointment at Stanford, Dr. Lim was on the faculty Johns Hopkins University in Baltimore, MD. In both Maryland and California, Dr. Lim built one of the world's largest trigeminal neuralgia practices and used the most advanced surgical technologies and techniques for his patients. Dr. Lim holds a myriad of honors and awards. He has written more than 300 scientific articles and 20 book chapters and monographs. In addition to being a member of the FPA's Medical Advisory Board, he is a member of the Congress of Neurological Surgeons, American Association of Neurological Surgeons, and Society for Neuro-Oncology. He generously shares his time and knowledge with people with neuropathic facial pain by being a frequent presenter at FPA conferences and webinars. He is a beloved mentor and teacher. His patients with trigeminal neuralgia describe him as brilliant and compassionate.

Brenda C. Lovette, MS, CCC-SLP, CBIS, is a speech-language pathologist and rehabilitation scientist based in the Boston, MA, area. She specializes in helping adults with communication, swallowing, and voice challenges, focusing on their healing and improved quality of life. Brenda's research centers on using mindfulness to enhance health and wellness, complementing standard interventions. She is dedicated to making a positive impact through her compassionate clinical practice and patient-centered research.

Jesse McClure, MD, PharmD, PhD, is currently a surgical resident at the Charles E. Schmidt College of Medicine at Florida Atlantic University. He earned his PharmD in 2014 from the Medical University of South Carolina (MUSC) and then continued on at MUSC to earn a PhD in Drug Discovery and Biomedical Sciences in 2017, after which he moved to the University of Virginia from which he graduated with an MD degree in 2023. His research efforts have led to a patent for a novel series of small-molecule inhibitors for the treatment of acute myeloid leukemia and, ultimately, to the formation of an NIH-funded biotech company, Lydex Pharmaceuticals.

Leesa Morrow, PhD, JD, LP, is an attorney and health psychologist. She maintains private practices in forensic psychology and clinical health psychology, treating chronic pain disorders. Dr. Morrow completed a doctorate in Clinical Health Psychology at the University of North Texas (Denton, TX) and an internship in Clinical Psychology at Indiana University School of Medicine. Dr. Morrow has expertise in the treatment of acute and chronic pain, as well as stress-exacerbated systemic illnesses. She uses a variety of treatment modalities, including biofeedback, hypnosis, and cognitive behavioral therapy. A clinical psychologist with extensive experience working with trigeminal neuralgia patients, Dr. Morrow is a frequent presenter at FPA conferences.

Navid Pourtaheri, MD, PhD, is a plastic surgeon practicing in California Pacific Medical Center's Sutter Santa Rosa Regional Hospital. Dr. Pourtaheri attended Duke University School of Medicine and completed his residency at Case Western Reserve University. Dr. Pourtaheri pursued a fellowship in Craniofacial Surgery at Yale University School of Medicine. He is board-eligible in Plastic Surgery. Dr. Pourtaheri practices both cosmetic and reconstructive plastic surgery, providing patient-centered, state-of-the-art care.

Julie Pilitsis, MD, PhD, MBA, is Chair of the Department of Neurosurgery at University of Arizona (Tucson, AZ) and the Physician Executive for Functional Neurosurgery for Banner Health System. Prior to this role, she served as Dean of the Charles E. Schmidt College of Medicine and Vice President for Medical Affairs Strategic Initiatives at Florida Atlantic University (FAU), where she led the FAU Health Network initiative. In addition to these roles, Dr. Pilitsis has maintained a busy functional neurosurgery practice and built a program from the ground up at each institution where she has worked. She maintains an NIH-sponsored research program focused on device optimization for neuromodulation with 3 active grants and has published more than 250 journal articles, 5 textbooks, and numerous chapters. In 2023 she was the president of the North American Neuromodulation Society (NANS), a 2000-member organization. She is a member of the FPA's Medical Advisory Board.

Xiang Qian, MD, PhD, is the Stanford Medicine Endowed Director and Clinical Professor of Pain Medicine and Neurosurgery (by courtesy). Dr. Qian's clinical interests include the treatment of acute and chronic pain, with a special interest in both facial pain and head and neck pain. Dr. Qian is the co-director of the Stanford Health Care Facial Pain Program. Dr. Qian is also the Medical Director of Stanford Health Care's International Medical Services (IMS), supervising the care of international patients and promoting international collaborations.

Araika Ramchandran is a student intern in the laboratory of Dr. Michael Lim, who investigates a variety of different immunological and neurosurgical research topics. She is interested in pursuing a neurosurgical career and has focused her research efforts on tumor immunology and trigeminal neuralgia.

Hannah K. Rasmussen, MD, received her undergraduate degree from Harvard and completed her medical training at Stanford School of Medicine. She is currently a resident physician in anesthesiology at Stanford, where she is pursuing interests in acute and chronic pain management, regional anesthesia, and medical education.

Mohan S. Ravi, MD, earned his MD degree from Northwestern University Feinberg School of Medicine, from which he embarked on a journey focused on pain medicine. He has served as a Clinical Instructor at Marian University School of Medicine (Indianapolis, IN) and is currently a resident physician in Anesthesiology, Perioperative, and Pain Medicine at Stanford University School of Medicine. Dr. Ravi has been invited to present his research at the meetings of various pain societies such as the American Association of Pain Medicine and the American Society of Regional Anesthesia and Pain Medicine. His clinical interests include advancing the accessibility of patient-centered pain care, and his research interests are in the areas of facial pain and neuromodulation.

Alexander Ren is a second-year Stanford medical student with interests in neuroscience, immunology, and oncology. He is currently conducting research on immune-stimulating agents for the treatment of glioma in the laboratory of Dr. Michael Lim. Prior to medical school, Alexander graduated with a BA in neuroscience from Harvard College and an MPhil in translational biomedical research from the University of Cambridge.

Christine Ryu is a student intern in the laboratory of Dr. Michael Lim, who investigates a variety of different immunological and neurosurgical research topics. She is interested in pursuing a neurosurgical career and has focused her research efforts on tumor immunology and trigeminal neuralgia.

Zahra Sarabadani, DDS, a second-year resident at Rutgers School of Dental Medicine, is passionate about orofacial pain research. Through roles as a Guest Instructor and keynote speaker in Australia and New Zealand, she has gained a global perspective on dental and orofacial pain knowledge. Her research integrates advanced technologies, shaping the future of orofacial pain research and leaving a lasting impact on the scientific community.

Raymond F. Sekula, Jr., MD, is one of the world's foremost leaders in minimally invasive brain surgery. His world-renowned practice is devoted exclusively to cranial nerve disorders including trigeminal neuralgia, hemifacial spasm, and glossopharyngeal neuralgia. Each year, he performs more than 500 neurosurgical operations, including 200 MVDs. During his career, he has performed more than 2000 MVD surgeries. Prior to his career at Columbia University Medical School, Dr. Sekula was Professor and Residency Program Director at the University of Pittsburgh, Department of Neurological Surgery. Dr. Sekula's prolific academic career includes writing more than 100 scientific manuscripts, including editing the textbook *Microvascular Decompression Surgery*. He is Principal Investigator of a study concerning trigeminal neuralgia investigating the fundamental mechanisms of facial pain that receives funding from the National Institutes of Health. He is the newly elected chair of the FPA's Medical Advisory Board.

Bijal Shah, DMD, is a Senior Postgraduate Resident in Orofacial Pain at the Center for Temporomandibular Disorders and Orofacial Pain, Rutgers School of Dental Medicine.

Pari Shah is a student interested in pursuing majors in global health and neuroscience in college and, ultimately, in having a career in medicine. Last year, she worked at Lisman Laboratory (The Bronx, NY), researching correlations between gene expression and dendrite morphology. Currently, she is interning with Dr. Raymond Sekula in the Neurosurgery Department at Columbia University.

Celine Shon is a young, aspiring, and driven neuroscientist. She has pursued a rigorous academic path, excelling in biology, psychology, and chemistry, and has research experience in neuroscience and psychology. She plans on continuing her path into neuroscience by engaging in more research opportunities and laboratory work.

Konstantin Slavin, MD, FAANS, is a Professor and Head of Section of Stereotactic and Functional Neurosurgery at the University of Illinois College of Medicine. He is the current president of the World Society for Stereotactic and Functional Neurosurgery and president-elect of the International Neuromodulation Society, as well as the past president of the American Society for Stereotactic and Functional Neurosurgery. He earned his medical degree from the Azerbaijan State Medical Institute in 1988, when he was just 18 years old. He completed a neurosurgery residency at the Russian Post-Graduate Medical Academy and then completed both his internship and residency at the University of Illinois Medical Center in Chicago, IL. Subsequently, he completed a fellowship program at the Oregon Health Sciences University School of Medicine. Professor Slavin's research interests include chronic pain, movement disorders, surgery for psychiatric disorders, stereotactic radiosurgery, and occipital nerve stimulation. His clinical interests include stereotactic and functional neurosurgery, facial pain, trigeminal neuralgia, Chiari malformation, and gamma knife stereotactic radiosurgery.

Derek Steinbacher, MD, DMD, FACS, is a world-renowned plastic surgeon located in Guilford, CT. Having trained as both a dentist and a plastic and reconstructive surgeon, Dr. Steinbacher is uniquely qualified to perform complex craniofacial surgery in both children and adults. He performs artistic and meticulous work for his patients, including jaw, nose, face, and body procedures to improve contours and appearance. He also performs MVD surgery for people with severe migraine disorders. Dr. Steinbacher is an Assistant Professor of Plastic Surgery and Craniomaxillofacial Surgery at Yale University and is a member of the FPA's Medical Advisory Board.

Janet (Jan) Stubbs started having health issues when she developed rheumatoid arthritis at 20 years of age. She developed peripheral neuropathy and TN 18 years ago. She also had a below-knee amputation of her left leg 15 years ago because of a methicillin-resistant *Staphylococcus aureus* (MRSA) infection. She has been a life-long volunteer with her church. Now in her 80s, she continues to volunteer at church and in clubs in her retirement village. An important volunteer activity is driving people to their health appointments. Her TN was under control with Neurontin for several years until the drug depleted her sodium to dangerously low levels. Through a member of her son's church, she found a brain surgeon who performed a successful MVD in 2018, and she has been pain-free from TN since then. She is a member of an online TN support group.

Margaret Tugend, BA, lives in New York City and is a medical student at Columbia University. She is currently working as a predoctoral research fellow with Dr. Raymond Sekula, studying trigeminal neuralgia and hemifacial spasm. After medical school, she plans to pursue a career in neurosurgery.

Sai Charitha Velamati, DMD, is a second-year postgraduate student and Chief Resident of Orofacial Pain at the Rutgers School of Dental Medicine. With a strong foundation in dentistry, Dr. Velamati has seamlessly blended clinical expertise with a commitment to understanding and alleviating the complexities of orofacial pain. Throughout her career, she has demonstrated dedication to patient well-being, using a patient-centered approach to provide compassionate and effective care. She envisions a future in which orofacial pain is comprehensively understood and effectively managed, and she is actively contributing to this vision through her ongoing education and clinical training.

Lindsey Wallace, MBA, R.T(R)(ARRT), CPhT, is cochair of the Young Patients Committee (YPC) of the FPA. She is a certified pharmacy technician and currently works as a pediatric radiologic technologist. Lindsey advocates for patients at work and for young patients who have facial pain. Seeing patients thrive despite their medical conditions brings her great joy.

Risheng Xu, MD, PhD, is a fellowship-trained neurosurgeon with expertise in cerebrovascular and endovascular neurosurgery, as well as skull base pathologies. He treats patients with a wide range of skull base tumors, cerebrovascular disorders, and pain disorders such as trigeminal neuralgia. Dr. Xu completed his undergraduate studies at Harvard College and attended medical school at the Johns Hopkins University School of Medicine, where he also obtained a PhD in Pharmacology and Molecular Sciences. He continued his residency training in Neurosurgery at Johns Hopkins and remained there to complete a fellowship in Cerebrovascular and Endovascular Neurosurgery. Dr. Xu's basic science research focuses on molecular mechanisms underlying trigeminal neuralgia. Clinically, he studies the long-term outcomes of patients with cerebrovascular disorders and trigeminal neuralgia.

Richard S. Zimmerman, MD, is a neurosurgeon at Mayo Clinic's Phoenix, AZ, campus and a member of the FPA's Medical Advisory Board. He completed a residency in Neurosurgery, followed by a fellowship in Cerebrovascular and Skull Base Surgery at Boston University School of Medicine. He has focused his patient-centered clinical practice on minimally invasive and microsurgical options to treat trigeminal neuralgia, hemifacial spasm, seizure disorders, aneurysms, arteriovenous malformations, carotid artery disease, and brain tumors. Dr. Zimmerman pioneered Teflon-free microvascular decompression surgical protocols for trigeminal neuralgia, and his expertise has been recognized nationally and internationally. As a professor of neurosurgery Dr. Zimmerman has held numerous leadership roles at Mayo Clinic in Arizona including Dean of Education and Medical Director of Mayo Clinic Hospital. As nothing is more important to him than excellent patient outcomes, he has also chaired the Mayo Quality Outcomes and Patient Safety Subcommittees and has received Mayo Clinic's Lifetime Achievement Award for his career-long dedication to quality improvement and patient safety activities at Mayo Clinic.

Appendix 3
References by Chapter

References by Chapter and Section

Chapter 1

1.3 Treatment with Topical Medications

André N. *Observations pratiques sur les maladies de l'urèthre.* Paris: Delaguette; 1756.

Benoliel R, Heir G, Eliav E. Neuropathic orofacial pain. In Sharav Y, Benoliel R, eds. *Orofacial Pain and Headache.* 2nd ed. Chicago, IL: Quintessence International, 2015:407–474.

Fothergill J. Of a painful affection of the face. *In Medical observations and inquiries. By a Society of physicians in London.* 1773;5:129–142. [This publication was funded privately by Fothergill from 1771 to 1776. It is included in *Complete Works of John Fothergill*, a copy of which is held in the library of the Royal College of Physicians of London.]

Baad-Hansen L, Benoliel R. Neuropathic orofacial pain: Facts and fiction. *Cephalalgia.* 2017 Jun;37(7):670–679. doi: 10.1177/0333102417706310. Epub 2017 Apr 12. PMID: 28403646.

Finnerup NB, Haroutounian S, Kamerman P, et al. Neuropathic pain: An updated grading system for research and clinical practice. *Pain.* 2016 Aug;157(8):1599–1606. doi: 10.1097/j. pain.0000000000000492. PMID: 27115670; PMCID: PMC4949003.

Haribabu PK, Eliav E, Heir GM. Topical medications for the effective management of neuropathic orofacial pain. *J Am Dent Assoc.* 2013 Jun;144(6):612–614. doi: 10.14219/jada.archive.2013.0172.

Haviv Y, Zadik Y, Sharav Y, Benoliel R. Painful traumatic trigeminal neuropathy: An open study on the pharmacotherapeutic response to stepped treatment. *J Oral Facial Pain Headache*. 2014;28(1):52–60. doi: 10.11607/jop.1154.

Heir G, Karolchek S, Kalladka M, et al. Use of topical medication in orofacial neuropathic pain: A retrospective study. *Oral Surg Oral Med Oral Pathol Oral Radiol Endod*. 2008 Apr;105(4):466–469. doi: 10.1016/j.tripleo.2007.09.030.

Heir GM, Katzmann G, Covalesky B, et al. Use of compounded topical medications for treatment of orofacial pain: A narrative review. *J Oral Maxillofac Anesth*. 2022;1:27. https://dx.doi.org/10.21037/joma-22-10.

Heir G, Karolchek S, Kalladka M, et al. Use of topical medication in orofacial neuropathic pain: a retrospective study. *Oral Surg Oral Med Oral Pathol Oral Radiol Endod*. 2008 Apr;105(4):466–469. doi: 10.1016/j.tripleo.2007.09.030. PMID: 18329583.

International Association for Study of Pain. IASP Terminology web page. https://www.iasp-pain.org/resources/terminology/. Accessed Sep 2023.

Korczeniewska OA, Kohli D, Benoliel R, Baddireddy SM, Eliav E. Pathophysiology of post-traumatic trigeminal neuropathic pain. *Biomolecules*. 2022 Nov 25;12(12):1753. https://doi.org/10.3390/biom12121753.

Hughes MA, Frederickson AM, Branstetter BF, Zhu X, Sekula RF Jr. MRI of the trigeminal nerve in patients with trigeminal neuralgia secondary to vascular compression. *AJR Am J Roentgenol*. 2016 Mar;206(3):595–600. doi: 10.2214/AJR.14.14.

Plaza-Villegas F, Heir GM, Markman S, et al. Topical pregabalin and diclofenac for the treatment of neuropathic orofacial pain in rats. *Oral Surg Oral Med Oral Pathol Oral Radiol*. 2012 Oct;114(4):449–456. doi: 10.1016/j.oooo.2012.05.002.

Raddant AC, Russo AF. Calcitonin gene-related peptide in migraine: Intersection of peripheral inflammation and central modulation. *Expert Rev Mol Med*. 2011 Nov 29;13:e36. doi: 10.1017/S1462399411002067.

Seddon HJ. Three types of nerve injury. *Brain*. 1943 Dec;66(4):237–288. https://doi.org/10.1093/brain/66.4.237.

Slettebø H. Is this really trigeminal neuralgia? Diagnostic re-evaluation of patients referred for neurosurgery. *Scand J Pain*. 2021 Aug 2;21(4):788–793. https://doi.org/10.1515/sjpain-2021-0045.

Woolf CJ, Mannion RJ. Neuropathic pain: Aetiology, symptoms, mechanisms, and management. *Lancet*. 1999 Jun 5;353(9168):1959–1964. doi: 10.1016/S0140-6736(99)01307-0.

1.4   *Ketamine Infusions for Pain Relief*

Afridi SK, Giffin NJ, Kaube H, Goadsby PJ. A randomized controlled trial of intranasal ketamine in migraine with prolonged aura. *Neurology*. 2013 Feb 12;80(7): 642–647. doi: 10.1212/WNL.0b013e3182824e66.

Benoliel R, Gaul C. Persistent idiopathic facial pain. *Cephalalgia*. 2017 Jun;37(7):680–691. doi: 10.1177/0333102417706349.

Burch R, Rizzoli P, Loder E. The prevalence and impact of migraine and severe headache in the United States: Figures and trends from government health studies. *Headache*. 2018 Apr;58(4):496–505. doi: 10.1111/head.13281.

Carter GT, Duong V, Ho S, Ngo KC, Greer CL, Weeks DL. Side effects of commonly prescribed analgesic medications. *Phys Med Rehabil Clin N Am*. 2014 May 25(2):457–470. doi: 10.1016/j.pmr.2014.01.007.

Chah N, Jones M, Milord S, Al-Eryani K, Enciso R. Efficacy of ketamine in the treatment of migraines and other unspecified primary headache disorders compared to placebo and other interventions: A systematic review. *J Dent Anesth Pain Med*. 2021 Oct;21(5):413–429. doi: 10.17245/jdapm.2021.21.5.413.

Cruccu G, Finnerup NB, Jensen TS, et al. Trigeminal neuralgia: New classification and diagnostic grading for practice and research. *Neurology*. 2016 Jul 12;87(2):220–228. doi: 10.1212/WNL.0000000000002840.

Curto M, Lionetto L, Capi M, et al. O066. Kynurenine pathway metabolites in cluster headache. *J Headache Pain*.

2015;16(Suppl 1):A87. doi: 10.1186/1129-2377-16-S1-A87. Erratum in: J Headache Pain. 2017 Dec;18(1):11. PMID: 28132301; PMCID: PMC4759328.

Di Stefano G, La Cesa S, Truini A, Cruccu G. Natural history and outcome of 200 outpatients with classical trigeminal neuralgia treated with carbamazepine or oxcarbazepine in a tertiary centre for neuropathic pain. J Headache Pain. 2014 Jun 9;15(1):34. doi: 10.1186/1129-2377-15-34.

Etchison AR, Bos L, Ray M, et al. Low-dose ketamine does not improve migraine in the emergency department: A randomized placebo-controlled trial. West J Emerg Med. 2018 Nov;19(6):952–960. doi: 10.5811/westjem.2018.8.37875.

Garcia R, Chen Q, Posadas E, Tran J, Kwon A, Qian X. Continuous ketamine infusion as a treatment for refractory facial pain. Cureus. 2023 Mar;15(3):e35638. doi: 10.7759/cureus.35638.

Goadsby PJ, Holland PR, Martins-Oliveira M, Hoffmann J, Schankin C, Akerman S. Pathophysiology of migraine: A disorder of sensory processing. Physiol Rev. 2017 Apr;97(2):553–622. doi: 10.1152/physrev.00034.2015.

Granata L, Niebergall H, Langner R, Agosti R, Sakellaris L. Ketamine i. v. for the treatment of cluster headaches: An observational study [Article in German]. Schmerz. 2016 Jun;30(3):286–288. doi: 10.1007/s00482-016-0111-z.

Green SM, Roback MG, Kennedy RM, Krauss B. Clinical practice guideline for emergency department ketamine dissociative sedation: 2011 update. Ann Emerg Med. 2011 May;57(5):449–461. doi: 10.1016/j.annemergmed.2010.11.030.

Guimarães Pereira JE, Ferreira Gomes Pereira L, Mercante Linhares R, Darcy Alves Bersot C, Aslanidis T, Ashmawi HA. Efficacy and safety of ketamine in the treatment of neuropathic pain: A systematic review and meta-analysis of randomized controlled trials. J Pain Res. 2022 Apr 9;15:1011–1037. doi: 10.2147/JPR.S358070.

Iqbal S, Rashid W, Ain QU, Atiq T, Noor R, Irfan F. Efficacy of carbamazepine and oxcarbazepine for treating trigeminal neuralgia. BMC J Med Sci. 2022;3(2):55–59.

Lauritsen C, Mazuera S, Lipton RB, Ashina S. Intravenous ketamine for subacute treatment of refractory chronic migraine: A case series. *J Headache Pain*. 2016 Dec;17(1):106. doi: 10.1186/s10194-016-0700-3.

Leis K, Mazur E, Szyperski P, et al. Carbamazepine - Hematologic effects of the use. *J Educ Health Sport*. 2018;8(8):51–60. http://dx.doi.org/10.5281/zenodo.1296993.

Mathisen LC, Skjelbred P, Skoglund LA, Øye I. Effect of ketamine, an NMDA receptor inhibitor, in acute and chronic orofacial pain. *Pain*. 1995 May;61(2):215–220. doi: 10.1016/0304-3959(94)00170-J.

Mogahed MM, Anwar AG, Mohamed RM. Comparative study between intravenous ketamine and lidocaine infusion in controlling of refractory trigeminal neuralgia. *J Anesth Clin Res*. 2017;8(8):746. doi: 10.4172/2155-6148.1000746.

Moisset X, Giraud P, Meunier E, et al. Ketamine–magnesium for refractory chronic cluster headache: A case series. *Headache*. 2020 Nov;60(10):2537–2543. doi: 10.1111/head.14005.

Nicolodi M, Sicuteri F. Exploration of NMDA receptors in migraine: Therapeutic and theoretic implications. *Int J Clin Pharmacol Res*. 1995;15(5–6):181–189. PMID: 8835616.

Niesters M, Martini C, Dahan A. Ketamine for chronic pain: Risks and benefits. *Br J Clin Pharmacol*. 2014 Feb;77(2):357–367. doi: 10.1111/bcp.12094.

Orhurhu VJ, Vashisht R, Claus LE, Cohen SP. Ketamine toxicity. In: *StatPearls [Internet]*. Treasure Island, FL: StatPearls Publishing; 2019. Accessed 11/1/2023.

Peeters M, Gunthorpe MJ, Strijbos PJLM, Goldsmith P, Upton N, James NF. Effects of pan- and subtype-selective N-methyl-d-aspartate receptor antagonists on cortical spreading depression in the rat: Therapeutic potential for migraine. *J Pharmacol Exp Ther*. 2007 May;321(2):564–572. doi: 10.1124/jpet.106.117101.

Peres M, Zukerman E, Senne Soares CA, Alonso EO, Santos BFC, Faulhaber MHW. Cerebrospinal fluid glutamate levels in chronic migraine. *Cephalalgia*. 2004 Sep;24(9):735–739. doi: 10.1111/j.1468-2982.2004.00750.x.

Petersen AS, Pedersen AS, Barloese MCJ, et al. Intranasal ketamine for acute cluster headache attacks—Results from a proof-of-concept open-label trial. *Headache*. 2022 Jan;62(1):26–35. doi: 10.1111/head.14220.

Sacco S, Lampl C, Maassen van den Brink A, et al. Burden and Attitude to Resistant and Refractory (BARR) Study Group. Burden and attitude to resistant and refractory migraine: A survey from the European Headache Federation with the endorsement of the European Migraine & Headache Alliance. *J Headache Pain*. 2021 May 18;22(1):39. doi: 10.1186/s10194-021-01252-4.

Schwenk ES, Goldberg SF, Patel RD, et al. Adverse drug effects and preoperative medication factors related to perioperative low-dose ketamine infusions. *Reg Anesth Pain Med*. 2016 Jul–Aug;41(4):482–487. doi: 10.1097/AAP.0000000000000416.

Schwenk ES, Torjman MC, Moaddel R, et al. Ketamine for refractory chronic migraine: An observational pilot study and metabolite analysis. *J Clin Pharmacol*. 2021 Nov;61(11):1421–1429. doi: 10.1002/jcph.1920.

Sessle BJ, Neural mechanisms and pathways in craniofacial pain. *Can J Neurol Sci*. 1999 Nov;26(Suppl 3):S7–S11. doi: 10.1017/s0317167100000135.

Shahani R, Streutker C, Dickson B, Stewart RJ. Ketamine-associated ulcerative cystitis: A new clinical entity. *Urology*. 2007 May;69(5):810–812. doi: 10.1016/j.urology.2007.01.038.

Storer RJ, Goadsby PJ. Trigeminovascular nociceptive transmission involves N-methyl-d-aspartate and non-N-methyl-d-aspartate glutamate receptors. *Neuroscience*. 1999;90(4):1371–1376. doi: 10.1016/s0306-4522(98)00536-3.

Srirangam S, Mercer J. Ketamine bladder syndrome: An important differential diagnosis when assessing a patient with persistent lower urinary tract symptoms. *BMJ Case Rep*. 2012;2012:bcr2012006447. doi: 10.1136/bcr-2012-006447.

Strous JFM, Weeland CJ, van der Draai FA, et al. Brain changes associated with long-term ketamine abuse, a systematic review. *Front Neuroanat*. 2022 Mar 18;16:795231. doi: 10.3389/fnana.2022.795231.

Tran K, McCormack S. Ketamine for chronic non-cancer pain: A review of clinical effectiveness, cost-effectiveness, and guidelines [Internet]. Ottawa (ON): Canadian Agency for Drugs and Technologies in Health; 2020 May 28. Accessed November 1, 2023.

Wei DY, Goadsby PJ. Cluster headache pathophysiology—Insights from current and emerging treatments. *Nat Rev Neurol.* 2021;17(5):308–324. doi: 10.1038/s41582-021-00477-w.

1.5   *What To Do If Pain Takes You To an Emergency Department or Urgent Care Facility*

Bergouignan M. Cures heureuses de nevralgies faciales essentielles par le diphenylhydantoinate de soude [Successful cure of essential facial neuralgias by sodium diphenylhydantoinate]. *Rev Laryngol Otol Rhinol (Bord).* 1942;63:34–41.

Cheshire WP. Fosphenytoin: An intravenous option for the management of acute trigeminal neuralgia crisis. *J Pain Symptom Manage.* 2001;21:506–510. doi: 10.1016/s0885-3924(01)00269-x.

DynaMedex: A Benefit of ACP Membership. American College of Physicians. http://smartmedicine.acponline.org/content. aspx?gbosid=299. Must be a member to access.

Ende M. Diphenylhydantoin in tic douloureux and atypical facial pain. *Va Med Mont (1918).* 1957;84(7):358–359.

Facial Pain Association Home Page. https://www.facepain.org/.

Jannetta PJ, Alksne JF, Barbaro NM, et al. Facial pain experts establish a new pain classification. *TNA Quarterly.* 2012 Winter;1(4):12.

Neuropathic pain in adults: Pharmacological management in non-specialist settings. *NICE Clinical Guidelines No. 173.* London: National Institute for Health and Care Excellence (NICE);2013:1–41. (Updated: 22 September 2020.)

Pilitsis JG, Khazen O. Trigeminal Neuralgia – Causes Symptoms and Treatments. *American Association of Neurological Surgeons.* 2019. https://www.aans.org/Patients/Neurosurgical-Conditions-and-Treatments/Trigeminal-Neuralgia.

Tate R, Rubin LM, Krajewski KC. Treatment of refractory trigeminal neuralgia with intravenous phenytoin. *Am J Health Syst Pharm.* 2011 Nov 1;68(21):2059–2061. doi: 10.2146/ajhp100636.

Vargas A, Thomas K. Intravenous fosphenytoin for acute exacerbation of trigeminal neuralgia: case report and literature review. *Ther Adv Neurol Disord.* 2015 Jul;8(4):187–188. doi: 10.1177/1756285615583202.

Zakrzewska JM, Linskey ME. Trigeminal neuralgia. *BMJ Clin Evid.* (online). 2014 Oct 6;2014:1207. PMID: 25299564. PMCID: PMC4191151.

Chapter 2

2.1   Glossopharyngeal Neuralgia

Chen J, Sindou M. Vago-glossopharyngeal neuralgia: A literature review of neurosurgical experience. *Acta Neurochir (Wien).* 2015 Feb;157(2):311–321. doi: 10.1007/s00701-014-2302-7.

Dandy WE. Trigeminal neuralgia and trigeminal tic douloureux. Lewis D, ed. *Practice of Surgery.* Hagerstown, MD: WF Prior CO, 1932: 177-200.

Du T, Ni B, Shu W, Hu Y, Zhu H, Li Y. Neurosurgical choice for glossopharyngeal neuralgia: A benefit–harm assessment of long-term quality of life. *Neurosurgery.* 2020;88(1):131–139. doi: 10.1093/neuros/nyaa325.

Guclu B, Sindou M, Meyronet D, Streichenberger N, Simon E, Mertens P. Cranial nerve vascular compression syndromes of the trigeminal, facial and vago-glossopharyngeal nerves: Comparative anatomical study of the central myelin portion and transitional zone; correlations with incidences of corresponding hyperactive dysfunctional syndromes. *Acta Neurochir (Wien).* 2011 Dec;153(12):2365–2375. doi: 10.1007/s00701-011-1168-1.

Resnick DK, Jannetta PJ, Bissonnette D, Jho HD, Lanzino G. Microvascular decompression for glossopharyngeal neuralgia. *Neurosurgery.* 1995 Jan;36(1):64–69. doi: 10.1227/00006123-199501000-00008.

Sindou M, Keravel Y. Neurosurgical treatment of vago-glossopharyngeal neuralgia [Article in French]. *Neurochirurgie.* 2009 Apr;55(2):231–235. doi: 10.1016/j.neuchi.2009.01.010.

Taylor RJ, Lowe SR, Ellis N, Abdullah E, Patel S, Halstead LA. Laryngeal manifestations of cranial nerve IX/X compression at the brainstem. *Laryngoscope.* 2019 Sep;129(9):2105–2111. doi: 10.1002/lary.27678.

Zheng W, Zhao P, Song H, et al. Prognostic factors for long-term outcomes of microvascular decompression in the treatment of glossopharyngeal neuralgia: A retrospective analysis of 97 patients. *J Neurosurg.* 2021 Dec 17:1–8. doi: 10.3171/2021.9.JNS21877.

2.2   *Geniculate Neuralgia*

Bentley JN, Sagher O. Geniculate neuralgia: The more we learn, the less we know. *World Neurosurg.* 2013 Dec;80(6):e209–e210. https://dx.doi.org/10.1016/j.wneu.2013.01.076.

Clifton WE, Grewal S, Lundy L, Cheshire WP, Tubbs RS, Wharen RE. Clinical implications of nervus intermedius variants in patients with geniculate neuralgia: Let anatomy be the guide. *Clin Anat.* 2020 Oct;33(7):1056–1061. https://dx.doi.org/10.1002/ca.23536.

Gupta K, Commentary: Bilateral nervus intermedius sectioning for geniculate neuralgia: Case report and operative video. *Oper Neurosurg (Hagerstown).* 2022 Jan 1;22(1):e64–e65. https://dx.doi.org/10.1227/ONS.0000000000000030.

Holste KG, Hardaway FA, Raslan AM, Burchiel KJ. Pain-free and pain-controlled survival after sectioning the nervus intermedius in nervus intermedius neuralgia: A single-institution review. *J Neurosurg.* 2018 Aug;131(2):352–359. https://doi.org/10.3171/2018.3.JNS172495.

Kenning TJ, Kim CS, Bien AG. Microvascular decompression and nervus intermedius sectioning for the treatment of geniculate neuralgia. *J Neurol Surg B Skull Base.* 2019 Jun;80(Suppl 3): S316–S317. https://dx.doi.org/10.1055/s-0038-1675151.

Lovely TJ, Jannetta PJ. Surgical management of geniculate neuralgia. *Am J Otol.* 1997 Jul;18(4):512–517. https://www.ncbi.nlm.nih.gov/pubmed/9233495.

Nanda A, Khan IS. Nervus intermedius and geniculate neuralgia. *World Neurosurg.* 2013 May–Jun;79(5–6): 651–652. https://dx.doi. org/10.1016/j.wneu.2012.05.002.

Nguyen VN, Basma J, Sorenson J, Michael LM 2nd. Microvascular decompression for geniculate neuralgia through a retrosigmoid approach. *J Neurol Surg B Skull Base.* 2019 Jun;80(Suppl 3):S322. https://dx.doi.org/10.1055/s-0038-1676837.

Ouaknine GE, Robert F, Molina-Negro P, Hardy J. Geniculate neuralgia and audio-vestibular disturbances due to compression of the intermediate and eighth nerves by the postero-inferior cerebellar artery. *Surg Neurol.* 1980 Feb;13(2):147–150. https://www.ncbi. nlm.nih.gov/pubmed/7355379.

Peris-Celda M, Oushy S, Perry A, et al. Nervus Intermedius and the Surgical Management of Geniculate Neuralgia. *J Neurosurg.* 2018 Aug 10;131(2):343–351. https://dx.doi.org/10.3171/2018.3. JNS172920.

Piper K, Zheng QV, Heller RS, Agazzi S. Bilateral nervus intermedius sectioning for geniculate neuralgia: Case report and operative video. *Oper Neurosurg (Hagerstown).* 2021 Nov 15;21(6):E566–E568. https://dx.doi.org/10.1093/ons/opab354.

Pulec JL. Geniculate neuralgia: Diagnosis and surgical management. *Laryngoscope.* 1976 Jul;86(7):955–964. https://dx.doi. org/10.1288/00005537-197607000-00008.

Pulec JL. Geniculate neuralgia: Long-term results of surgical treatment. *Ear Nose Throat J.* 2002 Jan;81(1):30–33. https://www. ncbi.nlm.nih.gov/pubmed/11816385.

Robblee J. A pain in the ear: Two case reports of nervus intermedius neuralgia and narrative review. *Headache.* 2021 Mar;61(3):414–421. https://doi.org/10.1111/head.14066.

Rupa V, Saunders RL, Weider DJ. Geniculate neuralgia: The surgical management of primary otalgia. *J Neurosurg.* 1991 Oct;75(4):505–511. https://dx.doi.org/10.3171/jns.1991.75.4.0505.

Tang IP, Freeman SR, Kontorinis G, et al. Geniculate neuralgia: A systematic review. *J Laryngol Otol.* 2014 May;128(5):394–399. https://dx.doi.org/10.1017/S0022215114000802.

Thirumala P, Meigh K, Dasyam N, et al. The incidence of high-frequency hearing loss after microvascular decompression for trigeminal neuralgia, glossopharyngeal neuralgia, or geniculate neuralgia. J Neurosurg. 2015 Dec;123(6):1500–1506. https://dx.doi.org/10.3171/2014.10.JNS141101.

Tsau P-W, Liao M-F, Hsu J-L, et al. Clinical presentations and outcome studies of cranial nerve involvement in herpes zoster infection: A retrospective single-center analysis. J Clin Med. 2020 Mar 30;9(4):946. https://doi.org/10.3390/jcm9040946.

Tubbs RS, Mosier KM, Cohen-Gadol AA. Geniculate neuralgia: Clinical, radiologic, and intraoperative correlates. World Neurosurg. 2013 Dec;80(6):e353–e357. https://dx.doi.org/10.1016/j.wneu.2012.11.053.

2.3   Occipital Neuralgia

Cesmebasi A, Muhleman MA, Hulsberg P, et al. Occipital neuralgia: Anatomic considerations. Clin Anat. 2015 Jan;28(1):101–108. doi: 10.1002/ca.22468.

Choi I, Jeon SR. Neuralgias of the head: Occipital neuralgia. J Korean Med Sci. 2016 Apr;31(4):479–488. doi: 10.3346/jkms.2016.31.4.479. Epub 2016 Mar 9. PMID: 27051229. PMCID: PMC4810328.

Djavaherian DM, Guthmiller KB. Occipital neuralgia. In : StatPearls [Internet]. Treasure Island, FL: StatPearls Publishing; 2021. PMID: 30855865.

Dougherty C. Occipital neuralgia. Curr Pain Headache Rep. 2014 May;18(5):411. doi: 10.1007/s11916-014-0411-x. PMID: 24737457.

Janjua MB, Reddy S, El Ahmadieh TY, et al. Occipital neuralgia: A neurosurgical perspective. J Clin Neurosci. 2020 Jan;71:263–270. doi: 10.1016/j.jocn.2019.08.102. Epub 2019 Oct 9. PMID: 31606286.

Slavin KV, Isagulyan ED, Gomez C, Yin D. Occipital nerve stimulation. Neurosurg Clin N Am. 2019 Apr;30(2):211–217. doi: 10.1016/j.nec.2018.12.004. Epub 2019 Feb 18. PMID: 30898272.

Slavin KV, Nersesyan H, Wess C. Peripheral neurostimulation for treatment of intractable occipital neuralgia. *Neurosurgery.* 2006 Jan;58(1):112–119. doi: 10.1227/01.neu.0000192163.55428.62. PMID: 16385335.

Sweet JA, Mitchell LS, Narouze S, et al. Occipital nerve stimulation for the treatment of patients with medically refractory occipital neuralgia: Congress of Neurological Surgeons systematic review and evidence-based guideline. *Neurosurgery.* 2015 Sep;77(3):332–41. doi: 10.1227/NEU.0000000000000872. PMID: 26125672.

2.4   Hemifacial Spasm

Auger RG, Whisnant JP. Hemifacial spasm in Rochester and Olmsted County, Minnesota, 1960 to 1984. *Arch Neurol.* 1990 Nov;47(11):1233–1234. https://doi.org/10.1001/archneur.1990.00530110095023.

Foster KA, Shin SS, Prabhu B, Fredrickson A, Sekula RF Jr. Calcium phosphate cement cranioplasty decreases the rate of cerebrospinal fluid leak and wound infection compared with titanium mesh cranioplasty: Retrospective study of 672 patients. *World Neurosurg.* 2016 Nov;95:414–418. https://doi.org/10.1016/j.wneu.2016.02.071.

Jankovic J, Schwartz K, Donovan DT. Botulinum toxin treatment of cranial–cervical dystonia, spasmodic dysphonia, other focal dystonias and hemifacial spasm. *J Neurol Neurosurg Psychiatry.* 1990 Aug;53(8):633–639. https://doi.org/10.1136/jnnp.53.8.633.

Kaufmann AM. Hemifacial spasm: A neurosurgical perspective. *J Neurosurg.* 2023 Jul 7;140(1):240–247. https://doi.org/10.3171/2023.5.JNS221898.

Lagalla G, Logullo F, Di Bella P, Haghighipour R, Provinciali L. Familial hemifacial spasm and determinants of late onset. *Neurol Sci.* 2010 Feb;31(1):17–22. doi: 10.1007/s10072-009-0153-4.

Lawrence JD, Frederickson AM, Chang Y-F, Weiss PM, Gerszten PC, Sekula RF. An investigation into quality of life improvement in patients undergoing microvascular decompression for hemifacial spasm. *J Neurosurg.* 2018 Jan;128(1):193–201. https://doi.org/10.3171/2016.9.JNS161022.

Nilsen B, Le K-D, Dietrichs E. Prevalence of hemifacial spasm in Oslo, Norway. *Neurology.* 63(8), 1532–1533. https://doi.org/10.1212/01. wnl.0000142080.85228.e8.

Sekula RF Jr. The preoperative evaluation of the patient considering microvascular decompression for hemifacial spasm. *Originally published in the Benign Essential Blepharospasm Research Foundation Newsletter.* 2011;30(4):5–6. Available at https:// blepharospasm.org/wp-content/uploads/2021/05/The-Preoperative-Evaluation-of-the-Patient-Considering-Microvascular-Decompression-for-Hemifacial-Spasm-Sekula-2011-1.pdf. Accessed Apr 22, 2024.

Sekula RF Jr, Frederickson AM, Arnone GD, Quigley MR, Hallett M. Microvascular decompression for hemifacial spasm in patients >65 years of age: An analysis of outcomes and complications. *Muscle Nerve.* 2013 Nov;48(5):770–776. https://doi.org/10.1002/mus.23800.

2.5   *Burning Mouth Syndrome*

Adamo D, Celentano A, Ruoppo et al. The Relationship Between Sociodemographic Characteristics and Clinical Features in Burning Mouth Syndrome. *Pain Med.* 2015;16:2171–2179. doi: 10.1111/ pme.12808.

Cephalalgia Reports Burning mouth syndrome: An update Huann Lan Tan and Tara Renton Volume 3: 1–18 The Author(s) 2020 DOI: 10.1177/2515816320970143 journals.sagepub.com/home/rep

Wu S, Zhang W, Yan J, Noma N, Young A, Yan Z. Worldwide prevalence estimates of burning mouth syndrome: A systematic review and meta-analysis. *Oral Dis.* 2021;28:1431–1440. doi: 10.1111/odi.13868.

2.6   *Postherpetic Neuralgia*

Yu J, Tu M, Shi Y, et al. Acupuncture therapy for treating postherpetic neuralgia: A protocol for an overview of systematic reviews and meta-analysis. *Medicine (Baltimore).* 2020 Nov 20;99(47):e23283. doi: 10.1097/MD.0000000000023283. PMID: 33217857; PMCID: PMC7676539.

2.7   Anesthesia Dolorosa

Giller C (2002). "Atypical facial pain and anesthesia dolorosa". In
   Burchiel KJ (ed.). *Surgical management of pain*. New York: Thieme.
   pp. 311–6. ISBN 0-86577-912-0.

2.10   Medical Causes of Facial Pain

Shakiba Houshi, Mohammad Javad Tavallaei, Mahdi Barzegar Alireza
   Afshara-SafaviSaeed Vaheb, Omid Mirmosayyeb, Vahid
   Shaygannejad. Multiple Sclerosis and Related Disorders.
   Prevalence of trigeminal neuralgia in multiple sclerosis: A
   systematic review and meta-analysis. Review Article| Volume 57,
   103472, January 2022. Published: December 28, 2021 DOI:https://
   doi.org/10.1016/j.msard.2021.103472

Chapter 3

3.1   What Makes a Neurosurgeon an Expert?

Kalkanis, Steven N. M.D., Eskandar, Emad N. M.D., Carter, Bob S. M.D.,
   Ph.D., Barker, Fred G. II, M.D. Microvascular Decompression
   Surgery in the United States, 1996 to 2000: Mortality Rates,
   Morbidity Rates, and the Effects of Hospital and Surgeon Volumes.
   Neurosurgery 52(6): 1251–1262, June 2003. | DOI: 10.1227/01.
   NEU.0000065129.25359.EE

3.2   Microvascular Decompression for TN

Zimmerman RS, Butterfield RJ, Turcotte EL, et al. Microvascular
   transposition without Teflon: A single institution's 17- year
   experience treating trigeminal neuralgia operative neurosurgery.
   Oper Neurosurg (Hagerstown). 2021 Mar 15;20(4):397–405. doi:
   10.1093/ons/opaa413.

3.4   An Algorithm for the Surgical Treatment of Classical Trigeminal Neuralgia

Bethamcharla R, Abou-Al-Shaar H, Maarbjerg S, Chang Y-F, Gacka
   CN, Sekula RF Jr. Percutaneous glycerol rhizolysis of the trigeminal

ganglion for the treatment of idiopathic and classic trigeminal neuralgia: Outcomes and complications. *Eur J Neurol.* 2023 Oct;30(10):3307–3313. https://doi.org/10.1111/ene.15977.

Hardaway FA, Gustafsson HC, Holste K, Burchiel KJ, Raslan AM. A novel scoring system as a preoperative predictor for pain-free survival after microsurgery for trigeminal neuralgia. *J Neurosurg.* 2020;132(1):217–224. https://doi.org/10.3171/2018.9.JNS181208.

Headache Classification Committee of the International Headache Society (IHS). The International Classification of Headache Disorders, 3rd edition (beta version). *Cephalalgia.* 2013 Jul;33(9):629–808. doi: 10.1177/0333102413485658.

Hughes MA, Branstetter BF, Taylor CT, et al. MRI findings in patients with a history of failed prior microvascular decompression for hemifacial spasm: How to image and where to look. *AJNR Am J Neuroradiol.* 2015 Apr;36(4):768–773. https://doi.org/10.3174/ajnr.A4174.

Hughes MA, Jani RH, Fakhran S, et al. Significance of degree of neurovascular compression in surgery for trigeminal neuralgia. *J Neurosurg.* 2019 Jun 14;133(2):411–416. https://doi.org/10.3171/2019.3.JNS183174.

Maarbjerg S, Wolfram F, Gozalov A, Olesen J, Bendtsen L. Significance of neurovascular contact in classical trigeminal neuralgia. *Brain.* 2015 Feb;138(2):311–319. https://doi.org/10.1093/brain/awu349.

Panczykowski DM, Jani RH, Hughes MA, Sekula RF. Development and evaluation of a preoperative trigeminal neuralgia scoring system to predict long-term outcome following microvascular decompression. *Neurosurgery.* 2020 Jul 1;87(1):71–79. https://doi.org/10.1093/neuros/nyz376.

Sekula RF Jr, Frederickson AM, Jannetta PJ, Quigley MR, Aziz KM, Arnone GD. Microvascular decompression for elderly patients with trigeminal neuralgia: A prospective study and systematic review with meta-analysis. *J Neurosurg.* 2011 Jan;114(1):172–179. https://doi.org/10.3171/2010.6.JNS10142.

3.5 Surgical Treatment of Migraine Headaches

2002 Pharmacy Benchmarks. Trends in Pharmacy Benefit Management for Commercial Plans. Sacramento, CA: Pharmaceutical Care Network; 2002.

Abu-Arafeh I, Razak S, Sivaraman B, Graham C. Prevalence of headache and migraine in children and adolescents: A systematic review of population-based studies. Dev Med Child Neurol. 2010 Dec;52(12):1088–1097. doi: 10.1111/j.1469-8749.2010.03793.x.

Ascha M, Kurlander David, Sattar A, Gatherwright J, Guyuron B. In-depth review of symptoms, triggers, and treatment of occipital migraine headaches (Site IV). Plast Reconstr Surg. 2017 Jun;139(6):1333e–1342e. doi: 10.1097/PRS.0000000000003395.

Dodick DW. Triptan nonresponder studies: Implications for clinical practice. Headache. 2005 Feb;45(2):156–162. doi: 10.1111/j.1526-4610.2005.05031.x.

Forootan Seyed NS, Lee M, Guyuron B. Migraine headache trigger site prevalence analysis of 2590 sites in 1010 patients. J Plast Reconstr Aesthet Surg. 2017 Feb;70(2):152–158. doi: 10.1016/j.bjps.2016.11.004.

Goldberg LD. The cost of migraine and its treatment. Am J Manag Care. 2005 Jun;11(2 Suppl):S62–S67. PMID: 16095269. https://pubmed.ncbi.nlm.nih.gov/16095269.

Guyuron B. Is migraine surgery ready for prime time? The surgical team's view. Headache. 2015 Nov–Dec;55(10):1464–1473. doi: 10.1111/head.12714.

Guyuron B, Kriegler JS, Davis J, Amini SB. Five-year outcome of surgical treatment of migraine headaches. Plast Reconstr Surg. 2011 Feb;127(2):603–608. doi: 10.1097/PRS.0b013e3181fed456.

Guyuron B, Kriegler JS, Davis J, Amini SB. Comprehensive surgical treatment of migraine headaches. Plast Reconstr Surg. 2005 Jan;115(1):1–9. PMID: 15622223.

Guyuron B, Lineberry K, Nahabet EH. A retrospective review of the outcomes of migraine surgery in the adolescent population. Plast Reconstr Surg. 2015 Jun;135(6):1700–1705. doi: 10.1097/PRS.0000000000001270.

Guyuron B, Pourtaheri N. Therapeutic role of fat injection in the treatment of recalcitrant migraine headaches. *Plast Reconstr Surg.* 2019 Mar;143(3):877–885. doi: 10.1097/PRS. 0000000000005353.

Guyuron B, Riazi H, Long T, Wirtz E. Use of a Doppler signal to confirm migraine headache trigger sites. *Plast Reconstr Surg.* 2015 Apr;135(4):1109–1112. doi: 10.1097/PRS.0000000000001102.

Guyuron B, Yohannes E, Miller R, Chim H, Reed D, Chance M. Electron microscopic and proteomic comparison of terminal branches of the trigeminal nerve in patients with and without migraine headaches. *Plast Reconstr Surg.* 2014 Nov;134(5):796e–805e. doi: 10.1097/ PRS.0000000000000696.

Hu XH, Markson LE, Lipton RB, et al. Burden of migraine in the United States: Disability and economic costs. *Arch Intern Med.* 1999 Apr 26;159(8):813–818. doi: 10.1001/archinte.159.8.813.

International Headache Society. International Classification of Headache Disorders (ICHD) (3rd Edition) web page. https://www. ihs-headache.org/ichd-guidelines.

Kurlander D, Ascha M, Sattar A, Guyuron B. In-depth review of symptoms, triggers, and surgical deactivation of frontal migraine headaches (Site I). *Plast Reconstr Surg.* 2016 Sep;138(3):681–688. doi: 10.1097/PRS.0000000000002479.

Kurlander D, Punjabi A, Liu M, Sattar A, Guyuron B. In-depth review of symptoms, triggers, and treatment of temporal migraine headaches (Site II). *Plast Reconstr Surg.* 2014 April;133(4):897–903. doi: 10.1097/PRS.0000000000000045.

Larson K, Lee M, Davis J, Guyuron B. Factors contributing to migraine headache surgery failure and success. *Plast Reconstr Surg.* 2011 Nov;128:1069–1075. doi: 10.1097/PRS.0b013e31822b61a1.

Lipton RB, Bigal ME, Diamond M, Freitag F, Reed ML, Stewart WF; AMPP Advisory Group. Migraine prevalence, disease burden, and the need for preventative therapy. *Neurology.* 2007 Jan 30;68(5):343–349. doi: 10.1212/01.wnl.0000252808.97649.21.

Lipton RB, Stewart WF, Diamond S, et al. Prevalence and burden of migraine in the United States: Data from the American Migraine

Study II. Headache. 2001 Jul–Aug;41:646–657. doi: 10.1046/j.1526-4610.2001.041007646.x.

Pourtaheri N, Guyuron B. Computerized tomographic evaluation of supraorbital notches and foramen in patients with frontal migraine headaches and correlation with clinical symptoms. *J Plast Reconstr Aesthet Surg.* 2018 Jun;71(6):840–846. doi: 10.1016/j.bjps.2018.01.040.

Stewart WF, Shechter A, Rasmussen BK. Migraine prevalence: A review of population-based studies. *Neurology.* 1994;44(6 Suppl 4):S17–S23. PMID: 8008222.

SynerMed Communications. 21st century prevention and management of migraine headaches. *Clin Courier.* 2001;19:1–15.

Chapter 4

4.2   Harm Avoidance: The Role of One Inherited Temperament Trait in Chronic Facial Pain

Cloninger, C. R., Svrakic, D. M., & Przybeck, T. R. (1993). A psychobiological model of temperament and character. *Archives of General Psychiatry, 50,* 975–990.

4.3   The Reality We Live With

Bergdahl J, Anneroth G, Perris H. Cognitive therapy in the treatment of patients with resistant burning mouth syndrome: A controlled study. *J Oral Pathol Med.* 1995 May;24(5):213–215. doi: 10.1111/j.1600-0714.1995.tb01169.x.

Blackwell B, Galbraith JR, Dahl DS. Chronic pain management. *Hosp Community Psychiatry.* 1984 Oct;35(10):999–1008. doi: 10.1176/ps.35.10.999.

Dueñas M, Salazar A, de Sola H, Failde I. Limitations in activities of daily living in people with chronic pain: Identification of groups using clusters analysis. *Pain Pract.* 2020;20(2):179–187. doi: 10.1111/papr.12842.

Durham J, Raphael KG, Benoliel R, Ceusters W, Michelotti A, Ohrbach R. Perspectives on next steps in classification of oro-facial pain

– part 2: Role of psychosocial factors. *J Oral Rehabil.* 2015 Dec 42(12):942–955. doi: 10.1111/joor.12329.

Engel GL. The need for a new medical model A challenge for biomedicine. *Science.* 1977 Apr 8;196(4286):129–136. doi: 10.1126/science.847460.

Goldthorpe J, Peters S, Lovell K, McGowan L, Aggarwal V. 'I just wanted someone to tell me it wasn't all in my mind and do something for me': Qualitative exploration of acceptability of a CBT-based intervention to manage chronic orofacial pain. *Br Dent J.* 2016 May 13;220(9):459–463. doi: 10.1038/sj.bdj.2016.332.

Greenberg J, Popok PJ, Lin A, et al. A mind–body physical activity program for chronic pain with or without a digital monitoring device: Proof-of-concept feasibility randomized controlled trial. *JMIR Form Res.* 2020 Jun 8;4(6):e18703. doi: 10.2196/18703.

Litt MD, Shafer DM, Kreutzer DL. Brief cognitive behavioral treatment for TMD pain: Long-term outcomes and moderators of treatment. *Pain.* 2010 Oct;151(1):110–116. doi: 10.1016/j.pain.2010.06.030.

Morales ME, Yong RJ. Racial and ethnic disparities in the treatment of chronic pain. *Pain Med.* 2021 Feb 4;22(1):75–90. doi: 10.1093/pm/pnaa427.

Noma N, Watanabe Y, Shimada A, et al. Effects of cognitive behavioral therapy on orofacial pain conditions. *J Oral Sci.* 2020 Dec 23;63(1):4–7. doi: 10.2334/josnusd.20-0437.

Obermann M, Katsarava Z. Update on trigeminal neuralgia. *Expert Rev Neurother.* 2009 Mar 1;9(3):323–329. doi: 10.1586/14737175.9.3.323.

Penlington C, Ohrbach R. Biopsychosocial assessment and management of persistent orofacial pain. *Oral Surg.* 2020;13(4):349–357. https//doi.org/10.1111/ors.12470.

Peters S, Goldthorpe J, McElroy C, et al. Managing chronic orofacial pain: A qualitative study of patients', doctors', and dentists' experiences. *Br J Health Psychol.* 2015;20(4):777–791. doi: 10.1111/bjhp.12141.

Robinson K, Kennedy N, Harmon D. Is occupational therapy adequately meeting the needs of people with chronic pain?

Am J Occup Ther. 2011 Jan–Feb;65(1):106–113. doi: 10.5014/ajot.2011.09160.

Tan G, Glaros A, Sherman R, Wong C. Integrative approaches to orofacial pain: role of biofeedback and hypnosis. In: Ferreira JNAR, Fricton J, Rhodus N, eds. *Orofacial Disorders: Current Therapies in Orofacial Pain and Oral Medicine.* Cham, Switzerland: Springer; 2017:317–324. doi: 10.1007/978-3-319-51508-3_27.

Zakrzewska JM, Akram H. Neurosurgical interventions for the treatment of classical trigeminal neuralgia. *Cochrane Database Syst Rev* [Internet]. 2011 Sep 7;2011(9):CD007312. doi: 10.1002/14651858. CD007312.pub2. PMID: 21901707; PMCID: PMC8981212.

4.4 Facing It: Mindfulness for Chronic Orofacial Pain—Mindfulness and Mindfulness-Based Interventions

Ball EF, Nur Shafina Muhammad Sharizan E, Franklin G, Rogozińska E. Does mindfulness meditation improve chronic pain? A systematic review. *Curr Opin Obstet Gynecol.* 2017 Dec;29(6):359–366. doi: 10.1097/GCO.0000000000000417.

Bertoli E, de Leeuw R. Prevalence of suicidal ideation, depression, and anxiety in chronic temporomandibular disorder patients. *J Oral Facial Pain Headache.* 2016;30(4):296–301. doi: 10.11607/ofph.1675.

Bishop SR, Lau M, Shapiro S, et al. Mindfulness: A proposed operational definition. *Clin Psychol (New York).* 2004;11(3):230–241. doi: 10.1093/clipsy.bph077.

Burgess EE, Selchen S, Diplock BD, Rector NA. A brief mindfulness-based cognitive therapy (MBCT) intervention as a population-level strategy for anxiety and depression. *Int J Cogn Ther.* 2021;14(2):380–398. doi: 10.1007/s41811-021-00105-x.

Casey M-B, Murphy D, Neary R, Wade C, Hearty C, Doody C. Individuals perspectives related to acceptance, values and mindfulness following participation in an acceptance-based pain management programme. *J Contextual Behav Sci.* 2020 Apr;16:96–102. doi: 10.1016/j.jcbs.2020.03.005.

Cayoun B, Simmons A, Shires A. Immediate and lasting chronic pain reduction following a brief self-implemented mindfulness-based interoceptive exposure task: A pilot study. *Mindfulness*. 2020;11(1):112–124. doi: 10.1007/s12671-017-0823-x.

Chesin M, Interian A, Kline A, Benjamin-Phillips C, Latorre M, Stanley B. Reviewing mindfulness-based interventions for suicidal behavior. *Arch Suicide Res*. 2016 Oct–Dec;20(4):507–527. doi: 10.1080/13811118.2016.1162244.

Chiesa A, Serretti A. Mindfulness-based interventions for chronic pain: A systematic review of the evidence. *J Altern Complement Med*. 2011 Jan;17(1):83–93. doi: 10.1089/acm.2009.0546.

Creswell JD, Irwin MR, Burklund LJ, et al. Mindfulness-Based Stress Reduction training reduces loneliness and pro-inflammatory gene expression in older adults: A small randomized controlled trial. *Brain Behav Immun*. 2012 Oct;26(7):1095–1101. doi: 10.1016/j.bbi.2012.07.006.

Dash S, Bourke M, Parker AG, Trott E, Pascoe MC. Mindfulness is associated with reduced barriers to exercise via decreasing psychological distress in help-seeking young adults: A cross-sectional brief report. *Early Interv Psychiatry*. 2022 Sep;16(9):1049–1054. doi: 10.1111/eip.13249.

de Souza ICW, de Barros VV, Gomide HP, et al. Mindfulness-based interventions for the treatment of smoking: A systematic literature review. *J Altern Complement Med*. 2015 Mar;21(3):129–140. doi: 10.1089/acm.2013.0471.

Dibello V, Panza F, Mori G, et al. Temporomandibular disorders as a risk factor for suicidal behavior: A systematic review. *J Pers Med*. 2022 Oct 28;12(11):1782. doi: 10.3390/jpm12111782.

Dreisoerner A, Junker NM, van Dick R. The relationship among the components of self-compassion: A pilot study using a compassionate writing intervention to enhance self-kindness, common humanity, and mindfulness. *J Happiness Stud*. 2021;22(1):21–47. doi: 10.1007/s10902-019-00217-4.

Dunn BD, Wiedemann H, Kock M, et al. Increases in external sensory observing cross-sectionally mediate the repair of positive affect following mindfulness-based cognitive therapy in individuals with residual depression symptoms. *Mindfulness.* 2023;14(1):113–127. doi: 10.1007/s12671-022-02032-0.

Frostadottir AD, Dorjee D. Effects of mindfulness based cognitive therapy (MBCT) and compassion focused therapy (CFT) on symptom change, mindfulness, self-compassion, and rumination in clients with depression, anxiety, and stress. *Front Psychol.* 2019 May 17;10:1099. doi: 10.3389/fpsyg.2019.01099.

Ghahari S, Mohammadi-Hasel K, Malakouti SK, Roshanpajouh M. Mindfulness-based cognitive therapy for generalised anxiety disorder: A systematic review and meta-analysis. *East Asian Arch Psychiatry.* 2020 Jun;30(2):52–56. doi: 10.12809/eaap1885.

Greenberg J, Bakhshaie J, Lovette BC, Vranceanu A-M. Association between coping strategies and pain-related outcomes among individuals with chronic orofacial pain. *J Pain Res.* 2022 Feb 11;15:431–442. doi: 10.2147/JPR.S350024.

Greenberg J, Reiner K, Meiran N. "Mind the trap": Mindfulness practice reduces cognitive rigidity. *PLoS One.* 2012;7(5):e36206. doi: 10.1371/journal.pone.0036206.

Greenberg J, Spyropoulos DC, Bakhshaie J, Vranceanu A-M. Mindfulness facets associated with orofacial pain outcomes. *J Integr Complement Med.* 2022;28(10):839-844. doi: 10.1089/jicm.2022.0479.

Grossman P, Van Dam NT. Mindfulness, by any other name…: Trials and tribulations of *sati* in western psychology and science. *Contemp Buddhism.* 2011;12(1):219–239. doi: 10.1080/14639947.2011.564841.

Hanley AW, Dehili V, Krzanowski D, Barou D, Lecy N, Garland EL. Effects of video-guided group vs. solitary meditation on mindfulness and social connectivity: A pilot study. *Clin Soc Work J.* 2022;50(3):316–324. doi: 10.1007/s10615-021-00812-0.

Hayes SC, Strosahl KD, Wilson KG. *Acceptance and Commitment Therapy: The Process and Practice of Mindful Change,* 2nd ed. New York: Guilford Press; 2012.

Hilton L, Hempel S, Ewing BA, et al. Mindfulness meditation for chronic pain Systematic review and meta-analysis. *Ann Behav Med.* 2017 Apr;51(2):199–213. doi: 10.1007/s12160-u016-9844-2.

Hölzel BK, Lazar SW, Gard T, Schuman-Olivier Z, Vago DR, Ott U. How does mindfulness meditation work? Proposing mechanisms of action from a conceptual and neural perspective. *Perspect Psychol Sci.* 2011 Nov;6(6):537–559. doi: 10.1177/1745691611419671.

Howarth A, Riaz M, Perkins-Porras L, et al. Pilot randomized controlled trial of a brief mindfulness-based intervention for those with persistent pain. *J Behav Med.* 2019 Dec;42(6):999–1014. doi: 10.1007/s10865-019-00040-5.

Kabat-Zinn J. *Full Catastrophe Living: Using the Wisdom of Your Body and Mind to Face Stress, Pain, and Illness,* 15th Anniversary ed. New York: Delta Trade Paperback/Bantam Dell; 2005.

Kabat-Zinn J. Mindfulness-based interventions in context: Past, present, and future. *Clin Psychol (New York).* 2003;10(2):144–156. doi: 10.1093/clipsy.bpg016.

Kabat-Zinn J. *Wherever You Go, There You Are: Mindfulness Meditation in Everyday Life.* New York: Hachette Books; 1994.

Kabat-Zinn J, Lipworth L, Burney R. The clinical use of mindfulness meditation for the self-regulation of chronic pain. *J Behav Med.* 1985 Jun;8(2):163–190. doi: 10.1007/BF00845519.

Lin T-H, Tam K-W, Yang Y-L, Liou T-H, Hsu T-H, Rau C-L. Meditation-based therapy for chronic low back pain management: A systematic review and meta-analysis of randomized controlled trials. *Pain Med.* 2022 Sep;23(10):1800–1811. doi: 10.1093/pm/pnac037.

Linehan MM. Dialectical behavioral therapy: A cognitive behavioral approach to parasuicide. *J Pers Disord.* 1987;1(4):328–333. doi: 10.1521/pedi.1987.1.4.328.

Long R, Halvorson M, Lengua LJ. A mindfulness-based promotive coping program improves well-being in college undergraduates. *Anxiety Stress Coping.* 2021 Nov;34(6):690–703. doi: 10.1080/10615806.2021.1895986.

Lovette BC, Bannon SM, Spyropoulos DC, Vranceanu A-M, Greenberg J. "I still suffer every second of every day": A qualitative analysis of the challenges of living with chronic orofacial pain. *J Pain Res.* 2022 Jul 29;15:2139–2148. doi: 10.2147/JPR.S372469.

Meadows GN, Shawyer F, Enticott JC, et al. Mindfulness-based cognitive therapy for recurrent depression: A translational research study with 2-year follow-up. *Aust N Z J Psychiatry.* 2014 Aug;48(8):743–755. doi: 10.1177/0004867414525841.

Nila K, Holt DV, Ditzen B, Aguilar-Raab C. Mindfulness-based stress reduction (MBSR) enhances distress tolerance and resilience through changes in mindfulness. *Ment Health Prev.* 2016 Mar;4(1):36–41. doi: 10.1016/j.mhp.2016.01.001.

Okvat HA, Davis MC, Mistretta EG, Mardian AS. Mindfulness-based training for women veterans with chronic pain: A retrospective study. *Psychol Serv.* 2022;19(Suppl 1):106–119. doi: 10.1037/ser0000599.

Poulin PA, Romanow HC, Rahbari, et al. N The relationship between mindfulness, pain intensity, pain catastrophizing, depression, and quality of life among cancer survivors living with chronic neuropathic pain. *Support Care Cancer.* 2016 Oct;24(10):4167–4175. doi: 10.1007/s00520-016-3243-x.

Reynolds A, Hamidian Jahromi A. Improving postoperative care through mindfulness-based and isometric exercise training interventions. Systematic review. *JMIR Perioper Med.* 2022 Jun 10;5(1):e34651. doi: 10.2196/34651.

Rezaei S, Hassanzadeh S. Are mindfulness skills associated with reducing kinesiophobia, pain severity, pain catastrophizing and physical disability? Results of Iranian patients with chronic musculoskeletal pain. *Health Psychol Rep.* 2019;7(4):1–10. doi: 10.5114/hpr.2019.84747.

Robin N, Toussaint L, Sinnapah S, Hue O, Coudevylle GR. Beneficial influence of mindfulness training promoted by text messages on self-reported aerobic physical activity in older adults: A randomized controlled study. *J Aging Phys Act.* 2019 Nov 21;28(3):406–414. doi: 10.1123/japa.2019-0002.

Segal ZV, Williams JMG, Teasdale JD. *Mindfulness-Based Cognitive Therapy for Depression: A New Approach to Preventing Relapse.* New York: Guilford Press; 2002.

Shankland R, Tessier D, Strub L, Gauchet A, Baeyens C. Improving mental health and well-being through informal mindfulness practices: An intervention study. *Appl Psychol Health Well Being.* 2021 Feb;.13(1):63–83. doi: 10.1111/aphw.12216.

Shapero BG, Greenberg J, Pedrelli P, de Jong M, Desbordes G. Mindfulness-based interventions in psychiatry. *Focus (Am Psychiatr Publ).* 2018 Winter;16(1):32–39. doi: 10.1176/appi.focus.20170039.

Shapiro SL. The integration of mindfulness and psychology. *J Clin Psychol.* 2009 Jun;65(6):555–560. doi: 10.1002/jclp.20602.

Strohmaier S, Jones FW, Cane JE. One-session mindfulness of the breath meditation practice: A randomized controlled study of the effects on state hope and state gratitude in the general population. *Mindfulness.* 2022;13(1):162–173. doi: 10.1007/s12671-021-01780-9.

Thertus K. The psychological impact and management of trigeminal neuralgia. In: Abd-Elsayed A, ed. *Trigeminal Nerve Pain: A Guide to Clinical Management.* Cham, Switzerland: Springer International Publishing; 2021:215–227. doi: 10.1007/978-3-030-60687-9_21.

Tickell A, Ball S, Bernard P, et al. The effectiveness of mindfulness-based cognitive therapy (MBCT) in real-world healthcare services. *Mindfulness (N Y).* 2020;11(2):279–290. doi: 10.1007/s12671-018-1087-9.

Turner JA, Anderson ML, Balderson BH, Cook AJ, Sherman KJ, Cherkin DC. Mindfulness-based stress reduction and cognitive behavioral therapy for chronic low back pain: Similar effects on mindfulness, catastrophizing, self-efficacy, and acceptance in a randomized controlled trial. *Pain.* 2016 Nov;157(11):2434–2444. doi: 10.1097/j.pain.0000000000000635.

Veehof MM, Trompetter HR, Bohlmeijer ET, Schreurs KMG. Acceptance- and mindfulness-based interventions for the treatment of chronic pain: A meta-analytic review. *Cogn Behav Ther.* 2016;45(1):5–31. doi: 10.1080/16506073.2015.1098724.

Williams K, Hartley S, Anderson IM, et al. An ongoing process of reconnection: A qualitative exploration of mindfulness-based cognitive therapy for adults in remission from depression. *Psychol Psychother*. 2022 Mar;95(1):173–190. doi: 10.1111/papt.12357.

Williams JMG, Duggan DS, Crane C, Fennell MJV. Mindfulness-based cognitive therapy for prevention of recurrence of suicidal behavior. *J Clin Psychol*. 2006 Feb;62(2):201–210. doi: 10.1002/jclp.20223.

Zhang N, Fan F-M, Huang S-Y, Rodriguez MA. Mindfulness training for loneliness among Chinese college students: A pilot randomized controlled trial. *Int J Psychol*. 2018 oct;53(5):373–378. doi: 10.1002/ijop.12394.

4.6   *Empowered Relief®: An Evidence-Based One-Session Pain Relief Skills Intervention*

Banerjee A, Mackey SC, Vest N, Darnall BD. Pain in US corrections settings: The promise of digital solutions for better data and treatment access. *Pain Med*. 2024 Mar 1;25(3):165–168. doi: 10.1093/pm/pnad150.

Burns JW, Glenn B, Bruehl S, Harden RN, Lofland K. Cognitive factors influence outcome following multidisciplinary chronic pain treatment: A replication and extension of a cross-lagged panel analysis. *Behav Res Ther*. 2003 Oct;41(10):1163–1182. doi: 10.1016/s0005-7967(03)00029-9.

Cherkin DC, Sherman KJ, Balderson BH, et al. Effect of mindfulness-based stress reduction vs cognitive behavioral therapy or usual care on back pain and functional limitations in adults with chronic low back pain: A randomized clinical trial. JAMA. 2016 Mar;315(12):1240–1249. doi: 10.1001/jama.2016.2323.

Dahlhamer J, Lucas J, Zelaya C, et al. Prevalence of chronic pain and high-impact chronic pain among adults – United States, 2016. *MMWR Morb Mortal Wkly Rep*. 2018 Sep 14;67(36):1001–1006. doi: 10.15585/mmwr.mm6736a2.

Darnall BD, Burns JW, Hong J, et al. Empowered Relief, cognitive behavioral therapy and health education for people with chronic pain: A comparison of outcomes at 6-month follow-up for a randomized controlled trial. *Pain Rep.* 2024 Jan; 9(1): e1116. doi: 10.1097/PR9.0000000000001116.

Darnall BD, Roy A, Chen AL, et al. Comparison of a single-session pain management skills intervention with a single-session health education intervention and 8 sessions of cognitive behavioral therapy in adults with chronic low back pain: A randomized clinical trial. JAMA Netw Open. 2021 Aug 2;4(8):e2113401. doi: 10.1001/jamanetworkopen.2021.13401.

Darnall BD, Scheman J, Davin S, et al. Pain psychology: A global needs assessment and national call to action. *Pain Med.* 2016 Feb;17(2):250–63. doi: 10.1093/pm/pnv095.

Darnall BD, Ziadni MS, Krishnamurthy P, et al. "My surgical success": *Effect of a digital behavioral pain medicine intervention on time to opioid cessation after breast cancer surgery-A pilot randomized controlled clinical trial. Pain Med.* 2019 Nov 1; 20(11):2228–2237. doi: 10.1093/pm/pnz094.

Davin S, Savage J, Schuster A, Darnall BD. Transforming standard of care for spine surgery. Integration of an online single-session behavioral pain management class for perioperative optimization. *Front Pain Res (Lausanne).* 2022 May 2;3:856252.;doi: 10.3389/fpain.2022.856252.

Foster NE, Anema JR, Cherkin D, et al, Lancet Low Back Pain Series Working Group. Prevention and treatment of low back pain: Evidence, challenges, and promising directions. Lancet. 2018 Jun 9;391(10137):2368–2383. doi: 10.1016/S0140-6736(18)30489-6.

Freburger JK, Holmes GM, Agans RP, et al. The rising prevalence of chronic low back pain. *Arch Intern Med.* 2009 Feb 9;169(3):251–258. doi: 10.1001/archinternmed.2008.543.

Institute of Medicine Committee on Advancing Pain Research, Care, and Education. *Relieving Pain in America: A Blueprint for Transforming Prevention, Care, Education, and Research.* Washington, DC: National Academies Press; 2011. doi: 10.17226/13172.

Interagency Pain Research Coordinating Committee. *National Pain Strategy: A Comprehensive Population Health-Level Strategy for*

Pain. Washington, DC: National Institutes of Health, US Department of Health and Human Services; 2016.

Lanoye A, Stewart KE, Rybarczyk BD, et al. The impact of integrated psychological services in a safety net primary care clinic on medical utilization. *J Clin Psychol.* 2017 Jun;73(6):681–692. doi: 10.1002/jclp.22367.

Maixner W, Fillingim RB, Williams DA, Smith SB, Slade GD. Overlapping chronic pain conditions: Implications for diagnosis and classification. *J Pain.* Sep 2016;17(9 Suppl):T93–T107. doi: 10.1016/j.jpain.2016.06.002.

Pain Management Best Practices Inter-Agency Task Force Report: Updates, Gaps, Inconsistencies, and Recommendations. Washington, DC: US Department of Health and Human Services; May 2019.

Patient-Centered Outcomes Research Institute (PCORI). Comparing Two Online Programs for Treating Chronic Pain—The PROGRESS Study web page. https//www.pcori.org/research-results/2021/comparing-two-online-programs-treating-chronic-pain-progress-study.

Schrepf A, Phan V, Clemens JQ, Maixner W, Hanauer D, Williams DA. ICD-10 codes for the study of chronic overlapping pain conditions in administrative databases. *J Pain.* 2020 Jan–Feb;21(1–2):59–70. doi: 10.1016/j.jpain.2019.05.007.

Task Force on Taxonomy. *Classification of Chronic Pain: Descriptions of Chronic Pain Syndromes and Definitions of Pain Terms.* 2nd ed. Washington, DC: IASP Press; 1994.

Turner JA, Anderson ML, Balderson BH, Cook AJ, Sherman KJ, Cherkin DC. Mindfulness-based stress reduction and cognitive behavioral therapy for chronic low back pain: Similar effects on mindfulness, catastrophizing, self-efficacy, and acceptance in a randomized controlled trial. *Pain.* 2016 Nov;157(11):2434–2444. doi: 10.1097/j.pain.0000000000000635.

Williams AC, Eccleston C, Morley S. Psychological therapies for the management of chronic pain (excludingheadache) in adults. *Cochrane Database Syst Rev.* 2012 Nov 14;11(11):CD007407. doi: 10.1002/14651858.CD007407.pub3.

Williams ACC, Fisher E, Hearn L, Eccleston C. Psychological therapies for the management of chronic pain (excluding headache) in adults. *Cochrane Database Syst Rev.* 2020 Aug 12;8(8):CD007407. doi: 10.1002/14651858.CD007407.pub4.

Ziadni MS, Gonzalez-Castro L, Anderson S, Krishnamurthy P, Darnall BD. Efficacy of a single-session "Empowered Relief" Zoom-delivered group intervention for chronic pain: Randomized controlled trial conducted during the COVID-19 pandemic. *J Med Internet Res.* 2021 Sep 10;23(9):e29672. doi: 10.2196/29672.

Ziadni MS, You DS, Keanne RT, et al. "My surgical success": Feasibility and impact of a single-session digital behavioral pain medicine intervention on pain intensity, pain catastrophizing, and time to opioid cessation after orthopedic trauma surgery—A randomized trial. *Anesth Analg.* 2022 Aug; 135(2): 394–405. doi: 10.1213/ANE.0000000000006088.

4.7 Virtual Reality for Orofacial Pain: Unlocking Its Potential in Pain Management

Althumairi A, Sahwan M, Alsaleh S, Alabduljobar Z, Aljabri D. Virtual reality: Is it helping children cope with fear and pain during vaccination? *J Multidiscip Healthc.* 2021;14:2625–2632. doi: 10.2147/JMDH.S327349.

Colloca L, Raghuraman N, Wang Y, et al. Virtual reality: Physiological and behavioral mechanisms to increase individual pain tolerance limits. *Pain.* 2020 Sep 1;161(9):2010–2021. doi: 10.1097/j.pain.0000000000001900.

Darnall BD, Krishnamurthy P, Tsuei J, Minor JD. Self-administered skills-based virtual reality intervention for chronic pain: Randomized controlled pilot study. *JMIR Form Res.* 2020 Jul;4(7):e17293. doi: 10.2196/17293.

Eccleston C, Fisher E, Liikkanen S, et al. A prospective, double-blind, pilot, randomized, controlled trial of an "embodied" virtual reality intervention for adults with low back pain. *Pain.* 2022 Sep 1;163(9):1700–1715. doi: 10.1097/j.pain.0000000000002617.

Garcia LM, Birckhead BJ, Krishnamurthy P, et al. An 8-week self-administered at-home behavioral skills-based virtual reality program for chronic low back pain: Double-blind, randomized, placebo-controlled trial conducted during COVID-19. *J Med Internet Res.* 2021 Feb 22;23(2):e26292. doi: 10.2196/26292.

Garcia LM, Birckhead BJ, Krishnamurthy P, et al. Three-month follow-up results of a double-blind, randomized placebo-controlled trial of 8-week self-administered at-home behavioral skills-based virtual reality (VR) for chronic low back pain. *J Pain.* 2022 May;23(5):822–840. doi: 10.1016/j.jpain.2021.12.002.

Garcia LM, Darnall BD, Krishnamurthy P, et al. Self-administered behavioral skills-based at-home virtual reality therapy for chronic low back pain: Protocol for a randomized controlled trial. *JMIR Res Protoc.* 2021 Jan 19;10(1):e25291. doi: 10.2196/25291.

Hoffman HG, Chambers GT, Meyer WJ III, et al. Virtual reality as an adjunctive non-pharmacologic analgesic for acute burn pain during medical procedures. *Ann Behav Med.* 2011 Apr;41(2):183–191. doi: 10.1007/s12160-010-9248-7.

Honzel E, Murthi S, Brawn-Cinani B, et al. Virtual reality, music, and pain: Developing the premise for an interdisciplinary approach to pain management. *Pain.* 2019 Sep;160(9):1909–1919. doi: 10.1097/j.pain.0000000000001539.

Huang T-K, Yang C-H, Hsieh Y-H, Wang J-C, Hung C-C. Augmented reality (AR) and virtual reality (VR) applied in dentistry. *Kaohsiung J Med Sci.* 2018 Apr;34(4):243–248. doi: 10.1016/j.kjms.2018.01.009.

Joda T, Gallucci G, Wismeijer D, Zitzmann N. Augmented and virtual reality in dental medicine: A systematic review. *Comput Biol Med.* 2019 May;108:93–100. doi: 10.1016/j.compbiomed.2019.03.012.

Jones T, Moore T, Choo J. The impact of virtual reality on chronic pain. *PLoS One.* 2016;11(12):e0167523. doi: 10.1371/journal.pone.0167523.

Keefe FJ, Huling DA, Coggins MJ, et al. Virtual reality for persistent pain: A new direction for behavioral pain management. *Pain.* 2012 Nov;153(11):2163–2166. doi: 10.1016/j.pain.2012.05.030.

Maddox T, Chmielewski C, Fitzpatrick T. Virtual reality in chronic kidney disease education and training. *Nephrol Nurs J.* 2022 Jul–Aug;49(4):329–381. PMID: 36054805.

Maddox T, Garcia H, Ffrench K, Maddox R, Garcia L, Krishnamurthy P, Okhotin D, Sparks C, Oldstone L, Birckhead B, Sackman J, Mackey I, Louis R, Salmasi V, Oyao A, Darnall BD. In-home virtual reality program for chronic low back pain: durability of a randomized, placebo-controlled clinical trial to 18 months post-treatment. *Reg Anesth Pain Med.* 2022 Nov 25:rapm-2022-104093. doi: 10.1136/rapm-2022-104093. Epub ahead of print. PMID: 36427904.

Maddox T, Sparks C, Oldstone L, et al. Durable chronic low back pain reductions to 24-months post-treatment for an accessible, 8-week, in-home behavioral skills-based virtual reality program: Aq randomized controlled trial. *Pain Med.* 2023 Oct 3;24(10):1200–1203. doi: 10.1093/pm/pnad070.

Morris NA, Wang Y, Felix RB, et al. Adjunctive virtual reality pain relief after traumatic injury: A proof-of-concept within-person randomized trial. *Pain.* 2023 Sep 1;164(9):2122–2129. doi: 10.1097/j.pain.0000000000002914.

National Academies of Sciences, Engineering, and Medicine; Health and Medicine Division; Board on Health Care Services; Board on Health Sciences Policy; Committee on Temporomandibular Disorders (TMDs): From Research Discoveries to Clinical Treatment. *Temporomandibular Disorders: Priorities for Research and Care.* Yost O, Liverman CT, English R, Mackey S, Bond EC, eds. Washington, DC: National Academies Press; 2020 Mar 12. PMID: 32200600.

Real FJ, DeBlasio D, Beck AF, et al. A virtual reality curriculum for pediatric residents decreases rates of influenza vaccine refusal. *Acad Pediatr.* 2017 May–Jun;17(4):431–435. doi: 10.1016/j.acap.2017.01.010.

Scapin S, Echevarría-Guanilo ME, Boeira Fuculo Junior PR, Gonçalves N, Rocha PK, Coimbra R. Virtual Reality in the treatment of burn patients: A systematic review. *Burns.* 2018 Sep;44(6):1403–1416. doi: 10.1016/j.burns.2017.11.002.

Smith V, Warty RR, Sursas JA, et al. The effectiveness of virtual reality in managing acute pain and anxiety for medical inpatients: Systematic review. *J Med Internet Res.* 2020 Nov 2;22(11):e17980. doi: 10.2196/17980.

Spiegel B, Fuller G, Lopez M, et al. Virtual reality for management of pain in hospitalized patients: A randomized comparative effectiveness trial. *PLoS One.* 2019 Aug 14;14(8):e0219115. doi: 10.1371/journal.pone.0219115.

Sullivan C, Schneider PE, Musselman RJ, Dummett C Jr, Gardiner D. The effect of virtual reality during dental treatment on child anxiety and behavior. *ASDC J Dent Child.* 2000 May–Jun;67(3):193–196, 160–161. PMID: 10902078.

Trost Z, France C, Anam M, Shum C. Virtual reality approaches to pain: Toward a state of the science. *Pain.* 2021 Feb 1;162(2):325–331. doi: 10.1097/j.pain.0000000000002060.

Vandeweerdt C, Luong T, Atchapero M, et al. Virtual reality reduces COVID-19 vaccine hesitancy in the wild: A randomized trial. *Sci Rep.* 2022 Mar 17;12(1):4593. doi: 10.1038/s41598-022-08120-4.

Wang Y, Massalee R, Beebe K, et al. A glimpse of the multiple applications of virtual reality: Analgesia, embodiment and rehabilitation, interactive education and communication. In: Colloca L, Noel J, Franklin PD, Seneviratne C, eds. *Placebo Effects Through the Lens of Translational Research.* New York: Oxford University Press; 2023. https://doi.org/10.1093/med/9780197645444.003.0026.

Chapter 5

5.1   Pain and Sleep

Beninati W, Harris CD, Herold DL, Shepard JW Jr. The effect of snoring and obstructive sleep apnea on the sleep quality of bed partners. *Mayo Clin Proc.* 1999 Oct;74(10):955–958. doi: 10.4065/74.10.955.

Cremaschi RC, Hirotsu C, Tufik S, Coelho FM. Chronic pain in narcolepsy type 1 and type 2 – An underestimated reality. *J Sleep Res.* 2019 Jun;28(3):e12715. doi: 10.1111/jsr.12715.

Cruz MME, Sousa B, De Laat A. Sleep and orofacial pain: Physiological interactions and clinical management. In: Rossi FH, Tsakadze H, eds. *Updates in Sleep Neurology and Obstructive Sleep Apnea*. London: IntechOpen; 19 July 2019. doi: 10.5772/intechopen.86770.

Devor M, Wood I, Sharav Y, Zakrzewska JM. Trigeminal neuralgia during sleep. *Pain Pract*. 2008 Jul–Aug;8(4):263–268. doi: 10.1111/j.1533-2500.2008.00214.x.

Frost & Sullivan. *Hidden Health Crisis Costing America Billions: Underdiagnosing and Undertreating Obstructive Sleep Apnea Draining Healthcare System*. Darien, IL: American Academy of Sleep Medicine; 2016.

Frost & Sullivan. *In an Age of Constant Activity, the Solution to Improving the Nation's Health May Lie in Helping it Sleep Better: What Benefits Do Patients Experience in Treating their Obstructive Sleep Apnea?* Darien, IL: American Academy of Sleep Medicine; 2016.

Guilleminault C, Eldridge FL, Dement WC. Insomnia with sleep apnea: A new syndrome. *Science*. 1973 Aug 31;181(4102):856–858. doi: 10.1126/science.181.4102.856.

Haack M, Simpson N, Sethna N, et al. Sleep deficiency and chronic pain: Potential underlying mechanisms and clinical implications. *Neuropsychopharmacology*. 2020 Jan;45(1):205–216. doi: 10.1038/s41386-019-0439-z.

Herschkowitz M, Whiton K, Albert SM, et al. National Sleep Foundation's sleep time duration recommendations: Methodology and results summary. *Sleep Health*. 2015 Mar;1(1):40-43. doi: 10.1016/j.sleh.2014.12.010.

Lavigne GJ, Sessle BJ. The neurobiology of orofacial pain and sleep and their interactions. *J Dent Res*. 2016 Sep;95(10):1109–1116. doi: 10.1177/0022034516648264.

Roehrs T, Hyde M, Blaisdell B, Greenwald M, Roth T. Sleep loss and REM sleep loss are hyperalgesic. *Sleep*. 2006 Feb;29(2):145–151. doi: 10.1093/sleep/29.2.145.

Šedý J, Rocabato M, Olate LE, Vina M, Žižka R. Neural basis of etiopathologies and treatment of cervicogenic orofacial pain. *Medicina (Kaunas)*. 2022 Sep 21;58(10):1324. doi: 10.3390/medicina58101324.

Sweetman A. Co-morbid insomnia and sleep apnoea (COMISA): Latest research from an emerging field. *Curr Sleep Med Rep.* 2023;9:180–189. https//doi.org/10.1007/s40675-023-00262-9.

Tang NKY, Goodchild CE, Sanborn AN, Howard J, Salkovskis PM. Deciphering the temporal link between pain and sleep in a heterogeneous chronic pain patient sample: A multilevel daily process study. *Sleep.* 2012 May 1;35(5):675–687. doi: 10.5665/sleep.1830.

Travell JG, Simons DG. Myofascial Pain and Dysfunction: The Trigger Point Manual. *Vol 1: The Upper Extremities.* Baltimore, MD: Williams & Wilkins; 1983.

Watson NF, Badr MS, Belenky G, et al. Recommended amount of sleep for a healthy adult: A joint consensus statement of the American Academy of Sleep Medicine and Sleep Research Society. *Sleep.* 2015 Jun 1;38(6):843–844. doi: 10.5665/sleep.4716.

Chapter 6

6.1 Our Stories

Allam AK, Sharma H, Larkin MB, Viswanathan A. Trigeminal Neuralgia. *Neurol Clin.* 2023 Feb;41(1):107–121. https//doi.org/10.1016/j.ncl.2022.09.001. Accessed Mar 30, 2023.

Boadway J. *Life with Trigeminal Neuralgia – Cathryn's Story. YouTube.* Oct 6, 2021. Accessed Aug 15, 2023. https//www.youtube.com/watch?v=bFVBR16jzrl.

Browne SJ. How to Combat the Stigma of Invisible Disabilities, by Sarah Jeanne Browne. *RAISE Center blog.* Feb 16, 2022. https//raisecenter.blog/2022/02/16/how-to-combat-the-stigma-of-invisible-disabilities-by-sarah-jeanne-browne/. Accessed Aug 15, 2023.

Facial Pain from Trigeminal Neuralgia. Nash Disability Law. https//www.nashdisabilitylaw.com/qualifying-impairments/facial-pain-trigeminal-neuralgia-and-disability-benefits/. Accessed Aug 15, 2023.

Facial Pain Research Foundation. *Billy Shipp- A Trigeminal Neuralgia Story*. YouTube. Jul 22, 2020. https//www.youtube.com/watch?v=4E-sRFWtH_g. Accessed Aug 15, 2023.

Facial Pain Research Foundation. *Cori Murdoch- A Trigeminal Neuralgia Story*. YouTube. Apr 29, 2019. https//www.youtube.com/watch?v=rkPrFDNIYg4. Accessed Aug 15, 2023.

Facial Pain Research Foundation. *Kristin McQueen- A Trigeminal Neuralgia Story*. YouTube. Jul 22, 2020. www.youtube.com/watch?v=nfTQZMXJYRY. Accessed Aug 15, 2023.

Facial Pain Research Foundation. *Nicole Ferguson- A Trigeminal Neuralgia Story*. YouTube. Oct 27, 2022. www.youtube.com/watch?v=wAU5IGdGa3I. Accessed Aug 15, 2023.

Facial Pain Research Foundation. *Trigeminal Neuralgia Patients Describe Life with TN*. YouTube. Apr 23, 2017. www.youtube.com/watch?v=8F8yfIGHTTk. Accessed Aug 15, 2023.

Hendry G, Wilson C, Orr M, Scullion R. 'I just stay in the house so I don't need to explain: A qualitative investigation of persons with invisible disabilities. *Disabilities*. 2022 Mar;2(1):145–163. https//doi.org/10.3390/disabilities2010012.

Institute of Medicine (US) Committee on Pain, Disability, and Chronic Illness Behavior. Conflicts and contradictions in the disability program. In: Osterweis M, Kleinman A, Mechanic D, eds. *Pain and Disability: Clinical, Behavioral, and Public Policy Perspectives*. Washington, DC: National Academies Press; 1987:chap 4. www.ncbi.nlm.nih.gov/books/NBK219259/. Accessed April 16, 2024.

Institute of Medicine (US) Committee on Pain, Disability, and Chronic Illness Behavior. The sociopolitical background of the pain issue. In: Osterweis M, Kleinman A, Mechanic D, eds. *Pain and Disability: Clinical, Behavioral, and Public Policy Perspectives*. Washington, DC: National Academies Press; 1987:chap 2. https://www.ncbi.nlm.nih.gov/books/NBK219240/. Accessed Aug 15, 2023.

Khan S. When Chronic Pain Makes It Difficult to Talk to People. *The Mighty*. Dec 16, 2022. https//themighty.com/topic/chronic-illness/being-unable-to-talk-with-people-because-of-chronic-pain/. Accessed Aug 15, 2023.

Kiz. What I Have Learned and Gained from Living with Trigeminal Neuralgia since 2015. *The Pain Corner blog.* Feb 21, 2018. https// thepaincorner.com/2018/02/21/from-trigeminal-neuralgia-with-love-what-i-have-gained-from-living-with-chronic-pain/. Accessed Aug 15, 2023.

Kiz. What to Expect When… You Don't Meet Any of the Criteria to Get PIP for Trigeminal Neuralgia: Stage Three, Tribunal. The Pain Corner blog. Jul 24 , 2023. https//thepaincorner.com/2023/07/24/ pip-tribunal/. Accessed Aug 15, 2023.

Lawrence JD, Frederickson AM, Chang Y-F, Weiss PM, Gerszten PC, Sekula RF. An investigation into quality-of-life improvement in patients undergoing microvascular decompression for hemifacial spasm. *J Neurosurg.* 2018 Jan;128(1):193–201. https//doi. org/10.3171/2016.9.jns161022. Accessed Apr 21, 2020.

Levy C. My Trigeminal Neuralgia Story. *YouTube.* Sep 7 , 2013. www.youtube.com/watch?v=zyd1YNDXgtg. Accessed Aug 15, 2023.

Maarbjerg S, Di Stefano G, Bendtsen L, Cruccu G. Trigeminal neuralgia – Diagnosis and treatment. *Cephalalgia.* 2017 Jun;37(7):648–657. https//doi.org/10.1177/0333102416687280. Accessed Dec 30, 2019.

Mafakheri M, Salehi A, Mansori K, Akbarian M, Danesh Sh, Habibi Askarabad M. Standardization and evaluation of psychometric properties of the self-perceived burden questionnaire in patients with chronic pain. *Qom Univ Med Sci J.* 2021 Jul;15(4):252–263. https//doi.org/10.32598/qums.15.4.252. Accessed Mar 11, 2022.

McPherson CJ, Wilson KG, Murray MA. Feeling like a burden: Exploring the perspectives of patients at the end of life. *Soc Sci Med.* 2007 Jan;64(2)417–427. https://doi.org/10.1016/j. socscimed.2006.09.013. Accessed Feb 24, 2021.

Morgan P. Invisible disabilities: Break down the barriers. *Forbes.* Mar 20, 2020. www.forbes.com/sites/paulamorgan/2020/03/20/ invisible-disabilities-break-down-the-barriers/?sh=45660ac4fa50. Accessed Aug 15, 2023.

MVD for Trigeminal Neuralgia, Kayla's Story. Mayfield Brain & Spine Clinic. https//mayfieldclinic.com/mc_hope/story_kayla.htm. Accessed Aug 15, 2023.

Pilitsis JG, Khazen O. Trigeminal Neuralgia – Causes, Symptoms and Treatments. *American Association of Neurological Surgeons.* 2019. https//www.aans.org/Patients/Neurosurgical-Conditions-and-Treatments/Trigeminal-Neuralgia. Accessed August 15, 2023.

Social Security Administration. Benefits Planner | Social Security Credits and Benefit Eligibility | SSA. *Number of Credits Needed for Disability Benefits.* https//www.ssa.gov/benefits/retirement/planner/credits.html#h3. Accessed Aug 15, 2023.

Social Security Administration. Disability Determination Process. https//www.ssa.gov/disability/determination.htm. Accessed Aug 15, 2023.

Social Security Administration. Disability Evaluation Under Social Security. *11.00 Neurological - Adult. 11.01 Category of Impairments, Neurological Disorders* https//www.ssa.gov/disability/professionals/bluebook/11.00-Neurological-Adult.htm#11_01. Accessed Aug 15, 2023.

Social Security Administration. How You Qualify | Disability Benefits | SSA. How We Decide If You Have a Qualifying Disability. https//www.ssa.gov/benefits/disability/qualify.html#anchor3. Accessed Aug 15, 2023.

Trigeminal Neuralgia. National Institute of Neurological Disorders and Stroke. https//www.ninds.nih.gov/health-information/disorders/trigeminal-neuralgia. Accessed Mar 13, 2023.

Chapter 7

7.2   *Basimglurant: A Drug Trial for Trigeminal Neuralgia*

Headache Classification Committee of the International Headache Society (IHS) The International Classification of Headache Disorders, 3rd edition. *Cephalalgia.* 2018 Jan;38(1):1-211. doi: 10.1177/0333102417738202. PMID: 29368949.

7.4   A Potential Therapeutic Target for Trigeminal Neuralgia

Vasavda C, Xu R, Liew J, et al. Identification of the NRF2 transcriptional network as a therapeutic target for trigeminal neuropathic pain. *Sci Adv.* 2022 Aug 5;8(31):eabo5633. doi: 10.1126/sciadv.abo5633.

7.5   Familial Trigeminal Neuralgia

Bendtsen L, Zakrzewska JM, Abbott J, et al. European Academy of Neurology guideline on trigeminal neuralgia. *Eur J Neurol.* 2019 Jun;26(6):831–849. doi: 10.1111/ene.13950.

Cervera-Martinez C, Martinez-Manrique JJ, Revuelta-Gutierrez R. Surgical management of familial trigeminal neuralgia with different inheritance patterns: A case report. *Front Neurol.* 2018 May 7;9:316. doi: 10.3389/fneur.2018.00316.

Cruccu G, Di Stefano G, Truini A. Trigeminal neuralgia. *N Engl J Med.* 2020 Aug 20;383(8):754–762. doi: 10.1056/NEJMra1914484.

Di Stefano G, De Stefano G, Leone C, et al. Real-world effectiveness and tolerability of carbamazepine and oxcarbazepine in 354 patients with trigeminal neuralgia. *Eur J Pain.* 2021 May;25(5):1064–1071. doi: 10.1002/ejp.1727.

Di Stefano G, Maarbjerg S, Nurmikko T, Truini A, Cruccu G. Triggering trigeminal neuralgia. *Cephalalgia.* 2018 May;38(6):1049–1056. doi: 10.1177/0333102417721677.

Di Stefano G, Yuan JH, Cruccu G, Waxman SG, Dib-Hajj SD, Truini A. Familial trigeminal neuralgia – A systematic clinical study with a genomic screen of the neuronal electrogenisome. *Cephalalgia.* 2020 Jul;40(8):767–777. doi: 10.1177/0333102419897623.

El Otmani H, Moutaouakil F, Fadel H, et al. Familial trigeminal neuralgia [in French]. *Rev Neurol (Paris).* 2008 Apr;164(4):384–387. doi: 10.1016/j.neurol.2007.10.010.

Faber CG, Lauria G, Merkies ISJ, et al. Gain-of-function Nav1.8 mutations in painful neuropathy. *Proc Natl Acad Sci U S A.* 2012 Nov 20;109(47):19444–19449. doi: 10.1073/pnas.1216080109.

Fleetwood IG, Innes AM, Hansen SR, et al. Familial trigeminal neuralgia. Case report and review of the literature. *J Neurosurg.* 2001 Sep;95(3):513–517. doi: 10.3171/jns.2001.95.3.0513.

Gualdani R, Gailly P, Yuan J-H, et al. A TRPM7 mutation linked to familial trigeminal neuralgia: Omega current and hyperexcitability of trigeminal ganglion neurons. *Proc Natl Acad Sci U S A.* 2022 Sep 20;119(38):e2119630119. doi: 10.1073/pnas.2119630119. Epub 2022 Sep 12.

Gualdani R, Yuan J-H, Effraim PR, et al. Trigeminal neuralgia TRPM8 mutation: Enhanced activation, basal $[Ca^{2+}]_i$ and menthol response. *Neurol Genet.* 2021 Jan 11;7(1):e550. doi: 10.1212/NXG.0000000000000550.

Katusic S, Beard CM, Bergstralh E, Kurland LT. Incidence and clinical features of trigeminal neuralgia, Rochester, Minnesota, 1945–1984. *Ann Neurol.* 1990 Jan;27(1):89–95. doi: 10.1002/ana.410270114.

Maarbjerg S, Gozalov A, Olesen J, Bendtsen L. Trigeminal neuralgia—A prospective systematic study of clinical characteristics in 158 patients. *Headache.* 2014 Nov–Dec;54(10):1574–1582. doi: 10.1111/head.12441.

O'Callaghan L, Floden L, Vinikoor-Imler L, et al. Burden of illness of trigeminal neuralgia among patients managed in a specialist center in England. *J Headache Pain.* 2020 Nov 10;21(1):130. doi: 10.1186/s10194-020-01198-z.

Panchagnula S, Sularz AK, Kahle KT. Familial trigeminal neuralgia cases implicate genetic factors in disease pathogenesis. *JAMA Neurol.* 2019 Jan 1;76(1):9–10. doi: 10.1001/jamaneurol.2018.3322.

Siqueira SRDT, Alves B, Malpartida HMG, Teixeira MJ, Siqueira JTT. Abnormal expression of voltage-gated sodium channels Nav1.7, Nav1.3 and Nav1.8 in trigeminal neuralgia. *Neuroscience.* 2009 Dec 1;164(2):573–577. doi: 10.1016/j.neuroscience.2009.08.037.

Chapter 8

Di Stefano G, Yuan JH, Cruccu G, Waxman SG, Dib-Hajj SD, Truini A. Familial trigeminal neuralgia - a systematic clinical study with a genomic screen of the neuronal electrogenisome. *Cephalalgia*. 2020 Jul;40(8):767–777. doi: 10.1177/0333102419897623. Epub 2020 Jan 13. PMID: 31928344; PMCID: PMC7366428

Eide PK. Familial occurrence of classical and idiopathic trigeminal neuralgia. *J Neurol Sci*. 2022 Mar 15;434:120101. doi: 10.1016/j.jns.2021.120101. Epub 2021 Dec 22. PMID: 34954619.

Gambeta, Eder., Gandini, Maria A., Souza, Ivana A., Zamponi, Gerald W. CaV3.2 calcium channels contribute to trigeminal neuralgia. *PAIN* 163(12): 2315-2325, December 2022. | Doi: 10.1097/j.pain.0000000000002651

Liedtke W. Mechanistic contribution of CaV3.2 calcium channels to trigeminal neuralgia pathophysiology not clarified. F1000Res. 2022 Jul 27;11:718. doi: 10.12688/f1000research.122997.2. PMCID: PMC9468618.

Mannerak MA, Lashkarivand A, Eide PK. Trigeminal neuralgia and genetics: A systematic review. *Mol Pain*. 2021 Jan-Dec;17:17448069211016139. doi: 10.1177/17448069211016139. PMID: 34000891; PMCID: PMC8135221.

Panchwagh, Jaydev, MD https//trigeminalneuralgiatreatment.org/is-trigeminal-neuralgia-hereditary/pAN Blog post August 13 , 2020.

Index